Adult-Gerontology Acute Care Nurse Practitioner Certification Practice Q&A

Adult-Gerontology Acute Care Nurse Practitioner Certification Practice Q&A

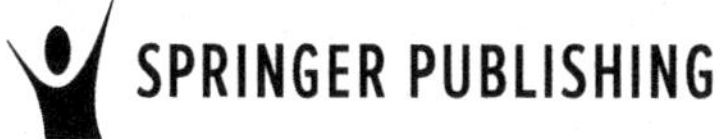

Springer Publishing Company

Springer Publishing Company, LLC
11 West 42nd Street, New York, NY 10036
www.springerpub.com

Acquisitions Editor: Elizabeth Nieginski
Compositor: diacriTech

ISBN: 978-0-8261-4571-0
ebook ISBN: 978-0-8261-4572-7
DOI: 10.1891/9780826145727

23 24 25 26 27 / 5 4 3 2 1

Medicine is an ever-changing science. Research and clinical experience are continually expanding our knowledge, in particular our understanding of proper treatment and drug therapy. The authors, editors, and publisher have made every effort to ensure that all information in this book is in accordance with the state of knowledge at the time of production of the book. Nevertheless, the authors, editors, and publisher are not responsible for any errors or omissions or for any consequence from application of the information in this book and make no warranty, expressed or implied, with respect to the content of this publication. Every reader should examine carefully the package inserts accompanying each drug and should carefully check whether the dosage schedules therein or the contraindications stated by the manufacturer differ from the statements made in this book. Such examination is particularly important with drugs that are either rarely used or have been newly released on the market. The publisher has no responsibility for the persistence or accuracy of URLs for external or third-party Internet websites referred to in this publication and does not guarantee that any content on such websites is, or will remain, accurate or appropriate.

Library of Congress Control Number: 2023931553

Contact sales@springerpub.com to receive discount rates on bulk purchases.

Note to Readers: **Publisher does not guarantee quality or access to any included digital components if book is purchased through a third-party seller.**

Printed in the United States of America by Gasch Printing.

Contents

Preface

Welcome to *Adult-Gerontology Acute Care Nurse Practitioner Certification Practice Q&A*! Congratulations on taking this important step on your journey to becoming a certified adult-gerontology acute care nurse practitioner (AGACNP). This resource is based on the most recent blueprints for the American Nurses Credentialing Center's (ANCC's) AGACNP-BC® examination and the American Association of Critical-Care Nurses's (AACN's) ACNPC-AG® examination and was developed by experienced AGACNPs. It is designed to help you sharpen your specialty knowledge with 350 practice questions organized by exam content subject areas, as well as strengthen your knowledge-application and test-taking skills with two 175-question practice exams. It also includes essential information about the AGACNP-BC and ACNPC-AG examinations, including eligibility requirements, exam content subject areas and question distributions, and tips for successful exam preparation.

PART I: PRACTICE QUESTIONS AND ANSWERS WITH RATIONALES

Part I includes three chapters based on the following exam content subject areas: Core Competencies, Clinical Practice, and Professional Role. Each chapter includes high-quality, exam-style questions and comprehensive answers with rationales that address both correct and incorrect answers. Part I is designed to strengthen your specialty knowledge and is formatted for ultimate studying convenience—answer the questions on each page and simply turn the page for the corresponding answers and rationales. No need to refer to the back of the book for the answers.

PART II: PRACTICE EXAMS AND ANSWERS WITH RATIONALES

Part II includes two 175-question practice exams that align with the exam content subject areas and question distributions on the most recent blueprints for the AGACNP-BC and ACNPC-AG examinations. These practice exams are designed to help you strengthen your knowledge-application and test-taking skills. Maximize your preparation and simulate the exam experience by setting aside 3.5 hours to complete one practice exam. Comprehensive answers and rationales that address both correct and incorrect answers are located in the chapters immediately following the practice exams.

We know life is busy, and being able to prepare for your exam efficiently and effectively is paramount. This resource will give you the tools and confidence you need to succeed. For additional exam preparation resources, including self-paced online courses, online QBanks, comprehensive review texts, and high-yield study guides, visit www.springerpub.com/examprep. Best of luck to you on your certification journey!

Introduction: Adult-Gerontology Acute Care Nurse Practitioner Certification Practice Exams and Tips for Preparation

AMERICAN NURSES CREDENTIALING CENTER

ELIGIBILITY REQUIREMENTS

The AGACNP-BC® examination is developed and administered by the American Nurses Credentialing Center (ANCC). To qualify to take the exam, you must meet the following requirements:

- Hold a current, active RN license in a state or territory of the United States or hold the professional, legally recognized equivalent in another country.
- Hold a master's, postgraduate certificate, or DNP from an AGACNP program accredited by the Commission on Collegiate Nursing Education, the Accreditation Commission for Education in Nursing, or the National League for Nursing Commission for Nursing Education Accreditation. A minimum of 500 faculty-supervised clinical hours must be included in the AGACNP program.
- Have completed three separate, comprehensive graduate-level courses in:
  - Advanced physiology/pathophysiology, including general principles that apply across the lifespan
  - Advanced health assessment, which includes assessment of all human systems, advanced assessment techniques, concepts, and approaches
  - Advanced pharmacology, which includes pharmacodynamics, pharmacokinetics, and pharmacotherapeutics of all broad categories of agents

Qualified applicants may submit an online application at https://ebiz.nursingworld.org/Login?returnurl=https://www.nursingworld.org/certapps/?certcode=AGACNP&SSOL=Y. Successful candidates will receive an Authorization to Test and must schedule the exam within a 90-day window. The exam fee is $395; the fee for members of the American Nurses Association is $295. Refer to the ANCC website for complete eligibility requirements, pricing, and certification information: www.nursingworld.org/our-certifications/adult-gerontology-acute-care-nurse-practitioner/.

ABOUT THE EXAMINATION

The AGACNP-BC examination takes 3.5 hours and consists of 175 multiple-choice questions with four answer options. You must select the single best answer. Only 150 questions are scored, and the remaining 25 questions are used as pre-test questions. It is impossible to know which questions are scored, so be sure to answer all of the questions to the best of your ability. See Table 1 for content domains and question distribution. For more detailed exam content information, refer to the AGACNP-BC exam blueprint at www.nursingworld.org/~4a8053/globalassets/certification/certification-specialty-pages/resources/test-content-outlines/exam-62-agacnp-tco-2020-01-13_for-web-posting.pdf.

Table 1 AGACNP-BC® Exam Content Domains and Question Distribution

Content Domain	Percentage of Questions
Core Competencies	23%
Clinical Practice	45%
Professional Role	32%

AMERICAN ASSOCIATION OF CRITICAL-CARE NURSES

ELIGIBILITY REQUIREMENTS

The ACNPC-AG® examination is developed and administered by the American Association of Critical-Care Nurses (AACN). To qualify to take the exam, you must meet the following requirements:

- A current, unencumbered U.S. RN or APRN license is required. An unencumbered license is not currently being subjected to formal discipline by the board of nursing in the state(s) in which the nurse is practicing and has no provisions or conditions that limit the nurse's practice. Provisions or conditions may include, but are not limited to, direct supervision of practice, drug administration limitations, and/or practice area exclusions. Nurses who do not hold an unencumbered license should email AACN at APRNcert@aacn.org.
- Candidates must complete a graduate-level advanced practice education program as an AGACNP at a nationally accredited school of nursing. The school's curriculum must include supervised clinical and didactic coursework consistent with competencies of AGACNP practice.

Qualified applicants may submit an online application at www.aacn.org/membership/signin?url=%252fcertification%252fget-certified%252facnpc-ag%252foverview&returnUrl=%2Fcertification%2Fget-certified%2Facnpc-ag%2Foverview. Candidate eligibility will be evaluated within 2 to 3 business days of the required documents being received. Upon approval, candidates receive a link the same day to schedule their exam appointment. The exam fee is $375; the fee for members of the AACN is $265. Refer to the AACN website for complete eligibility requirements, pricing, and certification information: www.aacn.org/certification/get-certified/acnpc-ag.

ABOUT THE EXAMINATION

The ACNPC-AG examination takes 3.5 hours and consists of 175 multiple-choice questions with four answer options. You must select the single best answer. Only 150 questions are scored, and the remaining 25 questions are used as pre-test questions. It is impossible to know which questions are scored, so be sure to answer all of the questions to the best of your ability. See Table 2 for content dimensions and question distribution. For more detailed exam content information, refer to the ACNPC-AG handbook at www.aacn.org/certification/preparation-tools-and-handbooks/~/media/aacn-website/certification/get-certified/handbooks/acnpcagexamhandbook.pdf?la = en.

Table 2 ACNPC-AG® Exam Content Dimensions and Question Distribution

Content Dimension	Percentage of Questions
Clinical Judgment	79%
Professional Caring and Ethical Practice	21%

TIPS FOR EXAM PREPARATION

You know the old joke about how to get to Carnegie Hall—practice, practice, practice! The same is true when seeking certification. Practice and preparation are key to your success on exam day. Here are 10 tips to help you prepare:

1. Allow at least 6 months to fully prepare for the exam. Do not rely on last-minute cramming sessions.
2. Thoroughly review the AGACNP-BC or ACNPC-AG blueprint so that you know exactly what to expect. Pay close attention to the question topics. Identify your strengths, weaknesses, and knowledge gaps so you know where to focus your studies. Review all of the supplementary resources available on the AGACNP-BC or ACNPC-AG website.
3. Create a study timeline with weekly or monthly study tasks. Be as specific as possible—identify *what* you will study, *how* you will study, and *when* you will study.
4. Use several exam prep resources that provide different benefits. For example, use a comprehensive review to build your specialty knowledge, use this resource and other question banks to strengthen your knowledge-application and test-taking skills, and use a high-yield review to brush up on key concepts in the days leading up to the exam. Springer Publishing offers a wide range of print and online exam prep products to suit all of your study needs; visit www.springerpub.com/examprep.

5. Assess your level of knowledge and performance on practice questions and exams. Carefully consider why you may be missing certain questions. Continually analyze your strengths, weaknesses, and knowledge gaps, and adjust your study plan accordingly.
6. Minimize distraction as much as possible while you are studying. You will feel more calm, centered, and focused, which will lead to increased knowledge retention.
7. Engage in stress-reducing activities, particularly in the month leading up to the exam. Yoga, stretching, and deep-breathing exercises can be beneficial. If you are feeling frustrated or anxious while studying, take a break. Go for a walk, play with your child or pet, or finish a chore that has been weighing on you. Wait until you feel more refreshed before returning to study.
8. Focus on your health in the weeks and days before the exam. Eat balanced meals, stay hydrated, and minimize alcohol consumption. Get as much sleep as possible, particularly the night before the exam.
9. Eat a light meal before the exam but limit your liquid consumption. The clock does not stop for restroom breaks! Ensure that you know exactly where you are going and how long it will take to get there. Leave with plenty of time to spare to reduce travel-related stress and ensure that you arrive on time.
10. Remind yourself to relax and stay calm. You have prepared, and you know your stuff. Visualize the success that is just ahead of you and make it happen. When you pass, celebrate!

Pass Guarantee

If you use this resource to prepare for your exam and do not pass, you may return it for a refund of your full purchase price, excluding tax, shipping, and handling. To receive a refund, return your product along with a copy of your exam score report and original receipt showing purchase of new product (not used). Product must be returned and received within 180 days of the original purchase date. Refunds will be issued within 8 weeks from acceptance and approval. One offer per person and address. This offer is valid for U.S. residents only. Void where prohibited. To initiate a refund, please contact Customer Service at csexamprep@springerpub.com.

Part I

Practice Questions and Answers With Rationales

1

Core Competencies

1. A patient in the intensive care unit is being treated for sepsis. Vital signs are blood pressure 75/42 mmHg, heart rate 102 bpm, respiratory rate 22 breaths/min, and temperature 101°F (38.3°C). Laboratory studies reveal an increase in baseline creatinine to 2.1 mg/dL. Which physical examination finding is most concerning for the AGACNP?

   A. Decreased level of consciousness
   B. Diminished lung sounds
   C. Poor skin turgor
   D. Hypoactive bowel sounds

2. A patient presents with right flank pain, nausea, and decreased urine output. CT of the abdomen and pelvis shows a 5-mm, obstructing right ureteral stone with associated hydronephrosis. Which physical examination finding by the AGACNP correlates with this diagnosis?

   A. Cardiac murmur
   B. Diminished pedal pulses
   C. Bradycardia
   D. Costovertebral angle tenderness

3. A patient with end-stage renal failure on hemodialysis is admitted with symptoms of diarrhea, nausea, and weakness. Laboratory studies reveal a potassium level of 6.5 mEq/L. Which physical examination finding correlates with this diagnosis?

   A. Bradycardia
   B. Hyperreflexia
   C. Bradypnea
   D. Tachycardia

(See answers next page.)

1. A) Decreased level of consciousness

The patient is being treated for septic shock and is showing signs of acute kidney injury secondary to sepsis and hypotension. Decreased level of consciousness is concerning for severe metabolic derangement, has the potential to lead to respiratory failure, and requires immediate intervention by the AGACNP. Diminished lung sounds, poor skin turgor, and hypoactive bowel sounds all need to be addressed but do not take priority over the patient's altered mentation and inability to protect their airway.

2. D) Costovertebral angle tenderness

The patient presents with obstructing renal calculi. The presence of costovertebral angle tenderness is supportive of this diagnosis. Auscultation of a cardiac murmur is an abnormal finding; however, it is unrelated to renal calculi. Diminished pedal pulses indicate a vascular flow problem, which is also unrelated to renal calculi. Bradycardia is unlikely in this patient population because they frequently have significant pain and are tachycardic.

3. A) Bradycardia

A patient with end-stage renal failure on hemodialysis is presenting with symptoms of hyperkalemia. Patients with hyperkalemia often suffer from bradycardia or complete heart block due to the negative action of excess potassium on cardiac function. In addition, they have decreased to absent deep tendon reflexes and tachypnea.

4. A patient with end-stage renal failure on hemodialysis presents to the emergency department with complaints of shortness of breath and lower extremity edema after missing a dialysis session. Which physical examination finding by the AGACNP is most concerning?

   A. Bilateral crackles
   B. Tachycardia
   C. Heart murmur
   D. Dry mucous membranes

5. A patient has just completed a course of antibiotics for an upper respiratory infection. They present to the office with complaints of oral burning and irritation. The AGACNP suspects oral candidiasis. Which physical examination finding supports this diagnosis?

   A. Facial edema
   B. Cervical lymphadenopathy
   C. White lesions coating the tongue
   D. Purulent nasal drainage

6. A patient with metastatic bone cancer presents with complaints of weakness, constipation, and polyuria. Laboratory studies reveal a calcium level of 10.6 mg/dL. Which physical examination finding supports this diagnosis?

   A. Altered mental status
   B. Wheezing
   C. Moist mucous membranes
   D. Positive Chvostek sign

7. A patient presents to the clinic with complaints of a burning sensation, discharge, and redness that began in one eye and is now affecting both. The AGACNP examines the patient and notes bilateral conjunctival erythema and purulent discharge. Which diagnosis is associated with these physical examination findings?

   A. Acute bacterial conjunctivitis
   B. Corneal abrasion
   C. Glaucoma
   D. Foreign object

(See answers next page.)

4. A) Bilateral crackles

This is a dialysis-dependent patient who reports missing a scheduled session. The patient's symptoms are consistent with volume overload. The presence of bilateral crackles is concerning for pulmonary edema, a complication of missing dialysis, and is top priority for the AGACNP. Tachycardia, a common secondary finding associated with volume overload, does not pose an immediate threat to the patient and will resolve with the removal of excess fluid. A heart murmur, although abnormal, does not take priority over the patient's ability to breathe. Dry mucous membranes are common in dialysis patients and do not warrant immediate action by the AGACNP.

5. C) White lesions coating the tongue

The patient presents with symptoms of oral candidiasis, a common complication associated with antibiotic use that is characterized by white lesions affecting the oral mucosa. Facial edema is not an expected finding with this diagnosis and would be more consistent with an inflammatory reaction. Cervical lymphadenopathy is a physical examination finding associated with bacterial infections and non-Hodgkin lymphoma. Purulent nasal drainage is indicative of an upper respiratory infection and does not support an oral candidiasis diagnosis.

6. D) Positive Chvostek sign

The patient has known metastatic bone cancer and presents with symptoms of hypercalcemia, a common complication of malignancy. Laboratory studies confirm hypercalcemia, and Chvostek sign is a physical examination finding specific to this diagnosis. Altered mentation and wheezing are broad physical examination findings that are not specific to hypercalcemia. It would be unusual for this patient to have moist mucous membranes; it is another vague physical examination finding that is not specific to hypercalcemia.

7. A) Acute bacterial conjunctivitis

The patient is presenting with symptoms of acute bacterial conjunctivitis. Purulent discharge and conjunctival erythema are hallmark physical examination findings associated with bacterial conjunctivitis. Corneal abrasions may produce discharge; however, it would not be purulent in nature and may only affect one eye. Symptoms of glaucoma include blurred vision, pressure, and redness, but not infection. The presence of a foreign object in the eye may produce erythema and discharge; however, it is unlikely to affect both eyes.

8. A patient presents with complaints of hearing loss, vertigo, and tinnitus. The AGACNP suspects Ménière disease. Which physical examination finding supports this diagnosis?

A. Positive Romberg test
B. Hemiplegia
C. Facial droop
D. Dysarthria

9. An 83-year-old bed-bound patient presents for evaluation. The AGACNP notes a sacral pressure injury with full-thickness skin loss. The AGACNP identifies this patient's injury as stage:

A. 1
B. 2
C. 3
D. 4

10. A patient with a peanut allergy presents with symptoms of shortness of breath, facial edema, and hives. Which physical examination finding by the AGACNP requires immediate intervention?

A. Tongue swelling
B. Periorbital edema
C. Tachycardia
D. Maculopapular rash

11. Which strains of human papillomavirus (HPV) are associated with genital warts?

A. 6 and 11
B. 16 and 18
C. 31 and 33
D. 45 and 52

12. An 84-year-old patient presents to the clinic with new confusion and inability to focus on tasks. The AGACNP suspects which condition?

A. Dementia
B. Delirium
C. Alzheimer disease
D. Attention deficit disorder (ADD)

(*See answers next page.*)

8. A) Positive Romberg test

The patient is presenting with symptoms of Ménière disease. A positive Romberg test is indicative of abnormal vestibular function, which is associated with this disease. Hemiplegia, facial droop, and dysarthria are all symptoms of cerebral vascular accidents.

9. C) 3

A stage 3 pressure injury is characterized by full-thickness skin loss. Stage 1 injuries present as nonblanchable erythema with intact skin. Stage 2 injuries have partial-thickness skin loss and exposed dermis. Stage 4 injuries have full-thickness skin loss plus tissue loss.

10. A) Tongue swelling

The patient is presenting with symptoms of anaphylaxis secondary to peanut ingestion. Tongue swelling should be addressed immediately due to its potential to cause airway obstruction. Periorbital edema will not affect the patient's respiratory or circulatory function; therefore, it is not the top priority. Tachycardia, although an abnormal finding, is a compensatory mechanism in response to the patient's anaphylaxis and will only worsen if the airway becomes obstructed. The presence of a maculopapular rash does not pose a threat to the respiratory or circulatory systems and is, therefore, not the top priority.

11. A) 6 and 11

HPV subtypes 6 and 11 are associated with genital warts. Subtypes 16, 18, 31, 33, 45, and 52 are associated with higher-grade dysplasia and genital cancers.

12. B) Delirium

Delirium should be suspected in an older patient with acute confusion and attention dicit. Dementia would present as a gradual onset of memory loss. Alzheimer's disease is an advanced form of dementia. ADD is not characterized by confusion and is less likely to begin in advanced age.

13. Which type of shock is associated with anaphylaxis characterized by urticaria, wheezing, and shortness of breath?

A. Cardiogenic
B. Septic
C. Hypovolemic
D. Distributive

14. The AGACNP is performing a visual examination and observes an abnormal eye movement of the patient's right eye, characterized by a rhythmical jerking movement. The AGACNP identifies the abnormal assessment findings as:

A. Disconjugate gaze
B. Conjugate gaze
C. Mydriasis
D. Nystagmus

15. Cisplatin (Platinol) is an antineoplastic that can potentially cause:

A. Nephrotoxicity
B. Hypercalcemia
C. Hepatotoxicity
D. Nephrotic syndrome

16. What is the safest parenteral route of administration for ketorolac (Toradol)?

A. Intravenous
B. Intramuscular
C. Subcutaneous
D. Epidural

17. A patient with end-stage liver disease (ESLD) presents to the emergency department 3 days prior to trans-jugular intrahepatic portosystemic shunt placement with agitation, nausea, reduced urinary output, lower-extremity edema, worsening ascites, and jugular venous distention. There are no drug allergies. The best choice for single-dose postoperative pain medication in this patient is:

A. Ketorolac (Toradol) injection, 30 mg intramuscularly (IM) once
B. Tramadol (Ultram) 50 mg tablet, 1 tablet orally once
C. Morphine (Astramorph PF) injection, 5 mg IM once
D. Fentanyl citrate (Sublimaze) solution, 25 mcg intravenous push once

(*See answers next page.*)

13. D) Distributive

These symptoms suggest anaphylactic shock, which is a type of distributive shock commonly resulting from an allergic reaction. Cardiogenic, sepsis, and hypovolemic shock are not characterized by urticaria, wheezing, and shortness of breath and can therefore be excluded.

14. D) Nystagmus

Nystagmus is the abnormal eye movement of one or both eyes characterized by rhythmical jerking movements. A disconjugate gaze involves misalignment of the eyes but is not characterized by any rhythmical movement. Conjugate gaze describes appropriate extraocular movements and is a normal examination finding. Mydriasis is dilation of the pupil.

15. A) Nephrotoxicity

Nephrotoxicity related to cisplatin (Platinol) is dose-related and can lead to renal failure. This drug can cause hypocalcemia. Hepatotoxicity is not a potential adverse effect related to cisplatin (Platinol). The nephrotoxicity that can be associated with cisplatin (Platinol) is not associated with a nephrotic syndrome.

16. A) Intravenous

Ketorolac (Toradol) is currently the only parenteral nonsteroidal anti-inflammatory drug available, and intravenous administration is the safest. When given intramuscularly, ketorolac (Toradol) is irregularly absorbed. Ketorolac (Toradol) should not be given via subcutaneous or epidural routes.

17. D) Fentanyl citrate (Sublimaze) solution, 25 mcg intravenous push once

Fentanyl citrate (Sublimaze) is a good option for acute pain management in ESLD. No dose adjustment is indicated for a single dose or infrequent bolus dosing. Nonsteroidal anti-inflammatory drugs, like ketorolac (Toradol), are contraindicated in ESLD due to increased risks of bleeding, interference with diuresis, hepatotoxicity, and drug toxicity. Tramadol (Ultram) is a possible option in well-compensated ESLD, but this patient's presentation suggests decompensated disease. The patient's symptoms also suggest concomitant renal failure, which is common in ESLD. While morphine (Astramorph PF) is an option for ESLD with preserved renal function, its use in patients with renal failure can lead to increased toxicity and respiratory depression.

18. Temozolomide (Temodar) is an alkylating chemotherapeutic drug commonly used to treat:

A. Acoustic neuroma
B. Glioblastoma
C. Colorectal cancer
D. Leukemia

19. What diagnosis is appropriate for a patient who presents with urticaria that has been present for 4 weeks?

A. Acute urticaria
B. Chronic urticaria
C. Chronic spontaneous urticaria
D. Autoimmune urticaria

20. What class of antiemetics is effective in preventing vertigo-induced nausea?

A. Antihistamines
B. Dopamine antagonists
C. Neurokinin receptor antagonists
D. Corticosteroids

21. What lab result is most helpful in diagnosing a 45-year-old patient who presents with several months of joint stiffness and bilateral pain in the hands?

A. Complete blood count (CBC)
B. Anti-cyclic citrullinated peptide (CCP) antibodies
C. Erythrocyte sedimentation rate (ESR)
D. C-reactive protein

22. A patient presents with atypical target lesions on the trunk and mucosal ulcerations totaling 8% body surface area (BSA) skin detachment following a course of allopurinol (Aloprim). The AGACNP suspects what diagnosis?

A. Stevens-Johnson syndrome
B. Toxic epidermal necrolysis
C. Erythema multiforme
D. Gout

(*See answers next page.*)

18. B) Glioblastoma

Temozolomide (Temodar) is a chemotherapeutic agent that is standard treatment for newly diagnosed and/or high-grade glioblastomas. It is not specific to a cell cycle and has good penetration of the blood-brain barrier. Temozolomide (Temodar) currently has no indication for acoustic neuroma, colorectal cancer, or leukemia.

19. A) Acute urticaria

Acute urticaria is classified as urticaria that lasts for less than 6 weeks. Urticaria that is present for 6 weeks or longer is chronic urticaria. If there is no identifiable cause, it is chronic spontaneous urticaria. While urticaria may be autoimmune, it is not characterized by duration.

20. A) Antihistamines

Antihistamines are effective in preventing nausea that occurs secondary to stimulation of the labyrinth, such as vertigo-induced nausea. Dopamine antagonists, neurokinin receptor antagonists, and corticosteroids are used for the prevention of acute and delayed chemotherapy-induced nausea.

21. B) Anti-cyclic citrullinated peptide (CCP) antibodies

Bilateral hand arthralgias and stiffness would raise suspicion for rheumatoid arthritis, particularly in a patient of this age. Anti-CCP antibody is the most specific test to diagnose rheumatoid arthritis with a specificity of about 95%. A CBC is most helpful to identify hematological abnormalities or infections. ESR and C-reactive protein may be abnormal in rheumatoid arthritis but are nonspecific because they are also elevated in other conditions.

22. A) Stevens-Johnson syndrome

Stevens-Johnson syndrome is a rare immune disorder that is triggered by certain medications or infections and is characterized by atypical target lesions on the trunk and mucosal ulcerations that total less than 10% BSA skin detachment. Toxic epidermal necrolysis is a similar disorder but is characterized by greater than 30% BSA detachment. Erythema multiforme is an inflammatory dermatological syndrome that is localized and usually presents on extensor surfaces rather than the trunk. Gout is characterized by erythematous, painful swollen joints.

23. A patient who is homeless presents to the emergency department with complaints of severe nocturnal itching and a rash affecting their palms and in between their fingers. The AGACNP examines the patient and notes erythematous papules in the genital area with evidence of burrows in the interdigital webs. These findings are consistent with which diagnosis?

A. Tinea cruris
B. Body lice
C. Herpes simplex virus (HSV)
D. Scabies

24. The AGACNP is examining a patient with newly diagnosed HIV. On inspection of the mouth, the AGACNP notices raised, white patches on the lateral aspect of the tongue. What is the cause of this?

A. Herpes simplex
B. Canker sore
C. Gingivostomatitis
D. Candida albicans

25. A synarthrosis joint is described as a joint that is:

A. Immovable
B. Slightly movable
C. Freely movable
D. Biaxial

26. While performing a thorough musculoskeletal assessment, the AGACNP evaluates arm abduction. Which of the following describes abduction?

A. Movement of a body part away from the body
B. Movement of a body part toward the body
C. Flexion of the head
D. Extension of the head

27. A patient presents to the emergency department with acute onset right-sided hemiparesis, aphasia, and altered mental status. What would the AGACNP suspect as the most likely diagnosis?

A. Sepsis
B. Acute cerebral vascular accident
C. Hypertensive emergency
D. Delirium

(*See answers next page.*)

23. D) Scabies

The patient is presenting with signs and symptoms of scabies, a mite infection affecting the skin that is prevalent in patients who are homeless. Tinea cruris, commonly known as jock itch, is a fungal infection of the genitals, inner thighs, and buttocks and is caused most often by trapped moisture due to tight clothing. It would not affect the patient's hands. Body lice are parasitic infections characterized by red noninflammatory lesions and the presence of eggs attached to the hair shafts. HSV is a viral infection that can affect oral or genital mucosa and is characterized by single or grouped painful vesicles and may be accompanied by a fever.

24. D) Candida albicans

Candida albicans, the type of fungus that causes what is commonly known as thrush, is an opportunistic yeast infection of the oral cavity that can occur in patients who are immunocompromised. Symptoms include raised, white, cottage cheese-like patches of the oral cavity. Herpes simplex virus presents as blisters or cold sores in the mouth; canker sores are less likely to be raised lesions; and gingivostomatitis is a more generalized medical term that encompasses infection of the mouth causing blistering and raw, bleeding gums.

25. A) Immovable

Synarthrotic joints are immovable, amphiarthrotic joints are slightly moveable, and diarthrodial joints are freely movable. The term *biaxial* refers to a joint's ability to flex/extend and abduct/adduct.

26. A) Movement of a body part away from the body

Abduction is the movement of a body part away from the body. Adduction is the movement of a body part toward the body. Flexion is the bending of a joint, and extension is the straightening of a joint.

27. B) Acute cerebral vascular accident

The patient is presenting with an acute onset neurologic deficit consistent with a cerebral vascular accident. Sepsis, an overwhelming systemic infection, may present with symptoms of altered mental status; however, it is not characterized by hemiparalysis or aphasia. Hypertensive emergency is a condition of severely elevated blood pressure and may be associated with headaches and blurred vision. Delirium is a disturbance in cognitive function that is characterized by altered mental status but does not include impairment of motor function.

28. A patient with a recent radial fracture and casting presents to the emergency department with complaints of severe pain and paresthesia in the affected limb. The AGACNP examines the patient and notes a palpable radial pulse with evidence of diminished reflexes. Which intervention is the priority for the AGACNP?

A. Remove the cast
B. Administer analgesic
C. Obtain arterial ultrasound
D. Obtain an x-ray of the affected limb

29. A key difference between bipolar I disorder and bipolar II disorder is that a diagnosis of bipolar II requires:

A. An episode of major depression
B. A suicide attempt
C. An episode of mania
D. Anxiety

30. A patient presents to the emergency department unresponsive after being involved in a motor vehicle crash. Emergency medical services reports that the patient had a period of lucidity followed by a decrease in consciousness. This clinical presentation is associated with which neurologic condition?

A. Subdural hematoma
B. Intracerebral hematoma
C. Epidural hematoma
D. Cerebral contusion

31. A patient presents to the clinic with complaints of abdominal pain, purulent vaginal discharge, and fever. The AGACNP examines the patient and notes adnexal tenderness and pain associated with the cervical examination. A culture is obtained and grows *Neisseria gonorrhoeae*. What does the AGACNP identify this condition as?

A. Polycystic ovarian syndrome
B. Ectopic pregnancy
C. Urinary tract infection
D. Pelvic inflammatory disease (PID)

(*See answers next page.*)

28. A) Remove the cast

The patient is presenting with symptoms of compartment syndrome, a serious complication associated with fracture and casting. Symptoms include severe pain (out of proportion to injury), sensation changes, diminished reflexes, and eventual loss of motor function. The priority for this patient is to remove the cast to relieve pressure and reestablish blood flow. Analgesic administration is necessary; however, it does not take priority over cast removal. Arterial ultrasound is not warranted at this time as the patient has a palpable pulse on examination. X-ray is not necessary as the patient has a known fracture and symptomology is concerning for vascular compromise.

29. A) An episode of major depression

A diagnosis of bipolar II requires the presence of major depression. Although it can be present in bipolar I, it is not required for that diagnosis. Mania is present in bipolar I; hypomania is the hallmark symptom of bipolar II. Suicide attempts and anxiety are not distinguishing factors between the two diagnoses.

30. C) Epidural hematoma

An episode of lucidity followed by neurologic decline is a hallmark finding for epidural hematoma. Intracerebral hematoma, subdural hematoma, and cerebral contusion all have similar neurologic presentations; however, they do not involve a period of lucidity.

31. D) Pelvic inflammatory disease (PID)

The patient's symptoms, physical exam findings, and culture results are consistent with PID, an infection affecting the upper reproductive tract caused by sexually transmitted organisms. Polycystic ovarian syndrome is an endocrine disorder that results in infrequent or absent ovulation. This condition does not involve purulent vaginal discharge, fever, abdominal pain, or adnexal tenderness on exam. An ectopic pregnancy occurs when an egg has been fertilized outside the uterus; it results in lower abdominal pain, adnexal tenderness, and dark brown (not purulent) discharge. A urinary tract infection is an infectious process involving the urinary system and is not associated with vaginal discharge or adnexal tenderness.

32. A patient presents to the AGACNP with complaints of excessive anxiety that interferes with activities of daily living and has been present for the past year. Which first-line pharmacologic treatment is indicated?

A. Analgesic
B. Selective serotonin reuptake inhibitor (SSRI)
C. Benzodiazepine
D. Tricyclic antidepressant

33. Which of the following clinical characteristics differentiates chronic obstructive bronchitis from emphysema?

A. Cyanosis
B. Shortness of breath
C. Cough
D. Sputum production

34. A 25-year-old patient presents to the clinic with complaints of excessive hair growth, irregular periods, and excessive weight gain. The AGACNP obtains laboratory studies that reveal a follicle-stimulating hormone (FSH) to luteinizing hormone (LH) ratio of 1:3. This is consistent with which diagnosis?

A. Polycystic ovarian syndrome
B. Hirsutism
C. Cushing syndrome
D. Adrenal tumor

35. The AGACNP is following up with a patient who was discharged from the hospital 2 weeks prior following a pneumonia diagnosis. The patient was treated with intravenous antibiotics while hospitalized. During the encounter, the patient complains of new onset nystagmus. What medication would the AGACNP suspect is the etiology of the patient's symptoms?

A. Amoxicillin (Amoxil)
B. Gentamicin (Garamycin)
C. Piperacillin (Pipracil)
D. Cefalexin (Keflex)

36. Which of the following is a schedule II medication?

A. Tramadol (Ultram)
B. Ketorolac (Toradol)
C. Morphine sulfate
D. Ketamine

(*See answers next page.*)

32. B) Selective serotonin reuptake inhibitor (SSRI)

The patient is presenting with symptoms of a generalized anxiety disorder (GAS). Selective SSRIs are first-line pharmacologic therapy for this disorder. Analgesics are not indicated for anxiety/mood disorders. Benzodiazepines and tricyclic antidepressants may be used for the treatment of GAS; however, they are not first-line therapy.

33. A) Cyanosis

In chronic obstructive bronchitis, inflammation in the bronchioles and the resulting mucous build-up restrict the movement of air into and out of the lungs. This restriction impacts the oxygenation of tissues, causing cyanosis in patients with the disorder. The hyperventilation typically present in patients with emphysema generally prevents cyanosis. Both conditions cause shortness of breath, cough, and sputum production.

34. A) Polycystic ovarian syndrome

The patient is presenting with signs and symptoms of the polycystic ovarian syndrome, an endocrine disorder characterized by male pattern hair growth, acne, irregular or absent periods, elevated serum testosterone, and weight gain. The presence of a 1:3 FSH to LH ratio in addition to symptomology is confirmatory of this syndrome. Hirsutism is male pattern hair growth that can occur in the absence of other symptoms and can be caused by multiple conditions. It does not involve a disruption in FSH or LH. Cushing syndrome is an endocrine disorder that results from excessive cortisol production. It is characterized by weight gain, acne, and infertility, but it does not cause a disproportionate FSH/LH ratio. The hormones attributed to an adrenal tumor are epinephrine and norepinephrine, not FSH or LH.

35. B) Gentamicin (Garamycin)

Aminoglycosides such as gentamicin (Garamycin) can cause ototoxicity. One of the potential adverse effects of this drug that can demonstrate itself days or weeks later after taking this medication is nystagmus. Thus, with a new complaint of nystagmus, the AGACNP may want to consider if this side effect is related to Garamycin. Amoxicillin (Amoxil), piperacillin (Pipracil), and cefalexin (Keflex) do not typically elicit nystagmus.

36. C) Morphine sulfate

Morphine sulfate is listed as a schedule II medication and carries a high potential for dependence. Tramadol (Ultram), a schedule IV medication, has small amounts of opioids and a low potential for dependence. Ketorolac (Toradol) is not a controlled substance; it is a nonsteroidal anti-inflammatory (NSAID), is non-habit forming, and is used for moderate to severe pain in adults. Ketamine, a schedule III medication, still carries the potential for dependence, but the risk is lower than that of schedule I or II medications.

37. The AGACNP working in an urgent care is seeing an oncology patient with complaints of new onset bone pain. The patient is scared that their cancer may be spreading and couldn't wait until the morning to call their oncologist. The patient states that they have been receiving chemotherapy and is scheduled for an autologous stem cell transplant next month. Knowing this, what medication would the AGACNP want to question the patient about that may be the cause of their bone pain?

A. Prazepam (Centrax)
B. Ondansetron (Zofran)
C. Fluconazole (Diflucan)
D. Granulocyte-colony stimulating factor (Neupogen)

38. The AGACNP is rounding on a patient admitted the previous night with *Clostridioides difficile*. When assessing the patient this morning, the RN called to report that the patient's face, neck, and anterior chest exhibited a red, flushed, and pruritic rash. Which medication does the AGACNP suspect was the cause of this adverse reaction?

A. Vancomycin (Vancocin)
B. Metronidazole (Flagyl)
C. Fidaxomicin (Dificid)
D. Nitazoxanide (Alinia)

39. The AGACNP is rounding on a patient admitted with diabetic ketoacidosis. In assessing the patient, the AGACNP recalls that the physiological reason for the patient's fruity breath smell is from which chemical compound response?

A. Increased nitrogen
B. Decreased chlorine
C. Increased acetone
D. Decreased magnesium

40. The AGACNP is rounding in the ICU on a patient with an admitting diagnosis of pheochromocytoma. The patient is hypertensive with a blood pressure reading of 190/110 mmHg, and the AGACNP needs to treat the blood pressure. Which antihypertensive drug would be the best choice considering this patient's diagnosis?

A. Phentolamine (OraVerse)
B. Benazepril (Lotensin)
C. Nifedipine (Adalat)
D. Candesartan (Atacand)

(*See answers next page.*)

37. D) Granulocyte-colony stimulating factor (Neupogen)

Granulocyte-colony stimulating factor (Neupogen) is used as a supportive medication with patients receiving antineoplastic drugs to stimulate the production of white blood cells. A classic side effect is bone pain. Therefore, the granulocyte-colony stimulating factor (Neupogen) is likely the culprit. Prazepam (Centrax), ondansetron (Zofran), and fluconazole (Diflucan) do not have this reported side effect.

38. A) Vancomycin (Vancocin)

Vancomycin flushing syndrome, or vancomycin infusion reaction, is an adverse reaction characterized by flushing, itching, and an erythema-like rash of the face, neck, and chest/abdomen. Metronidazole (Flagyl), fidaxomicin (Dificid), and nitazoxanide (Alinia) do not typically elicit this reaction.

39. C) Increased acetone

The smell is attributed to elevated levels of free acetone (a type of ketone), a byproduct of the metabolism of fat. Although nitrogen, chlorine, and magnesium are naturally occurring chemicals found in the body, they do not contribute to the fruity smell that can be associated with diabetic ketoacidosis.

40. A) Phentolamine (OraVerse)

In patients with a diagnosis of pheochromocytoma, phentolamine (OraVerse) is considered the drug of choice in treating hypertension attributable to the effects of noradrenaline and the ability to block alpha-adrenergic receptors. Benazepril (Lotensin), nifedipine (Adalat), and candesartan (Atacand) are not drugs of choice as they do not have this type of unique response that would be specific to the biochemistry related to an adrenal tumor diagnosis.

41. A patient presents with complaints of redness, swelling, and pain affecting bilateral lower extremities after encountering poison ivy. The AGACNP examines the patient and notes erythematous and edematous vesicles involving bilateral lower extremities. These findings are consistent with which diagnosis?

A. Acute contact dermatitis
B. Atopic dermatitis
C. Tinea pedis
D. Urticaria

42. Which of the following conditions is associated with poor wound healing?

A. Coronary artery disease
B. Diabetes mellitus
C. Hyperlipidemia
D. Pregnancy

43. A patient presents to the clinic appearing disheveled and reports symptoms of dyskinesia, mood swings, and chorea. The AGACNP obtains a CT scan of the brain that shows atrophy of the caudal nuclei and enlarged lateral ventricles. Which disease would the AGACNP first expect?

A. Lewy body disease
B. Frontotemporal degeneration
C. Prion disease
D. Huntington disease

44. A patient presents to the clinic with complaints of pain, numbness, and tingling affecting their right hand, primarily at night. Physical examination reveals positive Tinel's and Phalen's signs. These symptoms and physical examination findings are consistent with which diagnosis?

A. Carpal tunnel syndrome
B. Osteoarthritis
C. Cervical radiculopathy
D. Neuropathy

(*See answers next page.*)

41. A) Acute contact dermatitis

The patient is presenting with symptoms of acute contact dermatitis, a localized inflammatory skin reaction, after encountering poison ivy. Although acute contact dermatitis and atopic dermatitis are similar in appearance, atopic dermatitis is chronic in nature, characterized by exacerbations and remissions, and not localized to one area. Tinea pedis, also referred to by the term *athlete's foot*, is a fungal infection that presents as interdigital scaling, maceration, and, at times, erythema. Urticaria is also an acute allergic reaction; however, it is characterized by edematous wheals that can occur anywhere on the body.

42. B) Diabetes mellitus

Increased glucose levels associated with diabetes impair the body's ability to effectively heal wounds. There is no direct correlation between poor wound healing and coronary artery disease, hyperlipidemia, or pregnancy.

43. D) Huntington disease

The patient is exhibiting symptoms of Huntington disease and brain CT findings are confirmatory. Lewy body disease is the accumulation of protein in the nuclei of cortical neurons and is characterized by alteration in memory and motor control, which is like Alzheimer disease. This disease is diagnosed from symptomology and brain PET findings. Frontotemporal degeneration is caused by a mutation in genes, causes behavior and language disturbances, and is characterized by deterioration of the front and anterior lobes of the brain. Prion disease is a fatal disease that causes misfolding of endogenous proteins into infectious prion proteins, is characterized by personality and motor impairment, and is diagnosed after death via brain-tissue biopsy.

44. A) Carpal tunnel syndrome

Carpal tunnel syndrome is caused by compression of the median nerve and is characterized by hand numbness, tingling, and pain. Symptoms are more prominent when asleep due to redistribution of fluid and subsequent pressure on the median nerve. Positive Tinel's and Phalen's signs are confirmatory physical examination findings. Osteoarthritis is loss of articular cartilage and growth of osteophytes on the joints. This disease process is characterized by pain that increases with joint use. Cervical radiculopathy is characterized by continuous unilateral numbness, tingling, and pain due to compression of nerves in the cervical spine. Neuropathy is numbness and tingling that results from nerve damage and can affect hands and feet. Symptoms of neuropathy are no more prominent at night than they are during the day.

45. What structure secretes follicle-stimulating hormone (FSH) and luteinizing hormone (LH)?

A. Anterior pituitary
B. Posterior pituitary
C. Hypothalamus
D. Ovaries

46. Noncancerous enlargement of the prostate with symptoms of difficulty initiating stream and nocturia are characteristic of which reproductive disorder?

A. Erectile dysfunction (ED)
B. Benign prostatic hyperplasia (BPH)
C. Prostate neoplasm
D. Bacterial prostatitis

47. The AGACNP suspects that a patient has cystic fibrosis (CF). Which of the following diagnostic studies is considered the gold standard testing for diagnosis of CF?

A. Sweat chloride test
B. CF transmembrane regulator genetic analysis
C. CF transmembrane regulator functional testing
D. Immunoreactive trypsinogen

48. Which hormones stimulate the growth of ovarian follicles?

A. Follicle-stimulating hormone (FSH) and luteinizing hormone (LH)
B. Progesterone and FSH
C. LH and estrogen
D. Estrogen and progesterone

49. Naloxone (Narcan) is indicated for which drug overdose?

A. Acetaminophen (Tylenol)
B. Heroin
C. Metoprolol tartrate (Lopressor)
D. Alprazolam (Xanax)

(*See answers next page.*)

45. A) Anterior pituitary

FSH, LH, and prolactin are secreted from the anterior pituitary. The posterior pituitary secretes oxytocin and vasopressin. The hypothalamus releases gonadotropin-releasing hormone. The ovaries secrete estrogen and progesterone.

46. B) Benign prostatic hyperplasia (BPH)

BPH is a noncancerous overgrowth of the prostate that causes symptoms of difficulty initiating and maintaining urine stream and nocturia. ED is the inability to achieve and maintain an erection. Prostate neoplasm is cancerous overgrowth of the prostate that results in symptoms similar to BPH. Bacterial prostatitis is a bacterial infection of the prostate gland that causes symptoms of dysuria, frequency, and urinary retention.

47. A) Sweat chloride test

The sweat chloride test is considered the gold standard approach to diagnosing CF. CF transmembrane regulator genetic analysis, CF transmembrane regulator functional testing, and immunoreactive trypsinogen are all adjunctive testing methods; however, they are not the standard of care.

48. A) Follicle-stimulating hormone (FSH) and luteinizing hormone (LH)

FSH and LH stimulate the development and maturation of ovarian follicles. Progesterone is secreted by the corpus luteum after ovulation has occurred. Estrogen is produced by the theca interna, a layer within the ovarian follicle, which in turn provides negative feedback to FSH. Progesterone is produced by the corpus luteum in response to follicle rupture.

49. B) Heroin

Naloxone (Narcan) is an opioid antagonist used to reverse the effects of heroin and other opioids. The antidote for acetaminophen (Tylenol) overdose is acetylcysteine (Mucomyst). Glucagon is used in the treatment of metoprolol tartrate/beta-blocker overdose. Flumazenil (Romazicon) is a benzodiazepine receptor antagonist and is used in alprazolam (Xanax) overdose.

50. A patient being treated with amiodarone (Cordarone) presents to the clinic with complaints of progressive shortness of breath and nonproductive cough. The AGACNP examines the patient and notes tachypnea and fingernail clubbing. A pulmonary function test (PFT) is obtained and shows decreased vital capacity and total lung capacity with preserved expiratory flow rates. Which diagnosis does the AGACNP suspect?

A. Chronic obstructive pulmonary disease
B. Drug-induced interstitial lung disease
C. Hypersensitivity pneumonitis
D. Sarcoidosis

51. Which chamber of the heart pumps oxygenated blood out to the body?

A. Right atrium
B. Left atrium
C. Right ventricle
D. Left ventricle

52. Which patient-reported symptom will indicate to the AGACNP that the patient may have rheumatoid arthritis? Joint pain that:

A. Is worse in the morning and gets better with movement
B. Is progressive throughout the day and gets better with rest
C. Is constant and does not improve with movement or rest
D. Occurs only at night

53. A patient presents with dysphagia following a traumatic brain injury. The AGACNP suspects damage to which cranial nerve?

A. I
B. IV
C. VIII
D. IX

54. What is most likely to precipitate the development of diabetic ketoacidosis (DKA)?

A. Infection
B. Medication nonadherence
C. Newly diagnosed diabetes
D. Pancreatitis

(*See answers next page.*)

50. B) Drug-induced interstitial lung disease

The patient presents with symptoms of interstitial lung disease and is on a known causative agent, amiodarone (Cordarone). Chronic obstructive pulmonary disease is an inflammatory disease that results from recurrent exposure to noxious particles or gases. A PFT would show a decrease in expiratory flow rate in this patient population. Hypersensitivity pneumonitis results from repeated inhalation of dust. Sarcoidosis is a systemic disease that does not occur as a result of environmental exposure and is characterized by the presence of granulomas throughout the body.

51. D) Left ventricle

Blood returns from the body into the right atrium, and then to the right ventricle, and through the pulmonary arteries to the lungs. Oxygenated blood travels through the pulmonary veins into the left atrium and then into the left ventricle. Finally, the oxygenated blood leaves the ventricle to be dispersed to the body.

52. A) Is worse in the morning and gets better with movement

Rheumatoid arthritis, an immune-mediated disorder that leads to destruction of connective tissue, is characterized by pain that is worse in the morning and improves throughout the day with movement. Osteoarthritis, a degenerative joint disease, is associated with pain that worsens throughout the day and is relieved by rest. Joint pain that is chronic is not relieved by rest or activity, or only occurs at night is not characteristic of rheumatoid arthritis.

53. D) IX

Cranial nerve IX, also known as the glossopharyngeal nerve, plays a major role in the mechanics of swallowing. Cranial nerve I is involved with sense of smell, cranial nerve IV is responsible for eye movement and proprioception, and cranial nerve VIII is involved in hearing and balance.

54. A) Infection

Infection is the most common underlying cause of DKA because it increases stress on the body, which in turn triggers the release of glucose. Medication (namely, insulin) nonadherence, newly diagnosed diabetes, and pancreatitis are all possible triggers of DKA but to a lesser degree.

55. A patient presents with reports of right otalgia and otic discharge. On examination, there is pain with the traction of the right pinna, normal tympanic membrane, and debris noted in the right canal. The AGACNP suspects what diagnosis?

A. Otitis media with effusion
B. Acute otitis media
C. Acute otitis externa
D. Perichondritis

56. What is a manifestation of increased ocular pressure?

A. Glaucoma
B. Hypertension
C. Macular degeneration
D. Ptosis

57. The AGACNP reviews the complete blood count (CBC) and differential results of a patient: hemoglobin 9.2 g/dL, hematocrit 32.2 %, red blood cell count 3.1 million cells/mcL, mean corpuscular volume (MCV) 68 fl. The AGACNP informs the patient that this is considered:

A. Microcytic anemia
B. Macrocytic anemia
C. Iron-deficiency anemia
D. Normal CBC findings

58. The average life span of a red blood cell (RBC) is how many days?

A. 1
B. 7
C. 30
D. 120

59. What cells are part of the innate immune system?

A. T cells
B. B cells
C. Natural killer cells
D. Humoral cells

(*See answers next page.*)

55. C) Acute otitis externa

Acute otitis externa is characterized by otalgia, discharge, and pain with traction to the pinna. There is often debris in the ear canal as well. Otitis media with effusion is characterized by fluid in the middle ear. Perichondritis is characterized by redness in the pinna. Acute otitis media would exhibit a bulging, red tympanic membrane.

56. A) Glaucoma

Increased ocular pressure, largely influenced by the aqueous humor, causes glaucoma. It is not associated with hypertension, macular degeneration (retinal deterioration), or ptosis (drooping of the eyelid).

57. A) Microcytic anemia

This patient has low hemoglobin and low MCV, indicating microcytic anemia. In macrocytic anemia, the MCV would be greater than 100 fl. Iron-deficiency anemia is usually microcytic, but this diagnosis cannot be made without obtaining additional studies. The patient's CBC results are not normal.

58. D) 120

The average life span of an RBC is 120 days. Bone marrow regenerates RBCs as older ones are phagocytosed or broken down. Unless there is premature damage, the RBC lives longer than 1 day, 7 days, or 30 days.

59. C) Natural killer cells

Natural killer cells belong to the innate immune system. T cells and B cells are part of adaptive immunity. Humoral cells are not a type of cell related to immunity.

60. The term *pleiotropic* refers to the ability of cytokines to:

A. Have an effect on multiple cell types
B. Replicate indefinitely
C. Cause blood clots
D. Fight infection

61. The AGACNP examines a patient who presents with an acutely painful, erythematous left eye. Upon examination, a corneal ulcer is noted. What is the AGACNP's next step?

A. Prescription for ophthalmic dexamethasone (Dexasol)
B. Referral to ophthalmology
C. Prescription for ophthalmic neomycin (Gramicidin)
D. Flushing the eye with sterile water

62. The AGACNP is seeing a patient with HIV and explains that their CD4 count of 350 cells/mm^3 indicates a/an:

A. Diagnosis of AIDS
B. Higher risk of complications
C. Improvement to normal range
D. Active infection

63. The AGACNP is caring for a patient in the intensive care unit who is exhibiting signs of delirium on postoperative day 3. After reviewing the medication administration record, which class of medication should the AGACNP discontinue due to its potential to cause delirium?

A. Stool softeners
B. Benzodiazepines
C. Anticonvulsant
D. Vasopressors

(*See answers next page.*)

60. A) Have an effect on multiple cell types

The term *pleiotropic* refers to cytokines' ability to act on and enhance various types of cells in the immune response. Cytokines do not replicate indefinitely. While they are involved in fighting infections and can increase intravascular coagulation, this is not related to the term *pleiotropic.*

61. B) Referral to ophthalmology

A patient with a corneal ulcer should be referred to ophthalmology on an emergent basis to decrease the risk for permanent eye and vision issues. A prescription for ophthalmic dexamethasone (Dexasol) or neomycin (Gramicidin) may be indicated for bacterial conjunctivitis but not for corneal ulcers. Flushing the eye with water should not be done before the patient is evaluated by a specialist.

62. B) Higher risk of complications

A CD4 count of fewer than 400 cells/mm^3 puts the individual at higher risk for infectious complications. It is not diagnostic for AIDS or an active infection. The normal range for CD4 count is 500 to 1500 cells/mm^3.

63. B) Benzodiazepines

The patient is exhibiting signs of delirium. The AGACNP has been tasked with reviewing the medication administration record and determining which class of medication may contribute to the patient's altered mentation. Benzodiazepines are clinically shown to contribute to and/or worsen symptoms of delirium and should be discontinued if they are suspected to be the cause of altered mentation. Stool softeners treat constipation and do not affect neurologic or cognitive function. Although anticonvulsants affect the central nervous system, they generally do not contribute to delirium and are unlikely to be the culprit in this situation. Vasopressors are used to treat hypotension and do not have an adverse side effect of delirium.

64. A patient who underwent organ transplantation asks about when they will be able to receive the zoster vaccine recombinant, adjuvanted (Shingrix). Which is the AGACNP's response?

A. "You cannot receive the zoster vaccine recombinant, adjuvanted (Shingrix) because it is a live vaccine."
B. "You may receive the zoster vaccine recombinant, adjuvanted (Shingrix) 3 to 6 months after your transplant."
C. "You may receive the zoster vaccine recombinant, adjuvanted (Shingrix) anytime."
D. "You may receive the zoster vaccine recombinant, adjuvanted (Shingrix) once you stop your immunosuppressive medication."

65. A 45-year-old patient presents to the emergency department with complaints of difficulty speaking and right-sided weakness that abruptly began 30 minutes prior to arrival. CT of the brain is negative for tumors and hemorrhages. Repeat assessment reflects no change. Which pharmacologic intervention by the AGACNP is most appropriate?

A. Levetiracetam (Keppra)
B. Methylprednisolone sodium succinate (Solu-Medrol)
C. Mannitol (Osmitrol)
D. Tissue plasminogen activator (Alteplase)

66. A patient presents to the emergency department after being ejected from their vehicle during a motor vehicle crash. CT of the brain shows cerebral edema with midline shift. Which pharmacologic agent should the AGACNP order to aid in reduction of cerebral edema?

A. Mannitol (Osmitrol)
B. Levetiracetam (Keppra)
C. Alprazolam (Xanax)
D. Methylprednisolone sodium succinate (Solu-Medrol)

67. A patient presents to the emergency department with altered mental status, muscle rigidity, and fever. The AGACNP obtains a history and physical examination, which reveal that the patient takes fluoxetine (Prozac) and was recently treated with linezolid (Zyvox). Which diagnosis does the AGACNP suspect?

A. Sepsis
B. Serotonin syndrome
C. Delirium
D. Cerebral vascular accident

(*See answers next page.*)

64. B) "You may receive the zoster vaccine recombinant, adjuvanted (Shingrix) 3 to 6 months after your transplant."

Ideally, vaccines should be given before an organ transplantation. If that is not possible, vaccines should be given 3 to 6 months after transplantation. While it is true that live vaccines are contraindicated, the zoster vaccine recombinant, adjuvanted (Shingrix) is inactivated. An organ transplant patient will be on immunosuppressive medication indefinitely.

65. D) Tissue plasminogen activator (Alteplase)

The patient presents with acute-onset difficulty speaking and right-sided weakness, consistent with acute cerebral vascular accident (CVA). Intracranial hemorrhage and tumor have been ruled out via CT of the brain, leading the AGACNP to a diagnosis of acute ischemic CVA. The patient is older than 18 years, and symptoms have been present for less than 3 hours; therefore, they meet the criteria for administration of tissue plasminogen activator (Alteplase), a fibrinolytic agent used to treat acute ischemic events. Levetiracetam (Keppra), an anticonvulsant, is not the pharmacologic agent of choice as it does not aid in reperfusion therapy. Methylprednisolone sodium succinate (Solu-Medrol) and mannitol (Osmitrol) may be indicated for the management of cerebral edema but will not affect the occluded vessel.

66. A) Mannitol (Osmitrol)

Mannitol (Osmitrol) is the most commonly prescribed osmotic diuretic used to treat cerebral edema. Levetiracetam (Keppra), an anticonvulsant, is indicated to prevent seizures; however, it will have no effect on cerebral edema. Alprazolam (Xanax), a benzodiazepine, is contraindicated due to its potential to cause a decrease in level of consciousness in a patient who is already neurologically compromised. Methylprednisolone sodium succinate (Solu-Medrol), a corticosteroid, is not indicated for managing cerebral edema secondary to a traumatic brain injury.

67. B) Serotonin syndrome

The patient presents with signs and symptoms of serotonin syndrome. This occurs when a patient is taking fluoxetine (Prozac), a selective serotonin reuptake inhibitor, in conjunction with linezolid (Zyvox), an antibiotic. Although sepsis can cause altered mentation and fever, it does not cause muscle rigidity. A diagnosis of delirium would account for the patient's altered mental status but does not address the other presenting symptoms. Cerebral vascular accident does not result in fever and is unrelated to the use of these two medications.

68. A patient with psychosis is being seen after initiation of chlorpromazine (Thorazine). The patient complains of involuntary facial movements that began shortly after starting the medication. The AGACNP identifies these movements as:

A. Nervous tics
B. Seizure activity
C. Tardive dyskinesia
D. Muscle spasms

69. A patient has been diagnosed with pulmonary artery hypertension (PAH) and needs to be started on pharmacologic therapy. Which pharmacologic agent is indicated for treatment of PAH?

A. Metoprolol tartrate (Lopressor)
B. Sildenafil (Viagra)
C. Dobutamine (Dobutrex)
D. Pseudoephedrine (Sudafed)

70. A patient with chronic obstructive pulmonary disease (COPD) presents to the outpatient urgent care clinic with complaints of shortness of breath and sputum production. The AGACNP examines the patient and notes inspiratory wheezing, accessory muscle use, and pulse oximetry reading of 85%. Which initial pharmacologic intervention by the AGACNP is most appropriate?

A. Furosemide (Lasix)
B. Nebulized 3% normal saline (NS)
C. Albuterol (VoSpire ER)
D. Alprazolam (Xanax)

71. A patient recovering from repair of a hip fracture suddenly develops shortness of breath and tachycardia. The AGACNP orders a ventilation/perfusion study that reports multiple perfusion defects in the right lung. Which pharmacologic intervention by the AGACNP is indicated?

A. Clopidogrel (Plavix)
B. Unfractionated heparin (Heparin)
C. Vitamin K
D. Protamine sulfate (Protamine)

(*See answers next page.*)

68. C) Tardive dyskinesia

The patient has been diagnosed with psychosis and started on the antipsychotic chlorpromazine (Thorazine). A common side effect of this medication is tardive dyskinesia, which is characterized by involuntary movements of the face. A nervous tic is a compulsive disorder that can affect any part of the body and, although difficult to control, is voluntary. Seizure activity can present in a number of ways, including facial movements; however, psychosis, use of antipsychotics, and involuntary facial movements that are all associated with tardive dyskinesia. Muscle spasms are uncontrollable muscle contractions that are not specific to one muscle group or associated with antipsychotic use.

69. B) Sildenafil (Viagra)

Sildenafil (Viagra) is a phosphodiesterase inhibitor that is indicated for use in PAH patients. Metoprolol tartrate (Lopressor) is a beta-blocker and should be avoided due to its potential for decreasing right heart function. Dobutamine (Dobutrex) is a positive inotrope, and although it may help with left ventricular function, it will not affect decreasing pulmonary artery pressure. Pseudoephedrine (Sudafed), a decongestant, should be avoided in patients with PAH due to the risk of decreasing right heart function.

70. C) Albuterol (VoSpire ER)

The patient is presenting with an acute COPD exacerbation with signs of respiratory distress. The use of a short-acting beta-agonist is indicated for initial treatment of an acute COPD exacerbation. Although an acute COPD exacerbation involves airway edema, the use of furosemide (Lasix) will have no effect on airway obstruction resulting from inflammation. Nebulized 3% NS will assist in the mobilization of secretions but is not the initial pharmacologic agent of choice because it will not provide immediate relief of airway obstruction. Alprazolam (Xanax) is contraindicated because it acts on the central nervous system, causing respiratory depression and potential respiratory failure.

71. B) Unfractionated heparin (Heparin)

The patient's symptoms and radiologic findings are consistent with pulmonary embolism secondary to deep vein thrombosis. The patient needs to be started immediately on systemic anticoagulation with an agent such as heparin to prevent additional clot formation. Clopidogrel (Plavix), an antiplatelet agent, will not prevent additional clots from forming and is therefore not an appropriate form of anticoagulation therapy. Vitamin K and protamine sulfate (Protamine) reverse anticoagulation and promote clotting; therefore, they are contraindicated.

72. A patient presents to the emergency department with complaints of fever, cough, sputum production, and shortness of breath. The patient's chest x-ray shows a right lower lobe infiltrate. Which pharmacologic agent should the AGACNP order first?

A. Amoxicillin (Amoxil)
B. Methylprednisolone sodium succinate (Solu-Medrol)
C. Intravenous normal saline (NS)
D. Albuterol (VoSpire ER)

73. A patient presents to the emergency department and reports 9/10 substernal chest pain, jaw pain, shortness of breath, and diaphoresis. Vital signs are blood pressure 148/86 mmHg, heart rate 90 beats/min, respiratory rate 24 breaths/min, and pulse oximetry 92% on room air. Twelve-lead electrocardiogram shows ST-segment elevation in leads II, III, and aVF. Which physical examination finding would the AGACNP expect?

A. Rigid abdomen
B. Fingernail clubbing
C. Cool, clammy skin
D. Jaundice

74. The AGACNP is caring for a patient who presents to the outpatient setting with complaints of shortness of breath, lower extremity edema, and a 15-lb weight gain over 3 days. Physical examination reveals bilateral lower lobe crackles and 2+ pitting edema in the lower extremities. Which radiologic examination would initially be most appropriate for further assessment?

A. Chest radiograph
B. Chest CT
C. Abdominal CT
D. Abdominal radiograph

75. A patient with an iodine allergy has undergone percutaneous coronary intervention (PCI). The AGACNP is called to the bedside for evaluation. Which physical examination finding requires immediate intervention by the AGACNP?

A. Facial edema
B. Right femoral artery hematoma
C. Decreased breath sounds bilaterally
D. Irregular heart rhythm

(*See answers next page.*)

72. A) Amoxicillin (Amoxil)

The patient presents with signs and symptoms of community-acquired pneumonia (CAP). Initiation of broad-spectrum antibiotics is the immediate priority for the AGACNP while awaiting culture results. Per guidelines, amoxicillin (Amoxil), a broad-spectrum macrolide antibiotic, is first-line therapy for uncomplicated CAP. The use of methylprednisolone sodium succinate (Solu-Medrol), intravenous NS, and albuterol (VoSpire ER) may be indicated; however, they are not appropriate first-line pharmacologic interventions.

73. C) Cool, clammy skin

The patient presents with signs and symptoms of an acute inferior wall myocardial infarction (MI). The presence of cool, clammy skin is an expected physical examination assessment finding in a patient suffering from an MI. A rigid abdomen is indicative of an acute intra-abdominal process that is not supported by the patient's symptoms. Fingernail clubbing is a physical examination finding consistent with a chronic, rather than acute, disease process. Jaundice reflects a problem with the liver and would be considered a secondary finding associated with MI.

74. A) Chest radiograph

The patient presents with symptoms of heart failure and pulmonary edema. A chest radiograph is the least invasive and most cost-efficient radiologic examination to assess for the presence of pulmonary edema. Although chest CT is also capable of assessing for pulmonary edema, it provides more data than necessary to confirm this diagnosis. Abdominal CT and abdominal radiographs do not address the patient's pulmonary complaints.

75. A) Facial edema

The patient has a known iodine allergy and has just undergone PCI, which requires intravenous contrast. The presence of facial edema is concerning for iodine reaction and places the patient at immediate risk for airway compromise. Following the principle of ABCs (airway, breathing, and circulation), addressing the potential for airway compromise is top priority for the AGACNP. The presence of a femoral artery hematoma is concerning for arterial access complications; however, it is not top priority and can be addressed after the airway has been secured. Decreased breath sounds, although abnormal, do not pose an immediate danger to the patient and can be addressed after the airway is secured. Irregular heart rhythms are common postprocedure and, in this situation, can be addressed once the patient has been stabilized.

76. A patient is admitted to the telemetry unit with complaints of palpitations. The AGACNP is called to the bedside to evaluate an irregular rhythm with no discernable P waves noted on telemetry. Which physical examination finding would indicate that the patient is not tolerating the irregular heart rhythm?

A. Respiratory rate 30 breaths/min
B. Heart rate 110 bpm
C. Blood pressure 115/68 mmHg
D. Oral temperature 100.4°F (38.0°C)

77. A patient with a brain tumor has been hospitalized with complaints of decreased urine output, weight gain, and shortness of breath. Which physical examination finding does not correlate?

A. Bilateral crackles
B. Hyperthermia
C. Edema
D. Tachycardia

78. A patient is being evaluated in the clinic for complaints of weight loss, palpitations, and diaphoresis. Laboratory studies reveal elevated T3, elevated T4, and low thyroid-stimulating hormone. Which physical examination finding supports the patient's signs and symptoms?

A. Enlarged thyroid
B. Bradycardia
C. Lower extremity edema
D. Decreased deep tendon reflexes

79. A patient is admitted to the hospital with a small bowel obstruction. A nasogastric tube has been placed and has drained 1.5 L. Which physical examination finding alerts the AGACNP that the patient is clinically deteriorating?

A. Blood pressure 105/76 mmHg
B. Distended abdomen
C. Hypoactive bowel sounds
D. Rigid abdomen

(*See answers next page.*)

76. A) Respiratory rate 30 breaths/min

The patient is admitted with complaints of palpitations and is having irregular rhythm without discernable P waves noted on telemetry. The AGACNP identifies this rhythm as atrial fibrillation, and a common complication of this rhythm is flash pulmonary edema. Tachypnea is an examination finding consistent with flash pulmonary edema and is reflective of the patient's intolerance of the rhythm. A heart rate of 110 bpm, although elevated, does not indicate that the patient is not tolerating the change in rhythm. A blood pressure of 115/68 mmHg is within normal limits and does not alert the AGACNP of the patient's inability to tolerate the irregular rhythm. An elevated temperature is an unrelated finding.

77. B) Hyperthermia

The patient is presenting with symptoms of syndrome of inappropriate antidiuretic hormone secretion, a complication associated with brain tumors. As the patient's condition deteriorates, they lose their ability to regulate body temperature and develop hypothermia. The presence of crackles and edema are also common examination findings due to excess fluid retention. Tachycardia is a compensatory mechanism in response to excess fluid and will resolve with treatment of the underlying disease process.

78. A) Enlarged thyroid

The patient is presenting with signs and symptoms of hyperthyroidism. Due to overactive thyroid cells, the thyroid gland begins to enlarge, and this can be appreciated on examination. Patients with this diagnosis are frequently tachycardic rather than bradycardic. Lower extremity edema and decreased deep tendon reflexes are signs of hypothyroidism, not hyperthyroidism.

79. D) Rigid abdomen

The patient is being treated medically for a small bowel obstruction. The presence of a rigid abdomen is concerning for small bowel rupture, a clinical emergency. A blood pressure of 105/76 mmHg is on the lower side of normal; however, it does not indicate an acute abdomen or shock. Abdominal distention is common in these scenarios and does not alert the AGACNP of a potential problem. Hypoactive bowel sounds are to be expected and do not indicate a change in status.

80. A patient with end-stage liver disease has been admitted to the hospital for palliative paracentesis. Which physical examination finding would the AGACNP not expect with this patient?

A. Anicteric sclera

B. Abdominal distention

C. Altered mentation

D. Petechiae

(*See answers next page.*)

80. A) Anicteric sclera

The patient is presenting with end-stage liver disease. As the liver fails, it loses its ability to filter bilirubin, which results in icteric sclera. Abdominal distention is an expected finding and is the reason the patient has been admitted for palliative paracentesis. Altered mentation is common in this patient population due to increased ammonia levels. Petechiae develop due to hepatic disruption in the formation of clotting factors.

2

Clinical Practice

1. Which test is used to identify patients at risk for hip fracture secondary to osteopenia and osteoporosis?

A. Serum calcium
B. Hip x-ray
C. Dual-energy x-ray absorptiometry (DEXA) scan
D. Serum vitamin D

2. Which class of medication increases the risk of vertebral fracture?

A. Corticosteroids
B. Nonsteroidal anti-inflammatory drugs (NSAIDs)
C. Calcium supplements
D. Beta-blockers

3. A 72-year-old patient reports low back pain unresponsive to nonpharmacologic measures. Which medication should the AGACNP prescribe first?

A. Acetaminophen (Tylenol)
B. Ibuprofen (Advil)
C. Prednisone (Deltasone)
D. Oxycodone (OxyContin)

4. The AGACNP notes a positive lift-off test when examining an older adult patient. Which is the likely diagnosis for the patient?

A. Adhesive capsulitis
B. Patellar subluxation
C. Subscapularis tendon insufficiency
D. Sciatica

5. Which tool is best for an initial diagnosis of subarachnoid hemorrhage?

A. MRI of brain
B. CT of head
C. Carotid ultrasound
D. Cerebral arteriography

(See answers next page.)

1. C) Dual-energy x-ray absorptiometry (DEXA) scan

A DEXA scan is a test to evaluate bone density and is used to screen patients for osteopenia and osteoporosis, major risk factors for hip fractures. A hip x-ray can be used to diagnose fractures but is not used in screening. Calcium and vitamin D are important for bone health, but serum levels do not serve in screening patients for osteoporosis or osteopenia.

2. A) Corticosteroids

Chronic corticosteroid use can weaken bones and increase the risk for vertebral fractures. NSAIDs, calcium supplements, and beta-blockers have not been shown to increase the risk for vertebral fractures.

3. B) Ibuprofen (Advil)

If medication needs to be used for low back, nonsteroidal anti-inflammatory drugs (NSAIDs) are the preferred therapy of choice. Corticosteroids such as prednisone (Deltasone) and acetaminophen (Tylenol) are typically not effective for musculo-skeletal low back pain. Oxycodone (OxyContin) has a high risk for dependence, so it would not be the best initial choice of therapy.

4. C) Subscapularis tendon insufficiency

A lift-off test is a shoulder examination technique that can demonstrate whether the patient has subscapularis tendon insufficiency. A positive lift-off test is not indicative of adhesive capsulitis, or frozen shoulder. Patellar subluxation is a dis-location of the knee cap. Sciatica would be indicated by a positive straight leg raise.

5. B) CT of head

CT of the head (preferably with angiography) is the most sensitive in detecting cerebral hemorrhage within the first 24 hours following the incident. It is also quicker than MRI of the brain, so it allows for initiation of treatment sooner. Carotid ultrasound and cerebral arteriography may be indicated for a patient who has had a subarachnoid hemorrhage, but those tests would not be best for initial diagnosis.

6. A patient presents with neck pain and neuropathy in the right arm following a car crash. Which imaging study should the AGACNP order first?

   A. X-ray of cervical spine
   B. CT of neck
   C. MRI of cervical spine
   D. Ultrasound of the right arm

7. A patient with lung cancer presents with suspected leptomeningeal metastases. Which test should the AGACNP order to confirm the diagnosis?

   A. Cerebrospinal fluid analysis
   B. MRI of lumbar spine
   C. CT of brain
   D. CT of chest

8. A patient presents with bradykinesia, postural instability, rigidity, and tremors. The AGACNP suspects which clinical diagnosis?

   A. Parkinson disease
   B. Meningitis
   C. Alcohol intoxication
   D. Ischemic stroke

9. Which syndrome is characterized by the re-experience of previous trauma and avoidance of events related to that trauma?

   A. Generalized anxiety disorder (GAD)
   B. Major depressive disorder (MDD)
   C. Posttraumatic stress disorder (PTSD)
   D. Social anxiety disorder (SAD)

10. A 71-year-old patient presents to the emergency department with new-onset dysarthria and left-sided weakness. What imaging test should the AGACNP order first?

   A. MRI of the brain
   B. CT of the head
   C. X-ray of the left leg
   D. Ultrasound of the left leg

(*See answers next page.*)

6. C) MRI of cervical spine

A patient who presents with neck pain and neuropathy following a car crash raises concern for cervical radiculopathy. This is best evaluated with MRI of the cervical spine. An x-ray of the cervical spine or CT of the neck would not be as sensitive in identifying issues in the soft tissue or nerves. An ultrasound of the right arm does not address the likely root cause of the symptoms.

7. A) Cerebrospinal fluid analysis

An analysis of cerebrospinal fluid is the confirmatory examination for leptomeningeal metastases. While MRI of the lumbar spine may show signs of potential leptomeningeal spread, the diagnosis is confirmed with cerebrospinal fluid labs. CT of the brain is not as sensitive in detecting leptomeningeal spread. A CT of the chest would not show leptomeningeal disease, as this occurs in the brain and spinal cord.

8. A) Parkinson disease

Parkinson disease is characterized by bradykinesia, postural instability, rigidity, and tremors and can typically be diagnosed by examination and symptom review. A patient with meningitis would present with neck stiffness, fever, and infectious symptoms. Alcohol intoxication may present as lethargy, gait imbalance, and lack of coordination. An ischemic stroke has variable symptoms but may include unilateral weakness and dysarthria.

9. C) Posttraumatic stress disorder (PTSD)

PTSD is characterized by a history of exposure to a real or perceived threat/trauma and reexperience of that trauma. GAD, MDD, and SAD are not caused by specific traumatic events.

10. B) CT of the head

The patient's presentation is highly suspicious for a cerebral vascular accident. CT of the head is the gold standard for diagnostic imaging during the initial phase of care and should be performed as soon as possible after symptoms present. MRI of the brain should be ordered subsequently, but a CT of the head is preferably done first to show or rule out hemorrhage and can be done quickly. A left leg x-ray and left leg ultrasound do not address the most likely and critical etiology of the patient's symptoms.

11. Cervical cancer screening is appropriate for which patient?

A. A 34-year-old with a prior hysterectomy and cervix removal
B. A 59-year-old who had a normal Pap smear and negative human papillomavirus (HPV) test 3 years ago
C. A 20-year-old patient whose first sexual intercourse occurred at age 17 years
D. A 61-year-old patient who had a normal Pap smear 3 years ago

12. Which is a common symptom of cervical polyps?

A. Vaginal bleeding
B. Pelvic pain
C. Urinary incontinence
D. Vulvar pruritus

13. A 65-year-old postmenopausal patient presents with new vaginal bleeding. Which is the most appropriate next step?

A. Blood transfusion
B. Transvaginal sonography
C. Oral contraceptive taper
D. Referral to gynecologic oncology

14. A 58-year-old patient tells the AGACNP, "I do not need to have a Pap smear because I have previously received the human papillomavirus (HPV) vaccine." How should the AGACNP respond?

A. "Since you have received the vaccine, you will not need HPV co-testing but should still have a Pap smear."
B. "You are correct, you do not need cervical cancer screening since you are vaccinated."
C. "You should still undergo cervical cancer screening since the vaccine does not cover all carcinogenic HPV types."
D. "You should still have a Pap smear and HPV testing, but you will need it only every 10 years."

15. Which class of medication is used when performing spirometry for asthma evaluation?

A. Inhaled histamine
B. Methacholine (Provocholine)
C. Bronchodilator
D. Inhaled corticosteroid

(*See answers next page.*)

11. D) A 61-year-old patient who had a normal Pap smear 3 years ago

A 61-year-old patient who had a normal Pap smear 3 years ago is now due for a repeat screening. According to the U.S. Preventive Services Task Force, cervical cancer screening should be performed from age 21 to age 65 years. In patients age 30 to 65 years, cytology should be performed every 3 years or with HPV co-testing every 5 years. This excludes patients who have had a hysterectomy with cervix removal.

12. A) Vaginal bleeding

Vaginal bleeding and discharge are the most common symptoms of cervical polyps. Pelvic pain, urinary incontinence, and vulvar pruritus are not typically associated with cervical polyps.

13. B) Transvaginal sonography

Postmenopausal patients with abnormal uterine bleeding should undergo transvaginal sonography to measure endometrial thickness. A blood transfusion would only be indicated if the bleeding was profuse enough to cause severe anemia. An oral contraceptive taper is not appropriate before determining the cause of bleeding. Similarly, a referral to gynecologic oncology would not be indicated before knowing the etiology of the bleeding.

14. C) "You should still undergo cervical cancer screening since the vaccine does not cover all carcinogenic HPV types."

Patients should be counseled that cervical cancer screening is still important, as the HPV vaccine does not protect against all carcinogenic types of HPV. The testing should include both the Pap smear and HPV co-testing. Receiving the HPV vaccine does not change the frequency with which the screening is recommended.

15. C) Bronchodilator

When performing spirometry for asthma evaluation, measurements should be done before and after short-acting bronchodilator administration to determine whether airflow obstruction is reversible. Inhaled histamine and methacholine (Provocholine) are typically used in bronchial provocation testing. Inhaled corticosteroids are not used in this diagnostic setting.

16. The AGACNP reviews cervical screening results for a 62-year-old patient. The cytology shows atypical squamous cells of unknown significance, and the human papillomavirus (HPV) test is negative. Which is the AGACNP's next step?

A. Referral to colposcopy
B. Order for Pap smear and HPV co-testing in 1 year
C. Order for HPV 9-valent vaccine
D. Order for Pap smear and HPV co-testing in 3 years

17. The AGACNP is caring for a patient with chronic obstructive pulmonary disease (COPD). Which should prompt referral to a specialist?

A. COPD diagnosis at age 60 years
B. Two COPD exacerbations over the last year despite treatment
C. Use of supplemental oxygen for 3 weeks during an exacerbation
D. COPD managed on the current regimen

18. A patient reports nighttime awakenings from asthma and use of asthma reliever medication three times per week. How does the AGACNP classify this patient's asthma control?

A. Well-controlled
B. Partly controlled
C. Poorly controlled
D. Not controlled

19. Which is the treatment of choice for a thrombosed cardiac valve?

A. Unfractionated heparin
B. Clopidogrel (Plavix)
C. Aspirin
D. Warfarin (Coumadin)

20. Which is the target therapeutic international normalized ratio (INR) range for a 79-year-old patient with a mechanical aortic valve?

A. 1.0–2.0
B. 1.5–2.5
C. 2.0–3.0
D. 2.5–3.5

(*See answers next page.*)

16. B) Order for Pap smear and HPV co-testing in 1 year

A patient who has cytology showing atypical squamous cells of unknown significance with a negative HPV test should have a repeat Pap smear and HPV co-testing in 1 year. Colposcopy should be done only if the HPV test was positive. A 62-year-old patient would not be eligible for the HPV vaccine.

17. B) Two COPD exacerbations over the last year despite treatment

Referral to pulmonology or a COPD specialist should be made if a patient has two or more exacerbations within a year, has a diagnosis before age 40 years, requires long-term oxygen supplementation, or has severe COPD.

18. B) Partly controlled

Control of asthma is based on daytime symptoms, nighttime awakenings, interference with activity, and need for reliever medication. Because the patient has nighttime awakenings and uses reliever medication three times per week, this patient's asthma would be considered partly controlled. A well-controlled case of asthma would not produce any symptoms, and a case that is not controlled would be characterized by more symptoms. "Poorly controlled" asthma is not a classification.

19. A) Unfractionated heparin

All patients who develop a thrombosed valve should be treated with unfractionated heparin. Clopidogrel (Plavix), aspirin, and warfarin (Coumadin) are indicated in other cardiac conditions, but unfractionated heparin is indicated for all patients with thrombosed valves.

20. C) 2.0–3.0

The INR for a patient with a mechanical aortic valve should be maintained between 2.0 and 3.0. A level below this could increase the risk for thrombus formation, and a level above this could increase the risk of bleeding.

21. The AGACNP evaluates a patient with a low-density lipoprotein (LDL) level of 210 mg/dL. Which would be the most appropriate prescription for this patient?

A. Lovastatin (Altoprev) 20 mg daily
B. Pravastatin (Pravachol) 40 mg daily
C. Atorvastatin (Lipitor) 10 mg daily
D. Rosuvastatin (Crestor) 20 mg daily

22. Which is the appropriate statin treatment to prescribe for a 72-year-old patient with type 2 diabetes mellitus, an estimated 10-year atherosclerotic cardiovascular disease (ASCVD) risk of 6%, and a low-density lipoprotein (LDL) level of 120 mg/dL?

A. No statin therapy indicated
B. Low-intensity statin
C. Moderate-intensity statin
D. High-intensity statin

23. An 80-year-old patient presents to the emergency department with chest pain. The electrocardiogram shows ST-segment elevation. The patient reports an allergy to penicillin and aspirin. Which should the AGACNP order first?

A. Clopidogrel (Plavix)
B. Aspirin
C. Metoprolol (Lopressor)
D. Morphine (MS-Contin)

24. A patient reports recurrent chest pain that occurs with exertion but is promptly relieved with rest. Which medication should the AGACNP recommend the patient take first during these episodes?

A. Nitroglycerin (Nitrostat)
B. Ibuprofen (Advil)
C. Aspirin
D. Acetaminophen (Tylenol)

(*See answers next page.*)

21. D) Rosuvastatin (Crestor) 20 mg daily
A patient with an LDL level of 210 mg/dL requires high-intensity statin therapy, such as rosuvastatin (Crestor) 20 mg daily. Lovastatin (Altoprev) 20 mg daily is considered low-intensity statin therapy. Pravastatin (Pravachol) 40 mg daily and atorvastatin (Lipitor) 10 mg daily are moderate-intensity statin therapies.

22. C) Moderate-intensity statin
A patient age 40 to 75 years with type 2 diabetes should receive a moderate-intensity statin according to the ASCVD statin benefit algorithm. A low-intensity statin would not be sufficient for this patient's risk classification. A high-intensity statin should be prescribed only if the patient has an LDL level equal to or greater than 190 mg/dL or a 10-year ASCVD risk equal to or greater than 7.5%.

23. A) Clopidogrel (Plavix)
A patient who presents with chest pain and ST elevation on the electrocardiogram is experiencing myocardial infarction. Although aspirin is the first-line initial therapy for myocardial infarction, clopidogrel (Plavix) would be given because of the patient's reported allergy to aspirin. Metoprolol (Lopressor) may be ordered later for control of hypertension or arrhythmia but is not indicated as an initial treatment. Morphine (MS-Contin) can be used for pain relief but would not be the priority at this time.

24. A) Nitroglycerin (Nitrostat)
A patient who has chest pain with exertion that is relieved with rest likely has stable angina. Nitroglycerin (Nitrostat) is the treatment of choice for this condition. Ibuprofen (Advil) and acetaminophen (Tylenol) are pain relievers but would not be the best therapy of choice for angina. Aspirin is not recommended for acute management of angina.

25. A 79-year-old patient presents to the emergency department with chest pain and suspected myocardial infarction. Which medication should the AGACNP order first?

A. Aspirin
B. Clopidogrel (Plavix)
C. Morphine (MS-Contin)
D. Levofloxacin (Levaquin)

26. A patient in the intensive care unit (ICU) is exhibiting sustained ventricular tachycardia on the monitor and appears stable. Which is the AGACNP's next step?

A. Order electrical cardioversion
B. Order lidocaine (Xylocaine) bolus
C. Perform CPR
D. Continue to monitor

27. A patient is starting levothyroxine (Synthroid) for hypothyroidism. Which teaching does the AGACNP include in the patient's education?

A. Take levothyroxine (Synthroid) with food
B. Take levothyroxine (Synthroid) as needed for fatigue
C. Obtain blood work in 6 months
D. Take levothyroxine (Synthroid) at the same time each day

28. Adrenocorticotropic hormone (ACTH) deficiency results in decreased secretion of which hormones?

A. Cortisol and epinephrine
B. Growth hormone (GH) and aldosterone
C. Prolactin and thyroid-stimulating hormone (TSH)
D. Luteinizing hormone (LH) and follicle-stimulating hormone (FSH)

29. Which organism is responsible for many cases of peptic ulcer disease?

A. *Clostridioides difficile* (*C. difficile*)
B. *Helicobacter pylori* (*H. pylori*)
C. *Staphylococcus aureus* (*S. aureus*)
D. *Escherichia coli* (*E. coli*)

(*See answers next page.*)

25. A) Aspirin

All patients who have a suspected or confirmed myocardial infarction should receive aspirin 162 mg or 325 mg as soon as possible. Clopidogrel (Plavix) should be ordered only if a patient has a contraindication to aspirin. Morphine (MS-Contin) is a pain reliever but is not the priority treatment at this time. Levofloxacin (Levaquin) is indicated with suspected or confirmed infection, not with myocardial infarction.

26. B) Order lidocaine (Xylocaine) bolus

A patient with sustained ventricular tachycardia should be treated with lidocaine (Xylocaine) 1 mg/kg bolus if stable. If the patient is unstable, electrical cardioversion should be initiated. CPR is not indicated unless the patient is pulseless and not breathing. Ventricular tachycardia warrants intervention rather than observation.

27. D) Take levothyroxine (Synthroid) at the same time each day

It is important to educate patients to take levothyroxine (Synthroid) at the same time each day to achieve consistent serum levels. Levothyroxine (Synthroid) should be taken on an empty stomach rather than with food and should not be taken on an "as needed" basis. Blood work will need to be obtained after about 4 weeks.

28. A) Cortisol and epinephrine

ACTH deficiency leads to a decrease in the secretion of cortisol and epinephrine. It does not impact the level of GH, aldosterone, prolactin, TSH, LH, or FSH.

29. B) *Helicobacter pylori* (*H. pylori*)

H. pylori lives in the gastrointestinal tract and can cause damage to the stomach lining, resulting in peptic ulcer disease. *C. difficile, S. aureus,* and *E. coli* are causes of other infections but do not result in peptic ulcer disease.

30. An 82-year-old patient presents with confusion, hypothermia, and hypotension. Thyroid-stimulating hormone (TSH) level is 150 mU/L, and free T4 level is undetectable. Which is the AGACNP's first order?

A. Levothyroxine (Synthroid) 500 mcg intravenously (IV)
B. Levothyroxine (Synthroid) 500 mcg orally
C. 0.9% sodium chloride (NaCl) IV
D. MRI of brain

31. A 79-year-old patient is admitted with cirrhosis and a prothrombin time of 20 seconds. Which should the AGACNP order first to reduce bleeding risk?

A. Warfarin (Jantoven)
B. Vitamin K
C. Aspirin
D. Enoxaparin (Lovenox)

32. A patient presents with mild, nonbloody diarrhea and has remained afebrile. Which antidiarrheal agent should the AGACNP prescribe?

A. Bismuth subsalicylate (Pepto-Bismol, Kaopectate)
B. Diphenoxylate with atropine (Lomotil)
C. Loperamide (Imodium)
D. Ciprofloxacin (Cipro)

33. A patient treated for *C. difficile* colitis 4 weeks ago presents with recurrent diarrhea that tests positive for *C. difficile.* Which is the AGACNP's next step?

A. Order a prolonged vancomycin (Vancocin) taper
B. Refer the patient for fecal microbiota transplantation
C. Order loperamide (Imodium)
D. Refer the patient for colonoscopy

34. A patient presents with acute, uncomplicated appendicitis and is planned for appendectomy in 12 hours. Which order will the AGACNP issue first? Order for:

A. Stool culture
B. Acetaminophen (Tylenol)
C. Intravenous (IV) antibiotics
D. Chest CT

(*See answers next page.*)

30. A) Levothyroxine (Synthroid) 500 mcg intravenously (IV)
The patient's condition is consistent with a myxedema crisis, a state of severe hypothyroidism. Treatment focuses on immediate repletion of thyroid hormone, which should be done with levothyroxine (Synthroid) 500 mcg IV. Levothyroxine (Synthroid) should not be administered orally, as gastrointestinal absorption can be altered. IV hydration with 0.9% NaCl may be indicated but would not be the immediate priority. MRI of the brain is not indicated based because the patient's confusion is most likely due to a myxedema crisis.

31. B) Vitamin K
Patients presenting with cirrhosis and an elevated prothrombin time should be given vitamin K in order to decrease risk of bleeding. Warfarin (Jantoven), aspirin, and enoxaparin (Lovenox) are medications used to prevent thrombosis and can increase risk of bleeding.

32. C) Loperamide (Imodium)
Loperamide (Imodium) is the preferred antidiarrheal agent in uncomplicated, acute diarrhea. Bismuth subsalicylate (Pepto-Bismol, Kaopectate) is used for symptom relief with traveler's diarrhea as well as for upset stomach. Diphenoxylate with atropine (Lomotil) should not be used in cases of acute diarrhea due to possible toxic megacolon. Ciprofloxacin (Cipro) is not recommended in uncomplicated, noninfectious diarrhea.

33. A) Order a prolonged vancomycin (Vancocin) taper
A patient who has recurrent *C. difficile* infection within 8 weeks of initial treatment should be given either fidaxomicin (Dificid) or a prolonged taper and pulsed regimen of vancomycin (Vancocin). Fecal microbiota transplantation is used for patients who have three or more relapses of *C. difficile* colitis. Loperamide (Imodium) should not be given with active, untreated infection as it could slow motility and increase the severity of colitis. A colonoscopy or flexible sigmoidoscopy would be appropriate for a patient presenting with atypical symptoms, or symptoms despite appropriate therapy.

34. C) Intravenous (IV) antibiotics
Patients with appendicitis should be given a broad-spectrum antibiotic prior to appendectomy. Stool culture and chest CT are not typically indicated for appendicitis. Acetaminophen (Tylenol) may be given for pain but would not be the priority.

35. A patient with chronic bacterial prostatitis reports dysuria and perineal pain. Which medication should the AGACNP order for as-needed symptomatic relief?

A. Trimethoprim-sulfamethoxazole (Bactrim)
B. Indomethacin (Indocin)
C. Bisacodyl (Dulcolax)
D. Loratadine (Claritin)

36. Which antibiotic is indicated for the treatment of uncomplicated cystitis?

A. Ciprofloxacin (Cipro)
B. Nitrofurantoin (Macrobid)
C. Levofloxacin (Levaquin)
D. Cephalexin (Keflex)

37. A patient is admitted to the hospital with an obstructing urinary stone along with a temperature of 101.2°F (38.4°C) and leukocytosis. Which is the AGACNP's next step?

A. Make an urgent urology referral
B. Order intravenous (IV) antibiotics
C. Order IV fluids
D. Order Foley catheter insertion

38. A patient with acute bacterial prostatitis has received intravenous (IV) antibiotics for 4 days and has now been afebrile for 48 hours. Which is the AGACNP's next step?

A. Continue IV antibiotics for a total of 5 days
B. Discontinue antibiotics
C. Switch to oral antibiotics for 4 to 6 weeks
D. Order a pelvic CT scan

39. A patient presents to the emergency department with generalized myalgias. Labs reveal elevated creatinine, markedly elevated creatine kinase, and hypocalcemia consistent with rhabdomyolysis. Which is the AGACNP's next step?

A. Order continuous intravenous (IV) normal saline
B. Order calcium supplementation
C. Order CT of the chest
D. Make a referral to urology

(*See answers next page.*)

35. B) Bisacodyl (Dulcolax)

Patients with chronic bacterial prostatitis can be given anti-inflammatory agents such as indomethacin (Indocin) to relieve symptoms. Trimethoprim-sulfamethoxazole (Bactrim) is an antibiotic used to treat prostatitis but is not given for as-needed symptom relief. Bisacodyl (Dulcolax) is used for constipation, and loratadine (Claritin) is used for seasonal allergies.

36. B) Nitrofurantoin (Macrobid)

Treatment for uncomplicated cystitis should consist of single-drug therapy, preferably with fosfomycin (Monuril), nitrofurantoin (Macrobid), or trimethoprim-sulfamethoxazole (Bactrim). Fluoroquinolones such as ciprofloxacin (Cipro) or levofloxacin (Levaquin) are not recommended due to bacterial resistance. Cephalexin (Keflex) is indicated in other types of infection but is not the preferred medication for cystitis.

37. A) Make an urgent urology referral

An obstructing stone with associated infection is considered an emergency and requires an urgent referral to urology for renal drainage and stent or percutaneous nephrostomy tube placement. IV antibiotics may be needed but are inadequate as a monotherapy. Diuresis should be avoided, as it can exacerbate symptoms. A Foley catheter should not be placed if a patient has an infection and an obstructing stone.

38. C) Switch to oral antibiotics for 4 to 6 weeks

A patient with prostatitis should receive IV antibiotics with ampicillin and aminoglycoside and then transition to oral antibiotics once the patient has been afebrile for 24 to 48 hours. Antibiotics are continued for up to 6 weeks to ensure eradication of the infection. There is no need to continue IV antibiotics for 5 days. Discontinuing antibiotics at this point would likely not be sufficient treatment. A pelvic CT scan is only indicated if the patient is unresponsive to antibiotics.

39. A) Order continuous intravenous (IV) normal saline

Aggressive IV hydration with normal saline is the mainstay of treatment for rhabdomyolysis. Despite the presence of hypocalcemia, calcium supplementation should not be ordered unless the calcium level is extremely low and causing symptoms. A chest CT is not indicated in the workup of rhabdomyolysis. A referral to nephrology rather than urology should be obtained.

40. A patient with a history of nonobstructing renal calculi presents to urgent care with flank pain, a temperature of 102°F (38.4°C), and intractable nausea and vomiting. Which is the most appropriate next step?

A. Order oral trimethoprim-sulfamethoxazole
B. Order outpatient abdominal ultrasound
C. Admit the patient to the hospital
D. Refer the patient to urology

41. A patient reports a sense of fullness with decreased hearing in the right ear following an upper respiratory infection. The AGACNP suspects which diagnosis?

A. Eustachian tube dysfunction
B. Sensorineural hearing loss
C. Acoustic neuroma
D. Streptococcal pharyngitis

42. A patient presents with left-side hearing loss and is found to have cerumen impaction. What implement or measure would the AGACNP recommend to manage the impaction?

A. Cotton swab stick
B. Jet irrigator
C. Detergent ear drops
D. Cold water irrigation

43. A patient arrives at the emergency department following a car crash. The patient presents with labored breathing and the ability to move all their limbs. The AGACNP's first priority in assessing the patient is to:

A. Check for sources of bleeding
B. Assess airway patency and breathing
C. Ask the patient what occurred during the accident
D. Examine the patient for potential broken bones

44. A patient presents with left-side facial fullness and tenderness, nasal congestion, and malaise for 3 days. The AGACNP suspects rhinosinusitis. Which option should the initial treatment include?

A. Intranasal saline spray
B. Intranasal corticosteroids
C. Oral antibiotics
D. Oral corticosteroids

(See answers next page.)

40. C) Admit the patient to the hospital

Flank pain, along with fever and intractable vomiting, particularly in a patient with a history of renal calculi, should prompt significant concern and warrants hospitalization for further evaluation. Ordering oral antibiotics, an outpatient abdominal ultrasound, or a referral to urology negates the urgency of this clinical scenario.

41. A) Eustachian tube dysfunction

A sensation of fullness in the ear, along with decreased hearing following an upper respiratory infection, likely indicates Eustachian tube dysfunction, a condition that occurs from trapped air within the middle ear. Sensorineural hearing loss is a gradual loss of hearing from issues that arise in the cochlea. An acoustic neuroma is a tumor that can cause issues with hearing, but the clinical scenario presented points to Eustachian tube dysfunction as the more likely cause. Streptococcal pharyngitis is characterized by a sore throat.

42. C) Detergent ear drops

Management of cerumen impaction should begin with use of detergent ear drops such as 3% hydrogen peroxide or 6.5% carbamide peroxide. Irrigation can be done as well but should be done with water that is at body temperature, rather than cold water, to avoid vestibular caloric response. Cotton swab sticks and jet irrigation should be avoided because they can cause further impaction or damage to the tympanic membrane.

43. B) Assess airway patency and breathing

Assessment of the trauma patient focuses on "ABCDE"—*a*irway, *b*reathing, *c*irculation, *d*isability, and *e*xposure. The airway is the first priority and includes checking for obstruction and breathing. Checking for sources of bleeding, examining for broken bones, and interviewing the patient about the accident are also aspects of the nursing assessment, but none of these would be the first priority.

44. A) Intranasal saline spray

First-line treatment of rhinosinusitis includes intranasal saline spray, nasal decongestants, and nonsteroidal anti-inflammatory drugs. Intranasal corticosteroids should be used only if bacterial rhinosinusitis is suspected. Oral antibiotics are reserved for complicated cases or for symptoms lasting longer than 10 days that worsen rather than improve. Oral corticosteroids are not indicated in this condition.

45. The AGACNP notes a heart rate of 190 bpm, irregular rhythm, absence of P waves and PR interval, and no formed QRS complex on the patient's physiologic monitor. The AGACNP would immediately:

A. Provide CPR and cardiac defibrillation
B. Administer as-needed (PRN) metoprolol (Lopressor)
C. Contact the hospital cardiologist
D. Ensure correct placement of electrodes and adjust as necessary

46. A patient arrives to the emergency department after falling from a ladder and is placed in a cervical collar. When the patient inquires as to how long they will need to wear it, the AGACNP responds:

A. "You should wear the cervical collar for at least 2 weeks following your injury."
B. "Once your pain has subsided, I can remove the collar."
C. "You should wear the cervical collar until imaging of your cervical spine rules out injury."
D. "The cervical collar should remain in place until your surgery."

47. A patient presents following a car crash with significant bleeding from a suspected leg fracture. The trauma AGACNP prioritizes:

A. Splinting the leg for stability
B. Ordering an x-ray to evaluate the fracture
C. Applying external pressure to slow blood loss
D. Ordering pain medication to ease patient's discomfort

48. What diagnostic test should an AGACNP choose for suspected peptic ulcer disease (PUD)?

A. Endoscopy
B. Abdominal x-ray
C. Abdominal CT scan
D. Urea breath test

(*See answers next page.*)

45. A) Provide CPR and cardiac defibrillation

A heart rate of 190 bpm, irregular rhythm, absence of P waves and PR interval, and no formed QRS complex indicate ventricular fibrillation, which requires immediate defibrillation (with CPR until a defibrillator is available) as it is a life-threatening condition. Administering PRN metoprolol (Lopressor) is not the appropriate treatment for ventricular fibrillation. While the cardiologist may need to be contacted, this is not an immediate need as the abnormal rhythm is priority. Although checking electrode placement may be necessary in the case of suspected artifact or interruption of monitoring, the described characteristics do not support this intervention.

46. C) "You should wear the cervical collar until imaging of your cervical spine rules out injury."

Trauma patients should have their neck immobilized with a cervical collar until a cervical spine x-ray or CT rules out cervical injuries. No guidelines specify a need to wear a collar for 2 weeks following an injury. While a cervical collar may limit discomfort, a lack of pain does not justify removal of the cervical collar. Surgery is not always necessary and does not dictate how long a cervical collar should be worn.

47. C) Applying external pressure to slow blood loss

Hemorrhage is the most serious complication of limb trauma. Therefore, control of bleeding takes precedence in the initial evaluation and treatment of potential bone fractures. Splinting the limb may be indicated but is not the priority. Similarly, an x-ray and pain medication are likely necessary, but neither would be the first step in management.

48. A) Endoscopy

The endoscopy procedure allows for direct visualization of the upper gastrointestinal tract as well as biopsy, if necessary, to establish or rule out PUD. An abdominal x-ray does not show the esophageal, stomach, or intestinal mucosa and is not useful in diagnosing PUD. Abdominal CT scan is standard for identifying other abdominal conditions but not PUD. A urea breath test is a noninvasive test to detect *Helicobacter pylori* but is not a diagnostic examination for PUD.

49. A study assesses early-onset type 2 diabetes mellitus in female patients ages 15 to 25 years with a suspected diagnosis of polycystic ovary syndrome (PCOS). The AGACNP recalls the Rotterdam criteria and decides which patient is most appropriate for the study?

A. An 18-year-old patient who reports a last menstrual cycle more than 1 year ago and has hypothalamic dysfunction secondary to anorexia nervosa

B. A 25-year-old patient who shaves the coarse hair on their chin daily and has menstrual cycles every 60 to 90 days but has a normal pelvic ultrasound

C. A 22-year-old patient with a normal examination and normal menses but incidentally noted ovarian cysts on an abdominal ultrasound

D. A 16-year-old patient with chronic lower abdominal pain and self-diagnosed severe acne who has never had a menstrual cycle

50. The AGACNP evaluates a patient who complains of extreme weakness, weight loss, polyuria, and polydipsia. There is a history of a splenectomy 1 year prior. The patient expresses concern that diabetes could be the cause. The patient intermittently fasts but drank orange juice this morning. What test does the AGACNP order to screen for diabetes?

A. Glycosylated hemoglobin (HbA1C)

B. Oral glucose tolerance test (OGTT)

C. Random plasma glucose

D. Serum fructosamine level

51. An 86-year-old hospitalized patient with chronic cancer-related pain is diagnosed with opioid-induced constipation. What will the AGACNP prescribe?

A. Methylcellulose (Citrucel), four 500-mg caplets three times per day while taking opioids

B. Methylnaltrexone (Relistor) injection, 8 mg subcutaneously every other day for 10 days

C. Naltrexone (Vivitrol) injection, 380 mg intramuscularly once per week for 4 weeks

D. Naloxone (Narcan) injection, 0.04 mg (40 mcg) intravenous push once daily for 3 days

(*See answers next page.*)

49. B) A 25-year-old patient who shaves the coarse hair on their chin daily and has menstrual cycles every 60 to 90 days but has a normal pelvic ultrasound

The Rotterdam Criteria allow the diagnosis of PCOS based on the presence of two of the following criteria: presence of ovarian cysts on ultrasonography of the ovaries, clinical features or laboratory evidence of hyperandrogenism, and menstrual irregularities such as oligomenorrhea or anovulation. Coarse chin hair in a 25-year-old that requires daily removal is most likely hirsutism, or clinical hyperandrogenism. The prolonged menstrual cycle of up to 90 days is oligomenorrhea; these fulfill two of the Rotterdam Criteria that prompt the AGACNP to clinically diagnose PCOS. Anorexia nervosa causes hypothalamic suppression, which leads to a secondary amenorrhea. However, no other data provided for the patient with anorexia nervosa indicate the presence of ovarian cysts or hyperandrogenism. Incidentally noted, ovarian cysts alone do not fulfill the Rotterdam Criteria to diagnose PCOS because cysts can be seen in normal-cycling patients. Delayed menarche in the 16-year-old patient is not equivalent to anovulation and should prompt the AGACNP to evaluate other etiologies of symptoms.

50. C) Random plasma glucose

A single random plasma glucose at or above 200 mg/dL is diagnostic for diabetes for a patient with classic symptoms of hyperglycemia such as polydipsia, polyuria, weight loss, and/or fatigue. The HbA1C may be falsely elevated following a splenectomy due to alteration of red blood cell survival and should not be used to monitor or diagnose diabetes. An oral glucose tolerance test can be diagnostic for diabetes if the 2-hour glucose is greater than or equal to 200 mg/dL. However, the patient should consume at least 150 to 200 g of carbohydrates daily for 3 days prior to the test and fast for 8 hours the morning of the test. The OGTT and HbA1C must both be confirmed by a second test. A serum fructosamine level is best suited to be used as an alternative to the HbA1C if there are factors that alter part of the American Diabetes Association's diagnostic criteria for diabetes.

51. B) Methylnaltrexone (Relistor) injection, 8 mg subcutaneously every other day for 10 days

Methylnaltrexone (Relistor) is a peripherally acting opioid antagonist that inhibits the delayed gastric motility and reduced transit associated with opioids. Methylcellulose (Citrucel), a bulk-forming laxative, is not appropriate for older adults who may not adequately hydrate to move the laxative through the gastrointestinal tract. Naltrexone (Vivitrol) is an opioid antagonist but is not indicated for opioid-induced constipation. Intramuscular naltrexone (Vivitrol) administration would induce acute opioid withdrawal in the patient. Naloxone (Narcan) is also an opioid antagonist, but its primary use is the treatment of opioid intoxication and associated respiratory depression.

52. A patient complains of occasional diarrhea for 6 weeks with associated lower abdominal cramping and bloating. The patient has two to three loose, non-bloody stools some days and none other days. A chart review reveals that the following studies are normal to date: upper gastrointestinal endoscopy, colonoscopy, stool studies, CT can of abdomen and pelvis, complete blood count, complete metabolic panel, thyroid studies, inflammatory markers, rheumatologic studies, and autoimmune studies. The patient asks if the symptoms could be from irritable bowel syndrome (IBS) because that is what a friend has, and the symptoms are the same. The AGACNP states:

A. "You may have IBS, but it is a diagnosis of exclusion. The Rome IV criteria state that symptoms should be present for at least 3 months. I will refer you to a gastroenterologist to further evaluate you."
B. "The Rome IV consensus definition of IBS does not apply in this case because your stools seem to be predominantly loose. Current IBS definitions state that there must at least be occasional constipation."
C. "It is important to allow me to do a thorough history and examination before giving me your thoughts on a diagnosis. I cannot keep an open mind if you anchor your symptoms to a certain disease."
D. "To accurately diagnose IBS, the Rome IV criteria state that an 8-week stool diary should be used. Take this stool chart and note your symptoms for 2 weeks. Then you will need to return for follow-up."

53. An 85-year-old patient presents to the emergency department with a 5-day history of progressive exertional dyspnea, paroxysmal nocturnal dyspnea, lower-extremity edema, and cough. Physical examination reveals bilateral rales, 3+ pitting lower-extremity edema, tachypnea, and jugular venous distention. The AGACNP's first intervention is to order:

A. A chest radiograph
B. An echocardiogram
C. Furosemide (Lasix) 40 mg intravenously
D. B-type natriuretic peptide (BNP)

54. The most accurate definition of palliative inpatient care is:

A. Use of high-dose opioids to alleviate pain
B. Alleviation of bothersome symptoms
C. Decision to forego life-saving treatments
D. Care for a patient with more than 6 months expected survival

(*See answers next page.*)

52. A) "You may have IBS, but it is a diagnosis of exclusion. The Rome IV criteria state that symptoms should be present for at least 3 months. I will refer you to a gastroenterologist to further evaluate you."

The Rome IV consensus allows for a clinical diagnosis of IBS if a patient has abdominal pain for 1 or more days per week for 3 or more months and meets at least two of the following criteria: pain related to bowel movements, an associated change in the appearance of the stool, and an associated change in the frequency of stool. The stated symptoms seem consistent with IBS, but at least 3 months of symptoms establish a clinical diagnosis. Additionally, there is insufficient information regarding specific lab markers such as fecal calprotectin and celiac disease markers to rule out underlying causes, so referral to a gastroenterologist is appropriate. IBS's subtypes vary and include predominant constipation, predominant diarrhea, and mixed symptoms. It is important to remain empathetic during the patient interview to maintain a therapeutic relationship; discouraging the patient from expressing their thoughts is not appropriate. The Rome IV criteria do not include a stool diary or an 8-week option to make a clinical diagnosis.

53. C) Furosemide (Lasix) 40 mg intravenously

The patient is presenting with classic heart failure symptoms. The AGACNP recognizes the presenting symptoms and knows that the use of loop diuretics like furosemide (Lasix) is guideline-directed therapy for this condition. While chest radiography, echocardiogram, and BNP level are all part of the initial workup, the administration of diuretics is the priority to avoid clinical deterioration.

54. B) Alleviation of bothersome symptoms

The term *palliation* in the context of patient care refers to symptom management. Therefore, it is a component of all patient care. While patients receiving palliative care may require large doses of opioids, palliation is not limited to pharmacologic pain management. The decision to forego life-saving treatments can be a component of palliation but only if it helps to alleviate symptoms. Palliation is not dependent on expected survival.

55. A 29-year-old presents to the emergency department after a motor vehicle crash. Chest x-ray reveals a left-sided pneumothorax with evidence of mediastinal shift. What is the AGACNP's next intervention?

A. Needle decompression
B. Endotracheal intubation
C. Arterial blood gas (ABG)
D. CT of the chest

56. A 57-year-old patient is being treated for acute blood loss anemia in the setting of lower gastrointestinal bleeding. The patient has received four units of packed red blood cells (PRBC) and 2 L of normal saline (NS). Blood pressure is 80/54 mmHg, and heart rate is 108 bpm. When interventions appear to be unsuccessful, what is the AGACNP's next intervention?

A. Repeat complete blood count (CBC)
B. Administer 1 L of NS
C. Administer metoprolol (Lopressor) 5 mg intravenously
D. Start phenylephrine (Neo-Synephrine) infusion

57. The AGACNP is working in an emergency department where a patient is brought in via emergency medical services after experiencing blunt force trauma to the face. CT of the head reveals separation of the midfacial skeleton from the base of the cranium. The most appropriate action for the AGACNP to take is to:

A. Repeat head CT in 24 hours
B. Initiate transfer for urgent reduction in facial fracture
C. Assess for cerebral spinal fluid (CSF) leak
D. Perform an eye examination

58. A patient with a shellfish allergy presents to the emergency department with complaints of facial swelling and shortness of breath. The AGACNP administers epinephrine (Adrenalin) and methylprednisolone (Solu-Medrol) immediately. The patient then develops stridor, tachypnea, and a decrease in pulse oximetry to 85%. What action will the AGACNP take next?

A. Administer an additional dose of epinephrine (Adrenalin)
B. Administer normal saline (NS) fluid bolus
C. Perform endotracheal intubation
D. Obtain arterial blood gas (ABG)

(*See answers next page.*)

55. A) Needle decompression

This is a clinical emergency that can result in circulatory collapse if not treated immediately. The initial intervention is decompression of the pleural space followed by insertion of a chest tube on the affected side. Endotracheal intubation will not treat the underlying problem and may exacerbate hemodynamic instability. Obtaining an ABG will delay care and only confirm respiratory distress. A CT of the chest is not necessary as the pneumothorax has already been identified on chest x-ray.

56. D) Start phenylephrine (Neo-Synephrine) infusion

The patient is showing signs of hypovolemic shock in the setting of lower-gastrointestinal bleeding. After unsuccessful PRBC and hydration, the next appropriate intervention is to add a vasopressor such as phenylephrine (Neo-Synephrine). Repeating CBC is necessary to reassess hemoglobin and hematocrit; however, is not the priority intervention. Aggressive volume resuscitation has not improved hypotension; therefore, additional NS will not be beneficial. Tachycardia is a late clinical finding secondary to hypotension. Use of a beta-blocker like metoprolol (Lopressor) will only worsen hypotension.

57. B) Initiate transfer for urgent reduction in facial fracture

The patient's CT findings are consistent with Le Fort III fracture, which requires urgent reduction in facial fracture to improve airway function and prevent extension of intracranial hemorrhage. Repeat CT the following day does not address the immediate dangers of this injury. While assessing for CSF leak and performing a thorough eye examination are both integral to assessment of Le Forte fractures, the priority is to ensure airway patency through reduction of the facial fracture.

58. C) Perform endotracheal intubation

The patient presents with signs of anaphylaxis. After receiving epinephrine (Adrenalin) and methylprednisolone (Solu-Medrol), the patient shows signs of respiratory failure. Endotracheal intubation is the next appropriate intervention. Repeating epinephrine (Adrenalin) can be considered once an airway has been established. Obtaining an ABG will delay care and can be performed post intubation.

59. A 68-year-old patient with a past medical history of hypertension, type 2 diabetes mellitus, and hyperlipidemia is brought to the emergency department by their adult child after being found on the floor with right-sided weakness, right facial droop, and aphasia. The adult child reports that the patient was fine 2½ hours ago. On physical assessment, the patient is awake with right facial drooping and global aphasia and is unable to follow commands. The patient demonstrates spontaneous movement on the left side and is flaccid on the right with no movement to painful stimuli. The National Institutes of Health Stroke Scale score is 20, blood pressure is 180/95 mmHg, heart rate is 91 bpm, respiratory rate is 18 breaths/min, and oxygen saturation (SpO_2) is 96% on room air. The AGACNP's priority is to order:

A. Tissue plasminogen activator (tPA)
B. CT of the head
C. Anti-hypertensive medication given as intravenous (IV) push
D. A lumbar puncture

60. The patient reports to the AGACNP, "My last flu vaccine was 3 years ago. I don't need one this year." The AGACNP explains that the flu vaccine should be administered every:

A. 1 year
B. 5 years
C. 10 year
D. Season

61. A 75-year-old patient with medical history of hypothyroidism, type 2 diabetes mellitus, and previous stroke with no residual deficits is brought to the emergency department by a family member for worsening confusion and weakness over the past 2 days. The family member reports that at baseline the patient is "sharp," lives in an assisted living facility, is independent in basic activities of daily living, and uses a cane for walking. On physical assessment, the patient is somnolent but arousable to persistent verbal stimuli, oriented to person only, and mumbling incomprehensible words. There is spontaneous movement in all extremities with no obvious motor symmetry. Vital signs include heart rate 108 bpm, blood pressure 175/80 mmHg, respiratory rate 22 breaths/min, oxygen saturation (SpO_2) 93% on room air, and temperature 101.8°F (38.8°C) axillary. CT scan is negative for any acute intracranial process. Based on the patient's history and clinical findings, the AGACNP prepares the patient for:

A. CT with myelography
B. Lumbar puncture with biopsy
C. Spinal decompression
D. Radiation therapy

(See answers next page.)

59. B) CT of the head

The patient is presenting with stroke-like symptoms. A head CT is the highest priority diagnostic test in patients who present with stroke-like symptoms to determine whether there is an ischemic or hemorrhagic stroke or any other intracranial process. Further treatment and interventions are dependent on head CT findings. While the patient is within the time window for tissue plasminogen activator (tPA), it cannot be given until it is confirmed that there is no intracranial bleed. Before the patient is treated for hypertension, it must be determined whether this is an ischemic or a hemorrhagic stroke. Blood pressure goals for ischemic stroke include systolic blood pressure <185 mmHg; with hemorrhagic stroke, goals include systolic blood pressure <140 mmHg. Lumbar punctures are performed to obtain spinal fluid samples to be tested for bacterial infections and to determine possible causes for epilepsy. There is no clinical indication for a lumbar puncture in this patient.

60. A) 1 year

The influenza vaccine should be administered yearly for appropriate immune response. The pneumococcal vaccine should be received every 5 years for an appropriate immune response. The tetanus vaccine should be administered every 10 years.

61. B) Lumbar puncture with biopsy

The patient's clinical findings are indicative of central nervous system infection, which would warrant a lumbar puncture with aspiration and possible biopsy to determine exact etiology. A CT with myelography would be ordered in the event of spinal stenosis or congenital defects. Spinal decompression and radiation therapy are often combined in patients with metastatic cancer that has spread to spinal bone. Spinal decompression alone is often used in treating congenital compressions or injury/trauma in the spine.

62. A 55-year-old patient has past medical history of hypertension, hyperlipemia, and smoking one-half pack of cigarettes per day for 20 years. The patient presents to the emergency department with chest pain that started 2 to 3 days ago while they were walking up a hill and that proceeded to get worse last night. According to the patient, the pain is best described as discomfort in the middle of the chest that intermittently radiates to the jaw, comes on with increase in activity, and is relieved with rest. The patient also reports having had similar symptoms a few months ago. Physical examination reveals normal heart sounds, no murmurs or rubs, lungs clear to auscultation, palpable pulses, and no edema to extremities. Vital signs include heart rate 101 bpm, blood pressure 152/65 mmHg, respiratory rate 20 breaths/min, oxygen saturation (SpO_2) 95% on room air, and temperature 99.2°F (37.3°C) orally. Based on the patient's history and clinical assessment findings, the AGACNP anticipates which diagnostic test findings?

A. Normal troponin, T-wave inversion in anterior leads
B. Elevated troponin, ST-elevation in leads II, III, aVF
C. Elevated troponin, ST-depression in lateral leads
D. Normal troponin, ST-elevation in leads I, aVL

63. Which diagnostic test does the AGACNP order for preventive lung cancer screening?

A. CT with angiography of the chest
B. Low-dose CT of the chest
C. Two-view (posterior/anterior) chest radiograph
D. Low-dose CT of the chest with intravenous contrast

64. The AGACNP sees a patient on post stroke day 3 who is awaiting brain MRI before considering discharge. After completing the MRI checklist, the nurse reports to the AGACNP that the patient has an implanted insulin pump, pacemaker, nerve stimulator, and two peripheral intravenous (IV) catheters. Which device is known to be MRI safe?

A. Implanted insulin pump
B. Pacemaker
C. Nerve stimulator
D. Peripheral IV catheters

(See answers next page.)

62. A) Normal troponin, T-wave inversion in anterior leads

The patient's presenting symptoms are most suggestive of unstable angina, pain that is worsened with exertion and relieved with rest. Additional history also reveals chronicity of these symptoms, and past medical history and cigarette smoking also place the patient at risk for unstable angina related to coronary artery disease. In unstable angina, troponin levels are normal, and the electrocardiogram can have transient T-wave inversion in the anterior leads to the presence of chest pain. Elevated troponin and ST-elevation in leads II, III, aVF suggest acute inferior wall myocardial infarction (MI). Elevated troponin and ST-depression in lateral leads suggest non-ST-elevation MI. Normal troponin and ST-elevation in leads I, aVL suggest acute lateral wall MI.

63. B) Low-dose CT of the chest

Low-dose CT of the chest is used for preventive lung cancer screening because it is effective at detecting early lung cancer, and radiation exposure to the patient is reduced. Angiography reveals blood vessel anatomy. The priority is to visualize the lung parenchyma for early detection of a tumor. Angiography increases radiation exposure and uses intravenous contrast unnecessarily, increasing the risk of contrast nephropathy. Chest radiography is ineffective for detecting early evidence of lung cancer. Intravenous contrast is not needed for visualization of lung parenchyma.

64. D) Peripheral IV catheters

Of the patient's devices, only the peripheral IV catheters are known not to contain metal, meaning they cannot be damaged or affected by the MRI magnet. Implanted pumps, pacemakers, and nerve stimulators can potentially be damaged, and metal within them could become dislodged or heated while in the MRI, injuring the patient. Some implantable devices are designed to be "MRI safe" or "MRI conditional," meaning they can safely be introduced to the MRI environment as long as specific conditions are met. However, staff should assess each device for safety prior to the MRI procedure.

65. The most appropriate patient for a one-time abdominal aneurysm screening with an ultrasound is a:

A. 70-year-old woman with a history of tobacco use
B. 65-year-old woman with no history of tobacco use
C. 60-year-old man with a history of tobacco use
D. 70-year-old man with a history of tobacco use

66. The AGACNP is caring for a frail 75-year-old patient with multiple comorbidities whose last colonoscopy was 20 years ago. A fecal immunochemical test (FIT) was ordered, and the result was positive. What action does the AGACNP take next?

A. Refer for sigmoidoscopy
B. Refer for colonoscopy
C. Repeat fecal immunochemical test
D. Check stool for occult blood

67. The AGACNP is seeing a 38-year-old patient with no past medical history. The patient has a body mass index of 40 and reports that one parent has type 2 diabetes mellitus. What tests should be ordered to evaluate the patient for diabetes mellitus?

A. Hemoglobin A1C (HGA1C) and fasting plasma glucose
B. Complete blood count and urine for ketones
C. Urinalysis for glucose and ketones
D. C-peptide and urine for ketones

68. Which patient meets the current U.S. Preventive Services Task Force (USPSTF) criteria for lung cancer screening?

A. 50-year-old woman with a 10 pack-year history of smoking who quit 12 years ago
B. 60-year-old man with a 20 pack-year history of smoking who quit 20 years ago
C. 50-year-old woman who is an active smoker with a 30 pack-year history of smoking
D. 81-year-old man who is an active smoker with a 30 pack-year history of smoking

(See answers next page.)

65. D) 70-year-old man with a history of tobacco use

Routine screening is recommended by the U.S. Preventive Services Task Force (USPSTF) for men only, ages 65 to 75 years, who have smoked tobacco. The USPSTF recommends against screening for women who have never smoked. There is insufficient evidence to support routine screening for women ages 65 to 75 years who have smoked tobacco.

66. B) Refer for colonoscopy

Colonoscopy is the standard follow-up test for any abnormality found with stool testing. A sigmoidoscopy does not allow visualization of the right colon, only the left, so this would not be a comprehensive test. There is no additional information obtained from a stool for occult blood or FIT test, so these would not be performed or repeated.

67. A) Hemoglobin A1C (HGA1C) and fasting plasma glucose

HGA1C, fasting plasma glucose, and oral glucose testing are the standard of care for diagnosing diabetes. Urine ketones and urine glucose are not diagnostic for diabetes mellitus, and a complete blood count yields no information about diabetes. C-peptide levels are useful for differentiating type 1 from type 2 diabetes mellitus.

68. C) 50-year-old woman who is an active smoker with a 30 pack-year history of smoking

According to the USPSTF, lung cancer screening is appropriate for patients ages 50 to 80 years with a 20 pack-year history of smoking who currently smoke or who have quit within the last 15 years. A patient with a 10-pack-year history or one who quit smoking 20 years ago does not meet the screening criteria. An 81-year-old patient is outside of the age range for screening.

69. Which is an essential criterion for the diagnosis of dementia?

A. Compromise in three out of five cognitive domains as outlined by the *Diagnostic and Statistical Manual of Mental Disorders,* 5th edition (*DSM-5*)
B. Complete loss of short-term memory
C. Functional decline resulting in the loss of independent instrumental activities of daily living (IADLs)
D. Aphasia

70. Which is the most common form of dementia in the United States?

A. Alzheimer disease
B. Vascular dementia
C. Lewy body dementia
D. Delirium

71. A patient who is 72 years old presents with tonic-clonic status epilepticus. What is the AGACNP's first priority in managing the patient?

A. Ensure maintenance of airway patency
B. Order intravenous (IV) lorazepam (Ativan)
C. Order IV fosphenytoin (Cerebyx)
D. Keep patient in restraints to ensure safety

72. Which information would the AGACNP include in patient education after ordering donepezil (Aricept) for a patient with dementia?

A. "This drug slows functional decline."
B. "Continue taking the drug even without apparent benefit."
C. "This drug is used for mild cognitive impairment."
D. "You may experience diarrhea and nausea with this drug."

73. Which nonpharmacologic treatment has been shown to provide the greatest improvement in posttraumatic stress disorder (PTSD) symptoms?

A. Hypnosis
B. Acupuncture
C. Cognitive behavioral therapy
D. Electroconvulsive therapy

(*See answers next page.*)

69. C) Functional decline resulting in the loss of independent instrumental activities of daily living (IADLs)

A diagnosis of dementia requires that the individual have functional decline that is significant enough to result in loss of independent IADLs. Compromise in only one or more cognitive domains outlined by the DSM-5 is required. Loss of short-term memory may be present in dementia but is not an essential criterion for diagnosis. Aphasia may be present with dementia but is not necessary for diagnosis.

70. A) Alzheimer disease

Alzheimer disease makes up approximately two-thirds of dementia cases in the United States, while vascular dementia and Lewy body dementia account for the remaining cases. Delirium is not a form of dementia.

71. A) Ensure maintenance of airway patency

The initial priority in managing a patient with tonic-clonic status epilepticus is to stabilize and support the airway and breathing, place the patient on continuous cardiorespiratory monitoring and pulse oximetry, and establish IV or intraosseous access. The first dose of a benzodiazepine (IV lorazepam [Ativan]) should then be given, followed by antiseizure medication (such as fosphenytoin [Cerebyx]). Patients who are experiencing a seizure should not be restrained.

72. D) "You may experience diarrhea and nausea with this drug."

Diarrhea and nausea are common and bothersome side effects of donepezil (Aricept). Donepezil (Aricept) has not been shown to slow functional decline and should not be continued if the patient does not receive the apparent benefit. It is indicated for Alzheimer disease rather than mild cognitive impairment.

73. C) Cognitive behavioral therapy

Cognitive behavioral therapy, a form of psychotherapy, has shown evidence of significant improvement in PTSD symptoms when used either in conjunction with medication or as monotherapy. Hypnosis, acupuncture, and electroconvulsive therapy have not demonstrated the same degree of evidence.

74. A 58-year-old female patient presents to the ED with complaints of new-onset, intermittent heart palpitations over the last 36 hours. The patient is calm and talkative, with no signs or symptoms of shortness of breath. Other complaints include vague and occasional chest discomfort that feels like "shock waves" over the left breast. There is no history of heart disease or myocardial infarction. The patient's medications include hydrochlorothiazide (Microzide), citalopram (Celexa), and estradiol acetate (Femtrace). Medical history is relatively unremarkable except for hypertension and anxiety. EKG findings demonstrate sinus tachycardia at a rate of 110 beats/min and blood pressure of 160/86 mmHg. Initial lab results are normal except for an elevated D-dimer result. After reviewing these current findings, what will the AGACNP check next?

A. Abdomen
B. Thyroid
C. Lower extremities
D. Orthostatic blood pressure

75. Which hormone does the oral contraceptive minipill contain?

A. Estradiol
B. Norethindrone
C. Levonorgestrel
D. Testosterone

76. What is the primary mechanism of action of combined oral contraceptive pills?

A. Suppression of ovulation
B. Thickening of cervical mucus
C. Spermicide
D. Inhibition of endometrial thickening

77. Which information would the AGACNP include when educating a patient about the progestin minipill?

A. "There are 3 active weeks of pills and 1 inactive week of pills each cycle."
B. "The minipill should not be taken while breastfeeding."
C. "You may experience bleeding irregularities while on the minipill."
D. "There is a greater risk of cardiovascular events on the minipill compared with the combined oral contraceptive pill."

(*See answers next page.*)

74. C) Lower extremities

This postmenopausal patient on hormone replacement therapy presents with palpitations, mild chest discomfort, and tachycardia with an elevated D-dimer result. A positive D-dimer test indicates the presence of an abnormally high level of fibrin degradation products in the body. Thus, the next focus of the exam should be directed toward the patient's lower extremities to assess for signs or symptoms of a deep vein thrombosis (DVT), which may include unilateral swelling, redness/color changes, or tenderness/pain. Then, a CT pulmonary angiography should be ordered to determine if there is a pulmonary embolus as this is an urgent concern. A venous duplex ultrasound of the bilateral lower extremities to check for evidence of a DVT should also be included in the orders. The presenting symptoms and lab findings do not indicate a need to be concerned with an abdominal assessment. Given the elevated D-dimer result and the knowledge that all other lab results are normal (as a thyroid-stimulating hormone test would likely be included in initial lab orders with a chief complaint of heart palpitations and tachycardia), a thyroid exam would not be next in the sequencing of the physical assessment. And finally, orthostatic blood pressure measurements are irrelevant to the patient's current findings as there are no complaints of lightheadedness, dizziness, or indications of hypovolemia.

75. B) Norethindrone

The oral contraceptive minipill contains norethindrone, a form of progestin. It does not contain any form of estrogen such as estradiol. Levonorgestrel is a form of progestin used in injectable contraceptive methods. Testosterone is a hormone that is not involved in female contraceptive methods.

76. A) Suppression of ovulation

The main mechanism of action of combined oral contraceptives is the suppression of ovulation. Progestin-only pills typically cause thickening of cervical mucus. Contraceptive foam, creams, or jellies contain spermicide. Intrauterine devices cause inhibition of endometrial thickening.

77. C) "You may experience bleeding irregularities while on the minipill."

The progestin mini pill can cause bleeding irregularities such as spotting or amenorrhea. The minipill does not contain any inactive pills and can be taken during lactation. It lacks the cardiovascular risks that combined oral contraceptive pills carry.

78. A patient inquires about starting an oral contraceptive. Which would the AGACNP consider to be an absolute contraindication?

A. Cystic acne
B. Uncontrolled hypertension
C. Hirsutism
D. Migraine without aura

79. According to the CURB-65 assessment tool, which patient should the AGACNP admit to the hospital for management of pneumonia?

A. 80-year-old patient with a respiratory rate of 16 bpm
B. 52-year-old patient with altered mental status and blood pressure of 88/50 mmHg
C. 76-year-old patient with a blood pressure of 120/80 mmHg
D. 60-year-old patient with productive cough and uremia

80. Which statement would the AGACNP include in patient education for a patient with refractory asthma on daily prednisone (Deltasone)?

A. "It is important to take prednisone (Deltasone) on an empty stomach."
B. "You should take calcium and vitamin D supplements while on prednisone."
C. "You may stop taking the prednisone (Deltasone) once your breathing improves."
D. "Prednisone should be taken at bedtime."

81. The AGACNP visits the burn unit and examines a patient with second-degree burns to the left lower extremity who was readmitted from the skilled nursing facility due to poor wound healing. On examination, the AGACNP notes that the wound is primarily covered with eschar and prescribes which topical antimicrobial agent?

A. Silver sulfadiazine 1% cream (Silvadene)
B. Mafenide acetate 10% cream (Sulfamylon)
C. Silver nitrate 0.5% in water
D. Triamcinolone 0.025%

(See answers next page.)

78. B) Uncontrolled hypertension

Uncontrolled hypertension is considered an absolute contraindication to taking an oral contraceptive, as the medication can increase the risk of cardiovascular events. Cystic acne and hirsutism can be improved with the use of oral contraceptives. Migraine without aura is only a relative contraindication.

79. B) 52-year-old patient with altered mental status and blood pressure of 88/50 mmHg

The CURB-65 (confusion, uremia, respiratory rate, blood pressure, age older than 65 years) tool predicts increased mortality risk for patients with community-acquired pneumonia and can be used to aid in deciding which patients are appropriate for hospitalization. A patient with hypotension and altered mental status should be identified as high-risk and admitted for management. A patient who is older with a normal respiratory rate, a patient who is older and normotensive, and a patient with uremia only would not qualify as high-risk.

80. B) "You should take calcium and vitamin D supplements while on prednisone."

Individuals on chronic prednisone (Deltasone) treatment should take supplemental calcium and vitamin D because corticosteroids can affect bone mineral density. Prednisone (Deltasone) should be taken with food, not on an empty stomach, to avoid gastrointestinal upset. It is important not to stop prednisone (Deltasone) abruptly to avoid rebound effects. Prednisone (Deltasone) can cause insomnia, so it is best to avoid taking it at bedtime.

81. B) Mafenide acetate 10% cream (Sulfamylon)

Mafenide acetate 10% cream (Sulfamylon) is highly soluble and penetrates eschar well to allow for debridement while keeping infection management in mind. Silver sulfadiazine 1% cream (Silvadene) and silver nitrate 0.5% in water have poor eschar penetration and therefore would not facilitate debridement, which is necessary to establish good wound bed preparation for wound healing. Triamcinolone 0.025% is a topical steroid and does not facilitate debridement, which is required for the facilitation of healing in the presence of eschar.

82. A patient presents with a full-thickness pressure injury with tunneling and visible subcutaneous fat located on the coccyx. The AGACNP identifies the injury as which stage?

A. Stage 1
B. Stage 3
C. Unstageable
D. Stage 4

83. The AGACNP will recommend that patients begin yearly pneumococcal vaccination starting at how many years of age?

A. 55
B. 60
C. 65
D. 70

84. Review of an older adult patient's social history reveals they worked as a coal miner for 10 years. Which respiratory disease is this patient at risk of developing based on that history?

A. Chronic obstructive pulmonary disease (COPD)
B. Asthma
C. Cystic fibrosis (CF)
D. Tuberculosis

85. A 75-year-old patient with a history of hypertension presents to the clinic for an annual examination. The patient's laboratory data reveals uncontrolled hyperlipidemia, and their 10-year calculated cardiovascular disease event score is 12%. Which primary intervention will the AGACNP begin?

A. Encouraging dietary modification
B. Initiating low-dose statin therapy
C. Initiating high-dose statin therapy
D. Repeating lipid profile in 6 months

86. The AGACNP sees a 70-year-old male patient with a history of tobacco use for his yearly physical examination. Which radiologic tool will the AGACNP recommend to screen for cardiovascular disease?

A. Chest x-ray
B. CT scan of the chest
C. CT scan of the abdomen and pelvis
D. Abdominal aortic ultrasound

(*See answers next page.*)

82. B) Stage 3

Stage 3 is defined as an injury with full-thickness tissue loss, where subcutaneous fat may be visible and undermining and tunneling may occur. Slough may also be present; however, slough fully obstructing the view of the wound bed would make the pressure injury unstageable. Bone, tendon, and muscle are not exposed as would be found in Stage 4. Stage 1 pressure injuries are intact areas with non-blanchable erythema.

83. C) 65

Current guidelines recommend beginning yearly pneumococcal vaccination at age 65 years. Ages 55, 60, and 70 years are all outside the recommended treatment window.

84. A) Chronic obstructive pulmonary disease (COPD)

Patients with social histories that include extended exposure to environmental pollutants, such as coal dust, are at increased risk of developing COPD. The development of asthma in older adults is uncommon and is typically associated with a positive family history and tobacco use. CF is an inherited disorder that has no clinical correlation to environmental exposures. Tuberculosis is a pulmonary infection caused by *Mycobacterium tuberculosis* bacterium and is unrelated to exposure to coal dust.

85. B) Initiating low-dose statin therapy

The U.S. Preventive Services Task Force recommends initiating low-to-moderate–dose statins for primary prevention of cardiovascular disease in patients age 40 to 75 years who have one or more cardiovascular disease risk factors and a 10-year calculated cardiovascular disease event score of 10% or greater. Encouragement of dietary modification is an appropriate adjuvant therapy but should not stand alone as the primary intervention. Guidelines do not recommend use of high-dose statin therapy in patients with these risk factors in the absence of a documented history of cardiovascular disease. Repeating a lipid profile in 6 months would not address the patient's current risk factors.

86. D) Abdominal aortic ultrasound

The U.S. Preventive Services Task Force recommends a one-time screening for abdominal aortic aneurysm (AAA) by ultrasonography for men age 65 years or older with a history of tobacco use. Chest x-rays are not useful for assessing for the presence of an AAA. A CT scan of the chest would not completely visualize the abdominal aorta and is therefore insufficient. A CT scan of the abdomen and pelvis, although capable of detecting AAAs, is only clinically indicated if ultrasonography is suboptimal.

87. The AGACNP will recommend that a 70-year-old patient have a colonoscopy:

A. Annually
B. Every 5 years
C. Every 10 years
D. As needed

88. By which percentage would the AGACNP expect a patient's low-density lipoprotein (LDL) level to decrease after introduction of high-intensity statin therapy?

A. 10%
B. 25%
C. 40%
D. 50%

89. Based on practice guidelines, at what age can male patients stop having their prostate-specific antigen (PSA) checked?

A. 65 years
B. 69 years
C. 74 years
D. 80 years

90. Which diagnostic study does the AGACNP order for a 65-year-old patient with a positive fecal occult test?

A. PET scan
B. Flexible sigmoidoscopy
C. CT of the abdomen and pelvis
D. Colonoscopy

91. Which is classified as a primary risk factor for development of oral cancer?

A. Age
B. Recurrent oral bacterial infections
C. Human papillomavirus infection
D. Compromised immune system

(*See answers next page.*)

87. B) Every 5 years

The U.S. Preventive Services Task Force recommends that patients age 50 to 75 years undergo a screening colonoscopy every 5 years. Screening every 10 years or annually would be outside of treatment guidelines.

88. D) 50%

Research has shown that introduction of a high-intensity statin reduces LDL level by 50%.

89. B) 69 years

The U.S. Preventive Services Task Force recommends periodic PSA testing in male patients age 55 to 69 years. A 65-year-old patient should still undergo testing at their provider's discretion. Guidelines do not recommend testing for patients age 70 years and older.

90. D) Colonoscopy

Colonoscopy is considered the gold standard for colorectal cancer screening in cases where a stool test, imaging study, or flexible sigmoidoscopy has identified an abnormality. PET scans, which assess the metabolic function of normal and abnormal tissue, can be beneficial once a malignancy has been identified but are not indicated as the next step after stool testing has identified an abnormality. Flexible sigmoidoscopy is an alternative to screening with a fecal occult test. If colonoscopy were to identify a mass, a CT scan of the abdomen and pelvis would be a useful next step.

91. A) Age

Age is the primary risk factor for oral cancer. Recurrent oral bacterial infections, human papillomavirus infection, and a compromised immune system are all secondary risk factors for developing oral cancer.

92. How often should a patient with type 1 diabetes mellitus undergo screening for diabetic retinopathy?

A. Yearly
B. Every 2 years
C. Every 5 years
D. Every 10 years

93. The population most at risk for developing a folic acid deficiency is those patients with:

A. Chronic kidney disease
B. Diabetes mellitus
C. History of alcoholism
D. Liver failure

94. Which type of anemia will the AGACNP suspect in an adult patient of Mediterranean heritage with a family history of anemia and with current laboratory studies indicating decreases in hemoglobin, mean corpuscular volume (MCV), and mean corpuscular hemoglobin concentration (MCHC)?

A. Iron-deficiency anemia
B. Sickle cell anemia
C. Anemia of chronic disease
D. Beta-thalassemia

95. In addition to sunscreen use, the AGACNP will recommend an adjunctive intervention of supplementation with which vitamin for a patient with a history of osteopenia?

A. D
B. C
C. A
D. E

96. A patient with HIV has been compliant with antiretroviral treatment for the past 2 years, and their most recent CD4 count was 350 cells/mcL. How often will the AGACNP recommend reassessing the patient's CD4 count?

A. Monthly
B. Every 3 to 6 months
C. Every 4 to 6 months
D. Every 12 months

(See answers next page.)

92. C) Every 5 years

Guidelines recommend that patients with type 1 diabetes mellitus undergo diabetic retinopathy screening every 5 years after initial diagnosis. Screening performed yearly, every 2 years, or every 10 years would all be outside practice guidelines.

93. C) History of alcoholism

Folic acid deficiency is a malabsorption disorder most seen in patients with a history of alcoholism. While patients with chronic kidney disease are also at increased risk for developing a folic acid deficiency, the risk is lower in comparison with the risk for patients with a history of alcoholism. Diabetes has no correlation with the development of a folic acid deficiency. As in patients with chronic kidney disease, those with liver disease are at increased risk for folic acid deficiency; however, the risk is lower in comparison with the risk for patients with a history of alcoholism.

94. D) Beta-thalassemia

Patients of Mediterranean heritage are at increased risk for beta-thalassemia, a genetically inherited disorder characterized by decreased levels of hemoglobin, MCV, and MCHC. Iron-deficiency anemia is not an inherited disease. Sickle cell anemia, a genetically inherited disorder that results in misshapen red blood cells, is typically diagnosed in infancy or childhood. Anemia of chronic disease results from chronic health conditions such as renal failure or malignancy.

95. A) D

In patients with a history of or at increased risk for osteopenia, aggressive sunscreen application should be accompanied by vitamin D supplementation. Vitamins C, A, and E are not associated with the absorption of calcium and therefore do not influence the risk or progression of osteopenia.

96. D) Every 12 months

For patients with HIV infection who have been on antiretroviral medication for at least 2 years and whose CD4 counts are above 300 cells/mcL, current guidelines recommend assessing CD4 counts every 12 months.

97. A young adult presents to the emergency department after being bitten by a cat earlier in the day. Which antibiotic regimen will the AGACNP order?

A. Metronidazole (Flagyl) 500 mg orally every 6 to 8 hours for 7 to 14 days
B. Cephalexin (Keflex) 250 mg orally every 6 hours for 3 to 7 days
C. Amoxicillin/clavulanate (Augmentin) 500 mg orally every 8 hours for 5 to 7 days
D. Amoxicillin (Amoxil) 500 mg orally every 8 hours for 7 days

98. Which dose of amoxicillin (Amoxil) is appropriate for a patient with culture-confirmed streptococcal pharyngitis?

A. 1,000 mg by mouth daily
B. 500 mg by mouth daily
C. 1,000 mg by mouth twice daily
D. 500 mg by mouth three times daily

99. A patient presents to the emergency department reporting fever, flank pain, and dysuria. The AGACNP notes costovertebral angle tenderness during the physical examination and suspects acute pyelonephritis. Which diagnostic imaging study will the AGACNP order for further assessment?

A. Renal ultrasound
B. MRI of the abdomen and pelvis
C. Abdominal ultrasound
D. Renal angiography

100. A patient presents to the clinic after having an unprotected sexual encounter with an individual known to be positive for HIV. Which is the maximum number of hours postexposure that postexposure prophylaxis (PEP) with antiretroviral drugs can be administered to this patient for maximum benefit?

A. 24
B. 36
C. 48
D. 72

(*See answers next page.*)

97. C) Amoxicillin/clavulanate (Augmentin) 500 mg orally every 8 hours for 5 to 7 days

Amoxicillin/clavulanate (Augmentin) 500 mg orally for 5 to 7 days is guideline-directed therapy for animal bites. Metronidazole (Flagyl) is one of two antibiotics prescribed for infection with *Clostridioides difficile.* Cephalexin (Keflex) 250 mg orally every 6 hours for 3 to 7 days is indicated for bacterial skin infections. Amoxicillin (Amoxil) 500 mg orally every 8 hours for 7 days is indicated for standard bacterial infections nonspecific to animal bites.

98. A) 1,000 mg by mouth daily

Patients diagnosed with streptococcal pharyngitis should receive amoxicillin (Amoxil) 1,000 mg by mouth daily, whether as a single dose or as two 500-mg doses. A dosing regimen of 500 mg by mouth daily would be subtherapeutic, whereas 1,000 mg by mouth twice daily or 500 mg by mouth three times daily would be excessive.

99. A) Renal ultrasound

Renal ultrasound is a noninvasive diagnostic study that can be used to assess for renal obstruction and hydronephrosis in complicated pyelonephritis. Although MRI of the abdomen and pelvis allows for assessment of the renal system, it is both less cost-effective and more invasive than ultrasound. Abdominal ultrasounds are not specific to the renal system and would provide more information than necessary. Renal angiography is an invasive procedure performed to assess the renal vessels and does not provide information regarding renal obstruction or possible fluid accumulation.

100. D) 72

Guidelines for PEP recommend administration of a combination of antiretroviral drugs within 72 hours of unprotected, high-risk contact with an individual who is HIV positive for maximum benefit. PEP administered at 24, 36, or 48 hours post exposure would be well within the treatment window.

101. The AGACNP sees a new patient who was admitted early this morning through the emergency department with a preliminary diagnosis of hemolytic anemia. Which extrinsic factor does the AGACNP identify as a risk factor for this disorder?

A. Menorrhagia
B. Vegan diet
C. Medication reaction
D. Gastrointestinal bleed

102. As part of the differential diagnosis, an AGACNP suspects that the patient may have acute myeloid leukemia (AML). Other than the patient's recent complaint of increasing fatigue and the pancytopenia laboratory result, which physical examination finding would be a key indicator of this possible diagnosis?

A. White patches on the tongue
B. Ascites
C. Carotid bruit
D. Acanthosis nigricans

103. A patient presents with obstructing nephrolithiasis, a temperature of 100.9°F (38.3°C), and a blood pressure of 88/60 mmHg. Which is the AGACNP's best next step?

A. Admit the patient to the hospital
B. Refer to outpatient urology
C. Initiate antibiotics
D. Encourage increased hydration

104. A patient with a nephrolithiasis asks the AGACNP what they can do to decrease the risk of recurrence. Which dietary modification does the AGACNP recommend?

A. Increase lean protein intake
B. Increase hydration
C. Increase sodium intake
D. Decrease sugar intake

(See answers next page.)

101. C) Medication reaction

A drug-induced reaction can cause hemolytic anemia or the rapid destruction of red blood cells. Thus, the patient's medication list should be carefully reviewed. Menorrhagia or heavy menstrual bleeding, a diet low in iron-rich foods such as a strict vegan diet, or blood loss from the gastrointestinal tract may contribute to iron-deficiency anemia.

102. A) White patches on the tongue

The patient's new complaints of fatigue and the laboratory results of pancytopenia (a reduction in red blood cells, white blood cells, and platelets) are highly suspicious of AML. In addition, due to the low white cell blood count, the patient is susceptible to various infections such as thrush or an oral fungal (yeast) infection that presents as raised, white "cottage cheese-like" areas on the tongue and/or in the mouth. Other typical signs and symptoms of AML are associated with pancytopenia, such as pale skin, shortness of breath, bone pain, and fever. Ascites, carotid bruit, and acanthosis nigricans are not physical findings typically seen with AML.

103. A) Admit the patient to the hospital

An obstructing nephrolithiasis with signs and symptoms of infection is considered a medical emergency and will require inpatient management. While the patient will need a urology consult, this situation warrants urgent management. Antibiotics alone are insufficient, as a stent or nephrostomy tube will likely be needed. Increased hydration is also insufficient to address these issues.

104. B) Increase hydration

Increasing fluid intake to at least 3 L/day helps decrease the risk of nephrolithiasis development. Protein intake and sodium intake should be decreased. Sugar intake does not influence the formation of nephrolithiasis.

105. Which are the four features that make up the Centor criteria?

A. Fever over 100.4°F (38°C), tender anterior cervical nodes, pharyngotonsillar exudate, cough
B. Fever over 100.4°F (38°C), tender anterior cervical nodes, pharyngotonsillar exudate, absence of cough
C. Fever over 100.4°F (38°C), nasal discharge, maxillary sinus pressure, headache
D. Fever over 100.4°F (38°C), green phlegm, halitosis, sore throat

106. Which type of hearing acuity typically declines first?

A. High-pitched sounds
B. Middle-pitched sounds
C. Low-pitched sounds
D. Soft-pitched sounds

107. A patient presents with partial-thickness skin loss and visible dermis on the sacrum. Which stage does the AGACNP document for this pressure injury?

A. 1
B. 2
C. 3
D. 4

108. The AGACNP sees a patient who has had multiple recent sickle-cell crises. Which prescription by the AGACNP will reduce the frequency of these episodes?

A. Prophylactic antibiotics
B. Hydroxyurea (Hydrea)
C. Referral to physical therapy
D. Oxycodone-acetaminophen (Percocet)

109. Which is the most common cause of intracranial hemorrhage (ICH) in young adults?

A. Substance use
B. Uncontrolled hypertension
C. Motor vehicle crash
D. Arteriovenous malformation (AVM)

(*See answers next page.*)

105. B) Fever over 100.4°F (38°C), tender anterior cervical nodes, pharyngotonsillar exudate, absence of cough

The Centor criteria predict the likelihood that a person has group A beta-hemolytic streptococcal infection and include fever over 100.4°F (38°C), tender anterior cervical nodes, pharyngotonsillar exudate, and absence of cough. The Centor criteria do not include cough, nasal discharge, maxillary sinus pressure, headache, green phlegm, halitosis, or sore throat.

106. A) High-pitched sounds

Hearing acuity gradually lessens with age, and hearing acuity of high-pitched sounds typically declines earliest. As one ages, the acuity of middle-pitched sounds and then low-pitched sounds also decline sequentially. "Soft-pitched sounds" is not a category of sound quality.

107. B) 2

A stage 2 pressure ulcer is characterized by partial-thickness skin loss and exposed dermis. Stage 1 would have intact skin. Stage 3 would have full-thickness skin loss. Stage 4 would also have exposed fascia, muscle-tendon, bone, or cartilage.

108. B) Hydroxyurea (Hydrea)

Hydroxyurea (Hydrea) is a cytotoxic medication that can reduce the frequency of sickle-cell crisis episodes. While infection can trigger a crisis, prophylactic antibiotics are not indicated. Physical therapy will not lessen episodes. Pain medication such as oxycodone-acetaminophen (Percocet) may be necessary for patients with sickle cell anemia but will not lessen the frequency of episodes.

109. D) Arteriovenous malformation (AVM)

AVM is the most common cause of ICH among young adults. Hypertension is the most common cause of ICH among all ages. Substance use can cause ICH, but it is less common. Motor vehicle crashes do not typically cause ICH.

110. The AGACNP evaluates a patient who presents with pain following a traumatic injury to the right leg. Upon examination, the AGACNP notices pallor in the right lower extremity and cannot palpate a tibial pulse. Which is the AGACNP's next step?

A. Measure compartment pressure
B. Elevate the leg above the level of the heart
C. Order a Doppler ultrasound
D. Order a right tibia x-ray

111. The AGACNP witnesses a patient experiencing a seizure with alternating rhythmic muscle jerking and sustained muscle contractions. The AGACNP diagnoses this as which type of seizure?

A. Atonic
B. Clonic
C. Tonic
D. Tonic-clonic

112. The AGACNP witnesses a patient experiencing a seizure with rhythmic muscle jerking. The AGACNP diagnoses this as which type of seizure?

A. Atonic
B. Clonic
C. Tonic
D. Tonic-clonic

113. Which is the medication class of choice for posttraumatic stress disorder (PTSD)?

A. Benzodiazepines
B. Selective serotonin reuptake inhibitors (SSRIs)
C. Serotonin and norepinephrine reuptake inhibitors (SNRIs)
D. Tricyclic antidepressants (TCAs)

114. The AGACNP is interviewing a patient who describes a sudden onset, severely intense headache after having a bowel movement. Which will the AGACNP's next step be?

A. Prescribe stool softeners and laxatives as needed
B. Order noncontrast CT of the head
C. Encourage relaxation strategies to decrease stress headaches
D. Encourage a high-fiber diet with increased hydration

(*See answers next page.*)

110. A) Measure compartment pressure

The AGACNP would be concerned about compartment syndrome, a complication of traumatic injury that can present as pallor, pulselessness, paralysis, pain, and paresthesia. Direct measurement of compartment pressure is needed to confirm this diagnosis. Elevating the leg above the level of the heart would not be an appropriate intervention. Ordering a Doppler ultrasound would be helpful if a deep vein thrombosis were suspected. An x-ray would not confirm or rule out compartment syndrome.

111. D) Tonic-clonic

A tonic-clonic seizure is characterized by a combination of rhythmic muscle jerking and sustained contractions. Atonic seizures present as loss of muscle tone. A clonic seizure is characterized by rhythmic muscle jerking. Tonic seizures present as persistent muscle contractions.

112. B) Clonic

A clonic seizure is characterized by rhythmic muscle jerking. Atonic seizures present as loss of muscle tone. Tonic seizures present as persistent muscle contractions. A tonic-clonic seizure is characterized by a combination of rhythmic muscle jerking and sustained contractions.

113. B) Selective serotonin reuptake inhibitors (SSRIs)

SSRIs are the only medication approved by the U.S. Food and Drug Administration for PTSD and are, therefore, the drug class of choice for this disorder. Benzodiazepines are contraindicated in PTSD. SNRIs and TCAs may be helpful with the depression component of the disorder but are not specifically approved for this purpose.

114. B) Order noncontrast CT of the head

A sudden-onset, severe headache is often called a "thunderclap" headache and is concerning for intracranial hemorrhage. Therefore, the most appropriate step for workup is noncontrast CT of the head. Stool softeners and laxatives address constipation but not the headache. Relaxation strategies do not properly address the source of the headache. A high-fiber diet and increased hydration do not address a potentially dangerous headache.

115. A patient who started sertraline 10 days ago reports that the medication is not working and expresses a desire to stop taking it. Which is the AGACNP's best response?

A. "I respect your autonomy and your decision to stop taking the medication."
B. "I recommend switching to a different antidepressant that may work better."
C. "It can take 2 to 4 weeks to feel an effect from this antidepressant."
D. "I recommend increasing the dose so that it can work better."

116. A patient reports that they had a period of sadness and anhedonia following the death of their spouse, but it resolved after a grieving period of about 2 months. The AGACNP diagnoses this as:

A. Depression
B. Anxiety
C. Posttraumatic stress disorder (PTSD)
D. Adjustment disorder

117. A patient on a combined oral contraceptive pill presents to the clinic with elevated home blood pressure readings over the past month. Which is the AGACNP's best next step?

A. Continue the patient on the oral contraceptive pill
B. Decrease the dose of the oral contraceptive pill
C. Discontinue the oral contraceptive pill
D. Switch to a progestin-only pill

118. The AGACNP is reviewing lab results for a patient experiencing infertility. Which lab values indicate ovarian insufficiency?

A. Low follicle-stimulating hormone (FSH), low luteinizing hormone (LH), low estradiol
B. High FSH, high LH, high estradiol
C. High FSH, high LH, low estradiol
D. Low FSH, high LH, low estradiol

119. The AGACNP is auscultating the lung sounds of an adult patient post endotracheal intubation. Which assessment finding indicates a right mainstem bronchus intubation?

A. Absent breath sounds on the left
B. Absent breath sounds on the right
C. Decreased breath sounds on the left
D. Decreased breath sounds on the right

(See answers next page.)

115. C) "It can take 2 to 4 weeks to feel an effect from this antidepressant."
Selective serotonin reuptake inhibitors and certain other antidepressants typically take 2 to 4 weeks for an effect to be noted. It is important to educate patients so that they do not become discouraged or stop taking the medication. While it is important to respect a patient's autonomy, the AGACNP needs to give the patient proper education to make an informed decision. It would not be appropriate to switch to a different medication or to increase the dose at this point.

116. D) Adjustment disorder
Adjustment disorder is emotional distress that is a direct response to stress and is characterized by its temporary nature and ability to self-resolve. It occurs within 3 months of the stressor. While the syndrome might have overlapping symptoms similar to psychiatric disorders, it is specifically situational. This is unlike depression, anxiety, and PTSD, which tend to be more chronic issues.

117. D) Switch to a progestin-only pill
A patient who develops hypertension while on an oral contraceptive pill should be switched to a nonestrogen contraceptive method. The patient should not continue on the current pill with uncontrolled hypertension, and the dose cannot be decreased. Discontinuing the pill is an option but would not address the patient's need for contraception.

118. C) High FSH, high LH, low estradiol
Elevated FSH and LH levels accompanied by a decreased estradiol level indicate ovarian insufficiency. The other lab values do not correlate with ovarian insufficiency.

119. A) Absent breath sounds on the left
Absent breath sounds in the left lung field post intubation indicates a right mainstem bronchus intubation. Absent breath sounds on the right would be expected if the left mainstem bronchus were to be intubated. Decreased breath sounds in either lung field are not consistent with either left or right mainstem bronchus intubation.

120. The AGACNP follows which order when performing a respiratory examination?

A. Inspect, palpate, percuss, auscultate
B. Inspect, percuss, palpate, auscultate
C. Inspect, auscultate, palpate, percuss
D. Palpate, percuss, inspect, auscultate

121. A patient with a family history of premature coronary artery disease presents to the clinic for their yearly physical examination. Which action by the AGACNP is considered primary prevention of cardiovascular disease?

A. Hypertension screening
B. Prescribing an antihypertensive
C. Encouraging a nutritious diet and exercise
D. Scheduling a nuclear stress test

122. Gender expression is defined as the:

A. Sexual orientation of an individual
B. Sex assigned to an individual at birth
C. Sex an individual identifies as
D. Outward manner in which an individual expresses gender

123. Back pain associated with osteoporosis is classified as which type of pain?

A. Mechanical
B. Visceral
C. Neuropathic
D. Nonmechanical

124. Which statement by the AGACNP provides an adequate description of preventive measures for type 2 diabetes mellitus?

A. "Limit your daily sugar intake"
B. "Low-fat diet and 150 minutes of exercise weekly can reduce your risk of developing type 2 diabetes mellitus"
C. "If you don't have a family history of type 2 diabetes mellitus, then you have nothing to worry about."
D. "Start taking a multivitamin daily."

(*See answers next page.*)

120. A) Inspect, palpate, percuss, auscultate
Examination of the respiratory system begins with an inspection, followed by palpation, then percussion, and finally auscultation.

121. C) Encouraging a nutritious diet and exercise
Primary prevention aims at preventing disease. Encouraging a nutritious diet and frequent exercise reduces the risk of developing cardiovascular disease. Hypertension screening is considered a secondary intervention, as it involves screening for a disease before it has manifested any signs or symptoms. Prescribing an antihypertensive is considered a tertiary intervention, as it acknowledges a disease process is present and is aimed at slowing or stopping it. A nuclear stress test can be used as secondary or tertiary prevention, depending on the clinical scenario.

122. D) Outward manner in which an individual expresses gender
Gender expression is defined as the outward manner in which an individual expresses or displays gender. The term *sexual orientation* refers to a person's sexual attraction to others and is unrelated to their gender expression. The sex assigned to an individual at birth is typically female or male, but this does not refer to the individual's gender expression. The sex an individual identifies as is called their gender identity.

123. A) Mechanical
Pain related to osteoporosis, disk herniation, spinal stenosis, fractures, kyphosis, and spondylolysis is categorized as mechanical back pain. Causes of visceral back pain include abdominal aortic aneurysm, pancreatitis, nephrolithiasis, and pelvic inflammatory diseases. *Neuropathic* is not a classification of back pain. Sources of nonmechanical back pain include infections such as osteomyelitis, epidural abscess, paraspinal abscess, inflammatory arthritis, and osteochondrosis.

124. B) "Low-fat diet and 150 minutes of exercise weekly can reduce your risk of developing type 2 diabetes mellitus"
A low-fat diet and 150 minutes of exercise weekly have been clinically shown to decrease a patient's risk of developing type 2 diabetes mellitus. Limiting daily sugar intake may be helpful but would not significantly reduce risk. Although family history should be taken into consideration when determining risk factors for diabetes mellitus, a lack of family history does not mean a patient is unable to develop a disease. Taking a multivitamin is a beneficial intervention but does not have any effect on preventing type 2 diabetes mellitus.

125. A patient is diagnosed with a vertebral compression fracture secondary to osteoporosis. When reviewing the patient's history and physical assessment findings, what condition would the AGACNP identify as a potential contributing factor?

A. Gastric resection
B. Hypothyroidism
C. Rapid weight gain
D. Young age

126. A 59-year-old patient presents to the clinic with low back pain. Upon further examination, the patient is afebrile, with no tenderness with palpation along the lumbar spine and lower back region, and the pain improves with rest. What condition does the AGACNP suspect?

A. Kidney stones
B. Pancreatitis
C. Herniated disk
D. Osteomyelitis

127. A 68-year-old patient with a family history of stomach cancer presents with new onset dyspepsia. Which is the AGACNP's best next step?

A. Order famotidine (Pepcid) 20 mg daily
B. Educate the patient on dietary modifications
C. Order CT of the abdomen with contrast
D. Refer the patient for upper endoscopy

128. An 80-year-old bedridden patient enters the emergency department with altered mental status. Vital signs at the time of admission are blood pressure 102/61 mmHg, heart rate 105 bpm, respiratory rate 24 breaths/min, temperature 102°F (38.9°C), and oxygen saturation 95% on room air with clear breath sounds bilaterally and in all lobes. A family member reports that the patient is normally alert and oriented but is currently confused about place and time as of this morning. CT of the head does not show any emergent neurologic conditions, and a clean catch urine sample is negative for white blood cells. The patient presents with decubitus ulcers on the left heel. Which condition or diagnosis would be a priority for the AGACNP?

A. Dementia
B. Urinary tract infection
C. Pneumonia
D. Osteomyelitis

(See answers next page.)

125. A) Gastric resection

Patients post gastrectomy are at increased risk for osteoporosis. This is caused by nutritional intolerances and deficiencies such as dumping syndrome, fat maldigestion, gastric stasis, and lactose intolerance. Hyperthyroidism, not hypothyroidism, is a risk factor for osteoporosis. Rapid weight loss or malnourishment is associated with osteoporosis. Older age, not younger, increases the risk for osteoporosis.

126. C) Herniated disk

Disk herniation is a mechanical cause of back pain that improves with rest and is the most likely cause of the patient's low back pain. Kidney and pancreatitis stones are conditions of visceral back pain that can be identified by tenderness or pain upon palpation. The patient is afebrile, making nonmechanical or infectious causes of back pain, such as osteomyelitis, unlikely.

127. D) Refer the patient for upper endoscopy

A patient older than 60 years with new-onset dyspepsia and increased risk of malignancy should undergo an upper endoscopy to rule out malignancy. Famotidine (Pepcid) and dietary modifications may be indicated as well, but it is important to rule out other serious causes of dyspepsia. A CT of the abdomen is more useful in diagnosing disease in the pancreas, biliary tract, or intestines.

128. D) Osteomyelitis

The patient presents with symptoms of infection. After a negative head CT scan, the priority is to identify the source of infection causing the altered mental status. The decubitus ulcers may indicate osteomyelitis. The onset of the confusion is unlikely to be dementia, as rapidly progressive dementias can take weeks to months to progress. The patient has clear lung sounds and adequate oxygen saturation, lowering the suspicion of pneumonia. With no white blood cells present in the urine, urinary tract infection is unlikely.

129. A 73-year-old patient presents with new urinary incontinence secondary to detrusor overactivity. Which initial treatment does the AGACNP recommend?

A. Oxybutynin (Ditropan XL)
B. Pessary
C. Bladder training
D. Indwelling urinary catheter

130. Urinary leakage that occurs with sneezing, coughing, or standing is called:

A. Stress incontinence
B. Urge incontinence
C. Overflow incontinence
D. Positional incontinence

131. The AGACNP performs a whispered voice test on an older adult patient. The patient does not successfully identify all three numbers. Which is the AGACNP's next step?

A. Referral to audiogram
B. Prescription for hearing amplification device
C. Documentation of patient as having conductive hearing loss
D. Repeating the whispered voice test a second time

132. A patient is considering treatment with onabotulinum toxin A (Botox) for urinary incontinence. Which is the most important potential side effect the AGACNP should discuss with this patient?

A. The treatment can cause delirium or dry mouth
B. Benefit may not be noticeable for about 6 weeks
C. The treatment can cause sexual dysfunction
D. The treatment can cause severe urinary retention

133. A 68-year-old patient presents with new-onset idiopathic thrombocytopenia (ITP). Platelet count is 20,000/mcL, and the patient does not have active bleeding. Which is the AGACNP's next step?

A. Platelet transfusion
B. Corticosteroids
C. Observation only
D. Rituximab (Rituxan)

(See answers next page.)

129. C) Bladder training

Bladder training is the best initial treatment for detrusor overactivity and includes different behavioral techniques. Oxybutynin (Ditropan XL) should be reserved for cases in which bladder training is not effective. A pessary can be used in cases of urethral incompetence. Indwelling urinary catheterization is part of the treatment plan for overflow incontinence.

130. A) Stress incontinence

Stress incontinence is leakage of urine with certain actions such as coughing, sneezing, or standing up from a seated position. The term *urge incontinence* refers to urinary urgency with difficulty holding one's urine. Overflow incontinence can occur from a variety of causes, including urethral obstruction, and presents as dribbling post void. Postural, not positional, incontinence is associated with changes in body position.

131. D) Repeating the whispered voice test a second time

The whispered voice test is a simple screening test for hearing loss that involves whispering three numbers while standing behind a patient. If a patient cannot successfully identify the numbers on the first try, the test should be repeated once more with different numbers. Referral to audiogram should take place after two unsuccessful tests, and a prescription for a hearing amplification device should be reserved until further workup is completed. While documentation is important, this whisper test cannot definitively diagnose conductive hearing loss.

132. D) The treatment can cause severe urinary retention

Onabotulinum toxin A (Botox) is an effective treatment for detrusor overactivity but can cause urinary retention that necessitates self-catheterization. Antimuscarinic agents are more likely to cause dry mouth and delirium. Onabotulinum toxin A (Botox) typically takes 2 weeks to work. Sexual dysfunction is not a known side effect of onabotulinum toxin A (Botox).

133. B) Corticosteroids

The standard treatment for new-onset ITP is a short course of corticosteroids. Rituximab (Rituxan) is sometimes added to the corticosteroids but adds significant toxicity, so it is not considered standard. Platelet transfusion is indicated only with active bleeding. Treatment, rather than observation only, is indicated with platelet counts of less than 25,000/mcL or with active bleeding.

134. A 72-year-old patient is due for hip replacement surgery. When evaluating the patient, which is the most important part of the bleeding-risk assessment?

A. Directed bleeding history
B. Complete blood count (CBC)
C. Prothrombin time (PT)/international normalized ratio (INR)
D. Physical examination

135. A 70-year-old patient reports receiving neither the 23-valent pneumococcal polysaccharide vaccine (PPSV23) nor the 13-valent pneumococcal conjugate vaccine (PCV13). Which is the AGACNP's next step?

A. Explain that the pneumococcal vaccine is indicated only for high-risk patients
B. Order the PPSV23 followed by the PCV13 6 to 12 months later
C. Order the PCV13 followed by the PPSV23 6 to 12 months later
D. Order the PPSV23 only

136. The AGACNP is seeing a patient with a herpes zoster infection. Which advisory does the AGACNP include in this patient's education?

A. Herpes zoster is a sexually transmitted infection.
B. Herpes zoster may lead to chronic neuropathic pain.
C. There is currently no approved vaccine for herpes zoster.
D. Herpes zoster is no longer contagious 3 days after onset.

137. A 73-year-old patient presents with a chronic, nonhealing pressure injury that is draining pus. The patient is afebrile with a normal white blood cell count. Which is the AGACNP's next step?

A. Obtain a superficial wound culture
B. Admit patient to hospital
C. Order silver sulfadiazine to apply to the wound
D. Order an occlusive dressing to apply to the wound

138. Which tool can be used to assess the risk for development of pressure injuries?

A. Braden Scale
B. Banner Mobility Assessment
C. Karnofsky Performance Status Scale
D. Patient Health Questionaire-2

(See answers next page.)

134. A) Directed bleeding history

A reliable directed bleeding history is most valuable in determining whether a patient is at an increased risk for perioperative or postoperative bleeding. If abnormal bleeding is suggested from the history, a CBC and PT/INR would be warranted. Physical examination is not typically as valuable as an accurate bleeding history.

135. C) Order the PCV13 followed by the PPSV23 6 to 12 months later

All individuals who are 65 years or older are recommended to receive the pneumococcal vaccine. For patients who have not received any pneumococcal vaccine, the PCV13 should be administered first, followed by the PPSV23 6 to 12 months later. Patients who have received more than one dose of PPSV23 in the past should receive PCV13 more than 1 year after the last dose of PPSV23.

136. B) Herpes zoster may lead to chronic neuropathic pain.

Herpes zoster is fairly common in older individuals and in those who are immunosuppressed. It is important to make patients aware that it can cause chronic postherpetic neuralgia. It is not a sexually transmitted infection; it is a reactivation of the varicella zoster infection. Herpes zoster is considered contagious until all vesicles have crusted over.

137. C) Order silver sulfadiazine to apply to the wound

A pressure injury that appears infected without signs or symptoms of systemic infection should be treated with topical antiseptics such as silver sulfadiazine. Because bacteria contaminate all chronic pressure injuries, a superficial wound culture without signs of systemic infection would not be beneficial. Admitting the patient to the hospital would be necessary if the patient presented with signs and symptoms of systemic infection. An occlusive dressing will not manage the drainage nor treat the infection.

138. A) Braden Scale

The Braden Scale is a tool to help identify patients at risk for developing pressure injuries. The Banner Mobility Assessment aims to evaluate a patient's mobility level. The Karnofsky Performance Status Scale is a tool to measure performance status in oncology patients. Patient Health Questionaire-2 evaluates patients for risk of depression.

139. The AGACNP is teaching a patient how to use their new cane for ambulation. Which is an important point to include in this education?

A. The cane should be used on the stronger side.
B. The height of the cane should be set to reach the fingertips.
C. The cane should be used by the dominant hand.
D. The cane should be used only when ambulating outside the house.

140. Which is the best way to check gait and balance in the older adult?

A. Timed Up and Go Test
B. Romberg test
C. Exercise stress test
D. Range of motion test

141. Which is true regarding the *APOE-e4* allele?

A. Having two copies guarantees the development of Alzheimer disease.
B. Having no copies guarantees that Alzheimer disease will not develop.
C. Genetic testing for the *APOE-e4* allele is widely recommended.
D. It is associated with susceptibility for late-onset Alzheimer disease.

142. A 77-year-old patient presents with change in mood following an unwitnessed fall. Which should the AGACNP rule out first?

A. Substance use
B. Brain tumor
C. Subdural hematoma
D. Muscle sprain

143. Approximately what percentage of older adult men are affected by erectile dysfunction (ED)?

A. 10%
B. 25%
C. 50%
D. 75%

(*See answers next page.*)

139. A) The cane should be used on the stronger side.

A cane should be used on the stronger side for optimal benefit. The height of the cane should reach the wrist level. The hand used to hold the cane does not have to be the dominant hand. Canes should be used to ambulate both in and out of the house for safety.

140. A) Timed Up and Go Test

The Timed Up and Go test quickly and easily tests gait by having a patient demonstrate the ability to stand up from a seated position (without use of hands), ambulate, and return to a seated position. The Romberg test also checks balance but mainly checks the neurological component of gait. An exercise stress test checks cardiac function. A range of motion test assesses mobility rather than balance.

141. D) It is associated with susceptibility for late-onset Alzheimer disease.

The *APOE-e4* allele is associated with an increased risk of developing late-onset Alzheimer disease. Two copies do not guarantee the development of the disease, nor does a lack of copies guarantee that one will not develop the disease. Quantifying a risk for developing Alzheimer is difficult; therefore, genetic testing is not widely recommended.

142. C) Subdural hematoma

Subdural hematomas are a common and often undiagnosed complication of falls in older individuals. While a change in mood may indicate substance use or a brain tumor, the clinical picture should make the AGACNP suspect subdural hematoma. A muscle sprain may occur with a fall, but this would not be the priority diagnosis to address.

143. C) 50%

ED is defined as the inability to maintain an erection and affects approximately 50% of older adult men.

144. The AGACNP is discussing the use of acetylcholinesterase inhibitors with a patient. Which educational point does the nurse include?

A. They can delay progression of mild cognitive impairment to dementia.
B. The most common side effect is constipation.
C. They provide modest cognitive function improvement.
D. They should be continued long-term even if no benefit is noted.

145. The AGACNP is evaluating a patient with suspected fibromyalgia. Which finding would the AGACNP expect to see?

A. Elevated erythrocyte sedimentation rate (ESR)
B. Tender trigger points
C. Swollen joints
D. Decreased phosphate

146. A 65-year-old patient reports intermittent vaginal bleeding. The patient reports reaching menopause at age 51 years. Which is the AGACNP's most appropriate next step?

A. Reassure the patient that intermittent bleeding can occur after menopause
B. Order labs to check the patient's estrogen and progestin levels
C. Refer the patient for endometrial biopsy
D. Order hormonal replacement therapy for the patient

147. A 74-year-old patient presents with musculoskeletal back pain. Which medication should the AGACNP initially select for treatment?

A. Ibuprofen (Advil)
B. Celecoxib (Celebrex)
C. Diclofenac gel (Voltaren)
D. Oxycodone (OxyContin)

148. A 62-year-old patient presents with low back pain. Which associated symptom would the AGACNP identify as a "red flag"?

A. Increased pain with activity
B. Increased pain with sitting
C. Unexplained weight loss
D. Relief with ibuprofen (Advil)

(See answers next page.)

144. C) They provide modest cognitive function improvement.

Acetylcholinesterase inhibitors provide some improvement in cognitive function. They do not slow the progression of mild cognitive impairment to dementia. Diarrhea, rather than constipation, is a common side effect. The use of these medications should be re-evaluated after a 2-month trial and discontinued if no benefit is noted.

145. B) Tender trigger points

Presentation of fibromyalgia is typically unremarkable except for tender musculoskeletal trigger points. Elevated ESR and swollen joints may be seen with rheumatoid arthritis but not with fibromyalgia. A finding of hypophosphatemia would not be consistent with fibromyalgia.

146. C) Refer the patient for endometrial biopsy

Vaginal bleeding that occurs 6 months or more after menopause raises concern for endometrial cancer and warrants an endometrial biopsy. Reassuring the patient that bleeding after menopause can occur or ordering hormonal replacement therapy is inappropriate in this situation. Checking estrogen and progestin levels would not help to diagnose the issue as the patient requires a biopsy.

147. C) Diclofenac gel (Voltaren)

Diclofenac gel is a topical nonsteroidal anti-inflammatory drug (NSAID) that has fewer potential side effects as it has minimal systemic absorption. Ibuprofen (Advil) and celecoxib (Celebrex) can pose increased risk of renal damage and gastrointestinal bleed in older individuals. Oxycodone (OxyContin) is an opioid medication that should be reserved for select clinical scenarios only due to risk of dependence and respiratory depression.

148. C) Unexplained weight loss

Unexplained weight loss in conjunction with low back pain is concerning for cancer. Increased pain with activity and sitting can be seen with more benign etiologies of back pain. Relief of back pain with ibuprofen (Advil) does not specifically raise suspicion for alarming etiologies.

149. A patient presents with new-onset trigeminal neuralgia. Which medication should the AGACNP initially prescribe?

A. Phenytoin (Dilantin)
B. Carbamazepine (Tegretol)
C. Ibuprofen (Advil)
D. Metoprolol (Lopressor)

150. Which is the most common type of headache?

A. Tension
B. Cluster
C. Migraine
D. Thunderclap

151. A patient is starting escitalopram (Lexapro) for newly diagnosed generalized anxiety disorder. Which is an important educational point for the AGACNP to include in patient teaching?

A. You should avoid grapefruit juice while on this medication.
B. The medication may be taken on an as-needed basis.
C. This medication will cause weight loss.
D. The medication can take 4 weeks to show an effect.

152. A 71-year-old patient presents with suspected transient ischemic attack (TIA) that occurred 2 days ago. The patient has right lower extremity weakness, blood pressure of 160/95 mmHg, and history of diabetes mellitus. Which is the AGACNP's next step?

A. Prescribe warfarin (Coumadin)
B. Prescribe apixaban (Eliquis)
C. Admit patient to hospital
D. Refer patient to physical therapy

153. Which hormonal lab profile provides confirmation of menopausal transition?

A. High follicle-stimulating hormone (FSH), high estradiol
B. High FSH, low estradiol
C. Low FSH, low estradiol
D. Low FSH, high estradiol

(*See answers next page.*)

149. B) Carbamazepine (Tegretol)

Carbamazepine (Tegretol) is the first-line treatment for trigeminal neuralgia. Phenytoin (Dilantin) should be used only if carbamazepine (Tegretol) is ineffective or not tolerated. Ibuprofen (Advil) may be helpful in certain circumstances but is not a preferred treatment. Metoprolol (Lopressor) is used for certain cardiac conditions, not for trigeminal neuralgia.

150. A) Tension

Tension headache is the most common type of primary headache. Migraines and cluster headaches are less common. A thunderclap headache often occurs from a subarachnoid hemorrhage.

151. D) The medication can take 4 weeks to show an effect.

It is important to educate patients that selective serotonin reuptake inhibitors such as escitalopram (Lexapro) can take 2 to 4 weeks to take effect. Escitalopram (Lexapro) is not affected by grapefruit juice as are some other medications. The medication should be taken consistently and not "as needed." Weight gain, rather than weight loss, is a potential side effect.

152. C) Admit patient to hospital

The ABCD score (age 60 years and older, blood pressure 140/90 mmHg or higher, focal weakness, speech impairment, duration, diabetes mellitus) is used to identify patients who are at high risk for recurrent TIA or stroke, with a score of 4 or more indicating a need for hospitalization, particularly if the TIA occurred within the past week. The patient is older than 60 years, has a history of diabetes mellitus, and presents with focal weakness. Warfarin (Coumadin) and apixaban (Eliquis) may be used as anticoagulation therapy, but this should be managed once the patient is admitted. Physical therapy may be indicated once patient's clinical status is stabilized.

153. B) High FSH, low estradiol

A consistently elevated FSH combined with a low estradiol level can be used to confirm the menopausal transition. The other lab profiles shown are not indicative of menopause.

154. The AGACNP is evaluating a 57-year-old female patient's reproductive status. Which qualifies the patient for a diagnosis of menopause?

A. Irregular menstrual cycles for 1 year
B. Anovulatory menstrual cycles
C. No menstrual cycles for 1 year
D. Hot flushes and mood changes

155. The AGACNP is caring for a patient with an acute asthma exacerbation. Despite several doses of an albuterol (Ventolin) metered-dose inhaler, the patient continues to have dyspnea and wheezing. Which medication should the AGACNP prescribe next?

A. Levalbuterol (Xopenex)
B. Prednisone (Deltasone)
C. Montelukast (Singulair)
D. Salmeterol (Serevent)

156. When assessing an adult patient with acute asthma exacerbation, which finding should prompt the AGACNP to initiate systemic corticosteroids?

A. Pulse oximetry of 95% on room air
B. Peak flow measured at 75% of baseline
C. Lack of response to several short-acting beta-agonists (SABAs)
D. Ability to speak in phrases

157. Which is the best diagnostic tool for mitral valve stenosis?

A. Electrocardiogram
B. Echocardiogram
C. Chest x-ray
D. Cardiac catheterization

158. Which is the best diagnostic tool for pulmonary valve stenosis?

A. Electrocardiogram
B. Echocardiogram
C. Chest x-ray
D. Coronary angiogram

(*See answers next page.*)

154. C) No menstrual cycles for 1 year

Menopause is defined as a lack of menstrual cycles for one year. There may be irregular and anovulatory cycles as well as hot flashes and mood changes leading up to menopause, but these do not define the menopausal transition.

155. B) Prednisone (Deltasone)

If a patient is not responsive to several doses of a short-acting beta-agonist such as albuterol (Ventolin), a systemic corticosteroid such as prednisone (Deltasone) should be started. Levalbuterol (Xopenex) is a short-acting beta-agonist as well, so it would not be beneficial. Montelukast (Singulair) and salmeterol (Serevent) are indicated more for chronic, long-term control of asthma.

156. C) Lack of response to several short-acting beta-agonists (SABAs)

Lack of response to several SABA treatments should prompt initiation of systemic corticosteroids. Pulse oximetry of 95% on room air, peak flow at 75% of baseline, and ability to speak in phrases are more indicative of a mild to moderate asthma exacerbation.

157. B) Echocardiogram

An echocardiogram is best at identifying the presence of mitral valve stenosis. Electrocardiograms are best at identifying cardiac arrhythmias. Chest x-rays can show abnormalities in the lungs and cardiomegaly. Cardiac catheterization is used to identify coronary vessel disease.

158. B) Echocardiogram

An echocardiogram is best for identifying the presence, type, and gradient of pulmonary valve stenosis. Electrocardiograms are best for identifying cardiac arrhythmias. Chest x-rays can show abnormalities in the lungs and cardiomegaly. Coronary angiograms can evaluate for abnormalities in coronary blood vessels.

3

Professional Role

1. Which act passed in 2010 focused on providing or improving access to healthcare services, including new restriction on the ability of payers to limit coverage on the basis of preexisting conditions, an end to lifetime limits on coverage, and a requirement for payers to spend premium dollars on healthcare costs and not administrative costs?

   A. Affordable Care Act (ACA)
   B. Social Security Amendments–Public Law 89-97
   C. Emergency Medical Treatment and Active Labor Act (EMTALA)
   D. Health Insurance Portability and Accountability Act (HIPAA)

2. What determines an AGACNP's right to prescribe medications?

   A. The Drug Enforcement Agency
   B. The state where the AGACNP is practicing
   C. Nursing standards of practice
   D. The American Nurses Association

3. The AGACNP is asked by a friend to check on the friend's parent's lab results and share the information. The AGACNP explains that this is a violation of privacy and of which healthcare act?

   A. Emergency Medical Treatment and Active Labor Act (EMTALA)
   B. Affordable Care Act (ACA)
   C. Social Security Amendments–Public Law 89-97
   D. Health Insurance Portability and Accountability Act (HIPAA)

4. An organization has put together a performance improvement team to improve flow of patients from the emergency department (ED) to the inpatient units. The team is now analyzing data. Which of the following is an example of external benchmarking?

   A. Comparing information from the Joint Commission Core Measure data
   B. Reviewing flow data from the ED over the last 3 to 6 months
   C. Analyzing a survey that was performed in the hospital's inpatient unit
   D. Reviewing data from the most recent annual employee performance survey

(See answers next page.)

1. A) Affordable Care Act (ACA)

The ACA of 2010 tackled the issues of payment, access and insurance discrimination. Social Security Amendments–Public Law 89-97 established health insurance for those who are older or have disabilities in 1965; the programs established became known as Medicare and Medicaid. EMTALA, passed in 1986, requires hospitals participating in Medicare to screen and stabilize all persons who use their emergency departments regardless of ability to pay. HIPAA, passed in 1996, restricts use of pre-existing conditions in health insurance coverage determinations, sets standards for medical records privacy, and establishes tax-favored treatment of long-term care insurance.

2. B) The state where the AGACNP is practicing

Prescriptive authority is given by the state where the AGACNP is practicing.

3. D) Health Insurance Portability and Accountability Act (HIPAA)

The Health Insurance Portability and Accountability Act of 1996 sets standards for medical records privacy. Accessing healthcare records of people who are not patients by healthcare providers and disclosing test results and findings to other persons without patient consent is strictly forbidden. HIPAA also restricts use of pre-existing conditions in health insurance coverage determinations and establishes tax-favored treatment of long-term care insurance. The ACA of 2010 addresses the issues of payment, access, and insurance discrimination. The Social Security Amendments–Public Law 89-97 established programs that became known as Medicare and Medicaid. EMTALA, passed in 1986, requires hospitals participating in Medicare to screen and stabilize all patients who use their emergency departments regardless of ability to pay.

4. A) Comparing information from the Joint Commission Core Measure data

External benchmarking is the process of comparing an organization's performance with the performance of other organizations that provide the same types of services. The Joint Commission Core Measure data are an external benchmark that permits rigorous comparison of the actual results of care across hospitals. Reviewing hospital survey results or flow data from the ED involves analysis of data from the actual hospital system—a process that can help to establish an internal baseline or internal benchmarking.

5. Healthcare providers cite a number of barriers to evidence-based practice. Which of the following would help facilitate an evidence-based practice environment?

   A. Overwhelming patient loads
   B. Peer pressure to continue with practices that are steeped in tradition
   C. Time to critically appraise studies and implement their findings
   D. Demands from patients for a certain type of treatment

6. The AGACNP is considering adopting a new method of inserting central venous catheters after reading published studies. The AGACNP is aware that which of the following ranks highest on the hierarchy of evidence and would yield the strongest and least biased estimate of the effect of an intervention?

   A. Case control studies
   B. Cohort studies
   C. Opinion of expert committees
   D. Randomized controlled trial

7. The AGACNP wants to design a quantitative clinical study to measure the relationship between melatonin administration and hours of sleep in the ICU. Which of the following would be the independent variable in the study?

   A. Dose of melatonin administered
   B. Hours of sleep per patient in the ICU
   C. Number of ICU patients selected
   D. Other medications taken by the patients

8. An AGACNP is researching the Cochrane Reviews for strategies to decrease the incidence of decubitus ulcers in the unit. The AGACNP is aware that what types of studies are most likely to influence a practice change?

   A. Collection of systematic reviews or meta-analysis
   B. Collection of cohort studies
   C. Evidence from a collection of qualitative studies
   D. Reports of expert committees

(*See answers next page.*)

5. C) Time to critically appraise studies and implement their findings

For healthcare professionals to advance the use of evidence-based practice, knowledge and skills in this area must be enhanced, and time must be available to cultivate this learning. If time is constrained, as with overwhelming patient loads, there will be no opportunity for the practitioner to develop better methods. If the pressure is too strong to continue old habits, the practitioner will feel unsupported to implement a different practice. Finally, if patients demand treatment without justification, such as antibiotics for a viral infection, practitioners will find it difficult to implement evidence-based practice.

6. D) Randomized controlled trial

There are several rating systems for the hierarchy of evidence. Evidence from a randomized controlled trial is one of the highest as because randomized controlled trials use a rigorous process of well-defined, preset criteria to select for inclusion criteria, bias is overcome, and results are more credible. Evidence from case control and cohort studies is less robust, and evidence and opinion of authorities and/or reports of expert committees is lower still on the hierarchy of evidence. Of note, the best level of evidence comes from systematic reviews or meta-analysis of all relevant randomized controlled trials.

7. A) Dose of melatonin administered

The dose of melatonin is the independent variable in the study; it is the intervention being proposed. The hours of sleep per patient is the dependent variable, also known as the outcome. The number of ICU patients represents the sample size. The other medications the patients are taking could be seen as confounding or extraneous variables that could influence the outcome.

8. A) Collection of systematic reviews or meta-analysis

The Cochrane Review is a database of systematic reviews and meta-analyses that summarize and interpret the results of medical research. The highest level of evidence comes from systematic reviews or meta-analysis of all relevant randomized controlled trials. Ideally, practice changes would be based on these types of studies when available. Cohort studies, a collection of qualitative studies, and reports of expert committees are all lower-quality evidence when compared with collection of systematic reviews or meta-analysis.

9. An unexpected occurrence involves the death of a young adult patient the AGACNP was helping to care for. When analyzing this event to try to decrease risk recurrence, what is the best term to use to describe the occurrence?

   A. Sentinel event
   B. Near miss
   C. Medication error
   D. Breach of duty

10. An older adult patient is admitted to the hospital for congestive heart failure exacerbation. The patient is worried that their Medicare insurance will not cover the admission. The AGACNP knows that hospital admissions are covered under Medicare Part:

    A. A
    B. B
    C. C
    D. D

11. An AGACNP carelessly administers the wrong drug to a patient, but the patient is not hurt by this error. If a malpractice suit occurs as a result, the suit should not succeed because which two of the four elements of negligence are missing?

    A. Duty to use due care and breach of duty
    B. Breach of duty and damages
    C. Damages and causation
    D. Causation and duty to use due care

12. The AGACNP was granted permission by a healthcare organization to practice in a specific area of specialty within that organization after an in-depth application and interview. What is this agreement called?

    A. Degree
    B. License
    C. Certificate
    D. Credentials

(*See answers next page.*)

9. A) Sentinel event

A sentinel event is an unexpected occurrence involving death or serious physical or psychological injury, or the risk thereof. A medication error is a mistake that involves accidental drug overdose, administration of an incorrect substance, accidental consumption of a drug, or misuse of a drug. A near miss is an opportunity to improve patient safety. Breach of duty is a term used in a malpractice action when the issue is whether the practitioner exercised a standard of care that any reasonably prudent practitioner would have exercised under those circumstances.

10. A) A

Medicare Part A covers inpatient hospital stays, skilled nursing facility stays, some home health visits, and hospice care. Part B covers physician visits, outpatient services, preventive services, and some home health visits. Part C is the Medicare Advantage program, through which beneficiaries can enroll in a private health plan. Part D covers outpatient prescription drugs through private plans that contract with Medicare.

11. C) Damages and causation

The elements of malpractice that are absent in this case are damages and causation. No actual harm, or damage, occurred, and because no ill effect can be shown, no causation can be claimed that damage was caused by the act. Breach of duty is present because it is the issue of whether a practitioner exercised a standard of care that a reasonably prudent practitioner would have exercised under those same circumstances. Because the AGACNP acted carelessly, that breach of duty is present. Duty to use due care is the existence of a legal duty that the defendant owes to the patient to act in a reasonable manner.

12. D) Credentials

Credentials are a formal agreement granting permission through a regulatory mechanism to practice, whether by a national professional organization to a specific area of healthcare practice or by a healthcare organization to a licensed independent practitioner. A degree is a qualification awarded to students upon successful completion of a course of study in higher education, usually at a college or university. A license is the legal authority granted by a state to an entity to provide healthcare services within a specific scope of services. A certificate indicates that a healthcare professional has met certain predetermined standards as specified by that profession for specialty practice.

13. Which of the following is a characteristic of the quality improvement process in healthcare?

    A. Continuous process
    B. Chaotic structure
    C. Practice beyond scope of legal authority
    D. Criticism of nursing practice

14. Strategic planning for a performance improvement activity in healthcare may require a SWOT analysis to complete an assessment of the organization. In SWOT analysis, what does the S stand for?

    A. Strengths
    B. Standards
    C. Stop
    D. Student

15. The AGACNP would evaluate health literacy in a patient by asking:

    A. "How well do you speak, read, and write English?"
    B. "Do you have trouble reading and understanding your medication instructions?"
    C. "Do you feel comfortable talking about your symptoms with me?"
    D. "Would you like to receive your medical care in a specific language?"

16. The AGACNP instructs a patient with diabetes mellitus on how to control their blood glucose via diet and exercise. This is an example of which type of key component of the AGACNP role?

    A. Providing health promotion and health education counseling
    B. Performing comprehensive history and physical examination
    C. Assessing, educating, and providing referrals for the patient
    D. Ordering and interpreting diagnostic studies

(See answers next page.)

13. A) Continuous process

Quality improvement is a formal approach to the analysis of performance and systematic efforts to improve it. It is a continuous rather than an episodic process that is organized and seeks to recognize and reward nursing practice. It discourages practice beyond the scope of legal authority.

14. A) Strengths

SWOT analysis stands for Strengths, Weaknesses, Opportunities, and Threats.

15. B) "Do you have trouble reading and understanding your medication instructions?"

Health literacy is the degree to which an individual has the ability to understand and process basic healthcare information necessary to make appropriate healthcare decisions. Asking a patient if they have trouble reading their medication bottles and instructions evaluates the patient's health literacy because it assesses whether the patient can understand medical terms and follow directions for therapies. Asking a patient how well they communicate in English or if they would like to receive their medical care in a different language evaluates language barriers and assesses the need for an interpreter. Some patients may feel particularly sensitive about discussing issues openly; asking a patient if they feel comfortable recognizes that each patient may view certain sensitive issues differently and may require more communication or development of a deeper relationship.

16. A) Providing health promotion and health education counseling

A key component of the AGACNP role is mentoring and counseling the patient in how to successfully manage their own medications, conditions, and courses of treatment. Coaching the patient in how to manage their blood glucose via diet and exercise provides health promotion and health education. Performing a comprehensive history and physical examination involves a physical assessment of the patient. Assessing, educating, and providing referrals may involve referral to a diabetes educator or dietician. Ordering and interpreting diagnostic studies would likely involve assessment of the patient's glycosylated hemoglobin or other necessary laboratory values.

17. The AGACNP uses the technique of therapeutic communication by:

    A. Acknowledging that a quiet patient agrees with the treatment plan
    B. Using direct eye contact with all patients to ensure understanding of information
    C. Practicing assertiveness so the patient perceives confidence in the treatment plan
    D. Determining how the patient prefers to receive information before delivery of test results

18. Which school grade is the recommended reading level for patient educational materials?

    A. Fourth to fifth
    B. Fifth to sixth
    C. Sixth to eighth
    D. Eighth to tenth

19. Who is responsible for the process of credentialing and privileging for the Advanced Practice Registered Nurses (APRN)?

    A. State nurse practice acts
    B. Hospital credentialing committees
    C. Professional nursing organizations
    D. Certifying bodies

(*See answers next page.*)

17. D) Determining how the patient prefers to receive information before delivery of test results

Therapeutic communication involves using different styles of communication to establish rapport and negotiate for the best health outcome possible. Adapting to different communication styles and customs is important to establish a relationship with the patient. Determining how the patient prefers to receive information about results is important to establish because these preferences will differ from patient to patient. Personal and/or cultural preferences for a direct or indirect approach should be established before ordering tests. It should not be assumed that a quiet patient agrees with the treatment plan. Preferences around direct eye contact, touch, and personal space should be assessed for each patient; preferences may vary based on cultural background or for other reasons. Providers need to be sensitive to the preferences of their patients. While confidence in a treatment plan is necessary, being assertive and pushing views or treatment options on a patient can be overwhelming. The AGACNP should avoid passing judgment on patients, be flexible, get a sense for the patient's communication style, and be adaptable to fit best with the patient's preferences.

18. C) Sixth to eighth

Health literacy is an essential predictor of one's health status. Low health literacy is associated with more hospitalizations, greater need for emergent care, and less preventive care. Direct communication with medical professionals is important for healthcare education, but so is understanding of high-quality written educational materials. The American Medical Association and the National Institutes of Health recommend that patient materials be written at the sixth to eighth grade reading level.

19. B) Hospital credentialing committees

Credentialing and privileging involve the process by which an AGACNP is granted permission to practice in a certain institution. Based on the specific requirements of the institution to which the AGACNP requests access, the hospital credentialing committee will review and grant allowance for specific privileges, which must be congruent with the education preparation of the AGACNP and the APRN Consensus model. While state nurse practice acts, professional nursing organizations, and certifying bodies (e.g., American Nurses Credentialing Center, American Association of Critical-Care Nurses) guide the scope of AGACNP practice, they are not responsible for credentialing and privileging.

20. The scope of practice of the AGACNP, including the level of prescriptive authority, is regulated by which of the following?

A. State nurse practice acts
B. Professional nursing organizations
C. Institutional policy
D. Drug Enforcement Agency

21. A patient in the ICU acutely decompensates from sepsis. The patient is hypotensive, and the AGACNP orders the peripheral administration of vasopressors. The nurse continues to titrate up on the dose, surpassing the institutional protocol for the dosage limit of vasopressor administration through a peripheral line. The patient needs a central line, but the AGACNP is new to the facility. While they have submitted the appropriate paperwork, they have not received confirmation of approval for their specific privileges. The best action for the AGACNP is to:

A. Place the central line because the patient is acutely decompensating
B. Defer the central line placement until the next shift arrives
C. Ask the intensive care attending physician to supervise the procedure
D. Ask their manager if they are able to proceed given the emergent situation

22. A patient in the ICU acutely decompensates from sepsis. The patient is hypotensive and requires a central line to be inserted for the administration of vasopressors. After informed consent is obtained, a family member asks, "Are you qualified to insert a central line?" Which of the following is the best way for the AGACNP to respond?

A. "Of course, I am able to perform this procedure because of my APRN license."
B. "I can explain my licensure to you afterward, but right now I need to place this line."
C. "I am approved by the hospital's credentialing committee to perform this procedure."
D. "Would you like me to get my attending physician to talk to you?"

(*See answers next page.*)

20. A) State nurse practice acts

While the scope and standards are set by professional nursing organizations, AGACNP practice is externally regulated by the legal allowances in each state, according to and delineated by individual state nurse practice acts. These guidelines for nursing practice vary from state to state (e.g., some states allow full practice while others reduce and restrict practice). The Drug Enforcement Agency allows nurses in advanced practice to obtain registration numbers, but state practice acts dictate the level of prescriptive authority allowed. AGACNPs have a responsibility to understand their state's nurse practice act and be aware of their practice abilities. Institutional policies define practice within institutions.

21. C) Ask the intensive care attending physician to supervise the procedure

Institutional policies, procedures, and medical staff bylaws define practice within institutions. Starting at a new facility requires the AGACNP to obtain credentialing privileges for hospital practice. This grants the AGACNP permission to practice in a certain institution. Based on the specific requirements of the institution to which the AGACNP requests access, the hospital credentialing committee will review and grant allowance for specific privileges. Credentialing demonstrates that the AGACNP has the required education, licensure, and certification to practice. Privileging is the process by which a practitioner who is licensed for independent practice is permitted by law and the facility to practice independently and to provide specific medical and other patient care services within the scope of the individual's license. Because the AGACNP has not received approval yet, they cannot perform the procedure independently. They require supervision for central line placement until the proper credentialing process is completed. Even though the patient is becoming acutely hypotensive, the AGACNP should not place the line without appropriate supervision. The line should not be deferred until the next shift because the patient is already receiving above the maximum dose for peripheral administration based on the institutional protocol. The hospital credentialing committee, not the AGACNP manager, is responsible for granting privileges.

22. C) "I am approved by the hospital's credentialing committee to perform this procedure."

It is the responsibility of the hospital's credentialing committee to grant privileges and approve specific procedures that can be performed by the AGACNP. Having an advanced practice nursing license is not equivalent to automatic approval for invasive procedures. The APRN license validates meeting minimum education requirements, but credentialing may vary based on specific services at each institution. Putting off and ignoring the family member's question is not effective communication and does not invoke a therapeutic relationship. It is the duty of the AGACNP to engage as a communicator, facilitator, and collaborator to promote optimal patient care.

23. Which of the following grants authority for an AGACNP to practice in the advanced role?

A. Licensure
B. Postgraduate education
C. Institutional policies
D. Certification

24. AGACNP certification is obtained by which of the following processes?

A. Graduating with a Master of Science in Nursing degree
B. Receiving full privileges to practice at an institution by the hospital credentialing committee
C. Obtaining nursing licensure by the state board of nursing
D. Passing a national certification examination consistent with the role

25. A patient presents with a painless chancre, fever, sore throat, and fatigue. The patient reports a history of sexual activity without the use of protection. A sexually transmitted infection panel is significant for a positive treponemal immunoassay. Should the AGACNP report this disease to the health department?

A. Yes, chlamydia is a reportable disease.
B. No, herpes is not a reportable disease.
C. Yes, syphilis is a reportable disease.
D. No, most sexually transmitted infections do not have to be reported.

26. Certain infectious diseases require mandatory reporting by the AGACNP. Which of the following sexually transmitted infections is considered a reportable disease in every state?

A. Genital herpes
B. Gonorrhea
C. Bacterial vaginosis
D. Human papillomavirus

(*See answers next page.*)

23. A) Licensure

Licensure grants authority for an AGACNP to practice in the advanced role in the population for which they are educated and certified. While education and certification are necessary for practice, licensure establishes that a person is qualified to perform in a particular professional role and is defined by rules and regulations set forth by a governmental regulatory body (i.e., state board of nursing) to ensure public safety. Institutional policies define practice within specific institutions. While credentialing and privileging within the facility must be congruent with the educational preparation of the AGACNP, licensure grants authority for practice.

24. D) Passing a national certification examination consistent with the role

Certification establishes that a person has met certain standards in a particular profession that signify mastery of specialized knowledge and skills. After graduating from a masters, post-masters, or doctoral preparation in nursing, graduates must apply and sit for a national certification examination. Credentialing and privileging involve the process by which an AGACNP is granted permission to practice in a certain setting by a hospital credentialing committee. Obtaining nursing licensure from the state board of nursing is essential for practice, but certification is granted by nongovernmental agencies (e.g., American Nurses Credentialing Center, American Association of Critical-Care Nurses).

25. C) Yes, syphilis is a reportable disease.

This patient is presenting with signs and symptoms consistent with syphilis, which is confirmed by the serologic test (e.g., positive treponemal immunoassay). Syphilis is a reportable disease, and this case should be communicated to the health department. The requirements vary by state, but reportable diseases in every state include syphilis, gonorrhea, chlamydia, chancroid, and HIV.

26. B) Gonorrhea

In accordance with state and local statutory requirements, sexually transmitted infections should be reported. Reportable diseases in every state include syphilis, gonorrhea, chlamydia, chancroid, and HIV. Because the requirements for reporting other sexually transmitted infections vary by state, the AGACNP should be familiar with their specific reporting requirements.

27. The AGACNP patient practice population is based on which of the following?

A. Institution the AGACNP is working for

B. Specific practice environment

C. State regulations

D. Educational preparation of the AGACNP

28. A patient presents after being involved in a motor vehicle crash. The patient does not speak English but is accompanied by a family member who does. The AGACNP does not speak the patient's language. The patient appears nervous, appears to be in pain, and splints their chest. Which of the following is indicated for this patient?

A. Asking the patient's family member to translate

B. Allowing a nurse who speaks the patient's language to assist with translation

C. Arranging for a certified medical interpreter to be present or available by phone

D. Referring the patient to another provider who speaks the patient's language

29. An AGACNP who has completed an accredited, graduate-level AGACNP educational program with supervised clinical practice has the independent ability in all states to:

A. Pronounce and sign death certificates

B. Order and interpret diagnostic tests and procedures

C. Prescribe schedule II medications

D. Insert a central venous catheter in a patient in the ICU

30. An AGACNP graduate with an educational focus on the adult-gerontology acute care population is applying for jobs in the local area. Which of the following practice environments would be appropriate for this AGACNP?

A. An adult ICU that cares for patients with acute and/or complex chronic illnesses

B. A pediatric ICU that cares for children and adolescents with acute and/or complex illnesses

C. Any adult inpatient clinical setting, but the AGACNP cannot provide care in a telehealth setting

D. Any adult inpatient and outpatient setting, except for palliative care and/or hospice care

(*See answers next page.*)

27. D) Educational preparation of the AGACNP

The population served is determined by the education preparation of the AGACNP in a population focus (pediatric, late adolescent, or adult-gerontology). The practice population is not determined by the institution, the clinical practice setting, or the state. The institution and hospital credentialing committee will review and grant specific privileges and allow specific procedures in the clinical setting but will not determine the practice population. While AGACNP practice is regulated by the legal allowances in each state, the practice population is based on the educational preparation of the AGACNP.

28. C) Arranging for a certified medical interpreter to be present or available by phone

A medical interpreter should be available at all clinical institutions in the United States. It is the responsibility of the APRN to ensure that the medical interpreter and the patient understand what is being communicated during the conversation. The use of a certified medical interpreter ensures complete and accurate information and provides patients with the ability to fully participate in their healthcare. The use of bilingual staff or family members is strongly discouraged unless there is an imminent threat to the patient's life.

29. B) Order and interpret diagnostic tests and procedures

In all states, the formal educational preparation of the AGACNP allows them to independently perform comprehensive health assessments, order and interpret the full range of diagnostic tests and procedures, formulate a differential diagnosis to reach a diagnosis, plan and direct care, and order, provide, and evaluate the outcomes of interventions. The scope of practice of the AGACNP is governed by the laws in each state; it is vital to understand the scope of practice in the state in which the AGACNP is practicing. Regulations regarding pronouncing and signing death certificates and prescribing schedule II medications differ for each state. Inserting a central venous catheter in a patient in the ICU can be performed only once the AGACNP has gained credentialing and privileging at a certain facility.

30. A) An adult ICU that cares for patients with acute and/or complex chronic illnesses

The educational preparation of the AGACNP determines the patient practice population. In this case, the AGACNP has education in the adult-gerontology acute care population; therefore, the AGACNP can practice in any environment in which adult (not pediatric) patients have acute, chronic, and/or complex chronic illnesses or injuries. Examples include acute and critical care, emergency care for trauma stabilization, and procedural and interventional settings. Settings for acute care services include home care, ambulatory care, urgent care, long-term acute care, rehabilitative care, palliative care and/or hospice care, mobile environments, and virtual locations, such as tele-ICUs and areas using telehealth.

31. A patient with multiple comorbidities presents with elevated blood glucose and hypertension. The AGACNP reviews the patient's medication list and queries the patient about medication compliance. The patient admits that they have not been able to afford their medication with their current insurance. The AGACNP knows that the type of Medicare that may cover certain drugs is Part:

A. A
B. B
C. C
D. D

32. A patient with terminal lung cancer is concerned about medical costs. The patient is considering hospice but is worried about what Medicare insurance will cover. The AGACNP advises the patient that while there are many options, Medicare Part A does not cover:

A. Inpatient care in a hospital
B. Home healthcare
C. Durable medical equipment
D. Hospice care

33. In order to qualify to be a Medicare provider, an AGACNP must:

A. Hold a state license as an registered nurse
B. Be certified as an AGACNP by a recognized national certifying body
C. Possess a Doctor of Nursing practice degree
D. Be credentialed with hospital privileges

34. A patient who is hard of hearing is preparing for discharge after a same-level mechanical fall at home. Physical therapy recommends the use of a walker at home. The patient also has a history of diabetes mellitus and obstructive sleep apnea, for which the patient uses a continuous positive airway pressure (CPAP) device. Which of the following items of durable medical equipment is not covered by Medicare Part B?

A. Hearing aids
B. Crutches
C. Blood glucose test strips
D. CPAP device

(*See answers next page.*)

31. D) D

Medicare Part D helps pay for prescription drugs; it is optional and offered to everyone with Medicare, but a monthly premium is required. Medicare Part A covers inpatient care in a hospital, skilled nursing facility care, nursing home care (inpatient care in a skilled nursing facility that is not custodial or long-term care), hospice care, and home healthcare. Medicare Part B covers medically necessary services and preventive services. This includes clinical research, ambulance services, durable medical equipment, mental health (inpatient, outpatient, partial hospitalization), and limited outpatient prescription drugs. Medicare Advantage Plan (Part C) is available to patients enrolled in Medicare Parts A and B and provides the patient with the ability to receive all of their healthcare services through a provider organization under Part C.

32. C) Durable medical equipment

Medicare Part A covers inpatient care in a hospital, skilled nursing facility care, nursing home care (inpatient care in a skilled nursing facility that is not custodial or long-term care), hospice care, and home healthcare. Medicare Part B covers medically necessary services and preventive services. This includes clinical research, ambulance services, durable medical equipment, mental health (inpatient, outpatient, partial hospitalization), and limited outpatient prescription drugs. Medicare Parts A and B do not cover long-term care (custodial care), most dental care, eye exams (for prescription glasses), dentures, cosmetic surgery, massage therapy, routine physical exams, hearing aids and exams for fitting them, concierge care (e.g., boutique medicine), and covered items or services obtained from an opt-out physician or other provider.

33. B) Be certified as an AGACNP by a recognized national certifying body

AGACNPs applying for a Medicare billing number for the first time must meet the following requirements: be a registered professional AGACNP who is authorized by the state in which the services are furnished to practice as an AGACNP in accordance with state law; be certified as an AGACNP by a recognized national certifying body; and possess a master's degree in nursing or a Doctor of Nursing practice degree. Receiving credentialing and privileging at a hospital is not a requirement when applying for a Medicare billing number.

34. A) Hearing aids

Durable medical equipment is long-lasting and is used for a medical reason at home. Medicare covers blood glucose meters and test strips, canes, commode chairs, continuous passive motion devices, CPAP devices, crutches, hospital beds, home infusion services, infusion pumps and supplies, lancet devices, nebulizers, oxygen equipment, patient lifts, pressure-reducing support surfaces, suction pumps, traction equipment, walkers, wheelchairs, and scooters.

35. A patient in the ICU has developed hyperactive delirium and is attempting to pull at invasive lines and dressings. The nurse requests an order for restraints to prevent the patient from interfering with medical devices. Upon assessment, the AGACNP attempts verbal de-escalation of the patient's behavior and reorientation, but the patient continues to present as an imminent harm to themself. Which of the following is the next best action?

- **A.** Asking the collaborating physician to order the restraints because the AGACNP is not able to do so
- **B.** Call the patient's family to request permission to use restraints on the patient
- **C.** Continue to use verbal techniques because physical restraints should be avoided
- **D.** Order the restraints and safety checks, documenting the exact reason and rationale for their use

36. A patient reports with generalized bruising and a swollen eyelid. During the assessment, the patient remains quiet, jumpy, and nervous. After appropriate treatment, the patient requests to be discharged. The patient says, "I'm going to take him out tonight before he goes after my mom." The AGACNP sees a gun in the patient's bag. The next best action of the AGACNP is to:

- **A.** Call hospital security to confiscate the gun
- **B.** Call the local police department
- **C.** Warn the patient's potential victim
- **D.** Call the patient's mother

37. Which of the following is true regarding credentialing and privileging?

- **A.** Privileges are granted in full by a hospital credentialing committee.
- **B.** Credentialing comprises required education, licensure, and certification to practice as an AGACNP.
- **C.** Clinical privileges are specific to the provider but are the same at each facility.
- **D.** Only credentialing involves screening and evaluating of qualifications.

(See answers next page.)

35. D) Order the restraints and safety checks, documenting the exact reason and rationale for their use

Ordering and managing physical restraints is within the scope and practice of the AGACNP; a physician is not required to order restraints. Keeping family updated is important, but permission from the family is not required for use of restraints because the patient presents imminent harm to themself and would significantly disrupt important treatment or damage the environment without them. Verbal techniques should be attempted first because nearly all patients who present with agitation or violent behavior deserve the chance to calm down with soothing communication and approach. However, if the patient continues to present an imminent threat of harm to themself or others, physical restraints or chemical sedation may be necessary with the appropriate frequent checks and assessments.

36. C) Warn the patient's potential victim

The patient has shown intention to take the life of another. The AGACNP must uphold patient confidentiality but also has a duty to warn, which requires the AGACNP to warn any person whose life may be in danger from a patient. Failure to warn may make the AGACNP liable for injury to the third party. The duty to protect a patient from self-harm and harm to others supersedes the right to confidentiality. While a call to the police department may be necessary, the AGACNP first has a duty to warn the patient's potential victim. A call to hospital security may set the patient more on edge and lead to a dangerous situation. Calling the patient's family may help but is not the priority at this time.

37. B) Credentialing comprises required education, licensure, and certification to practice as an AGACNP.

Credentialing involves the process of screening and evaluating qualifications and other credentials, including licensure, required education, certification, relevant training and experience, and current competence and health status. Privileging involves a practitioner, licensed for independent practice, who is permitted by law and the facility to practice independently and to provide specific medical and patient services within the scope of the practitioner's license. The decision is based on screening from peer references, professional experience, health status, education, training, and licensure. Clinical privileges are specific to both the facility and the provider. Privileges may be granted in part or in full by the credentialing committee.

38. The AGACNP works in an ICU and participates in multidisciplinary rounds every morning, reviewing patient data and discussing patient treatment plans with the intensive care attending physician, pharmacist, registered dietician, respiratory therapist, and physical therapist. This provides an example of which standard of AGACNP professional performance?

A. Collaboration

B. Patient advocacy

C. Diversity

D. Reflective learning

39. Which of the following enforces the Health Insurance Portability and Accountability Act (HIPAA)?

A. Office of the Surgeon General

B. Practice protocols of the institution

C. Office for Civil Rights

D. Occupational Safety and Health Administration (OSHA)

40. A patient with a past medical history of anxiety presents to the emergency department with chest pain. The EKG is significant for ST segment elevation in two contiguous leads. The patient reports recently losing their job, and they are worried about how they will pay for medical costs. The patient has two children, who are 10 and 12 years old. The AGACNP reassures the patient and recommends which of the following health benefits?

A. Employee Retirement Income Security Act (ERISA)

B. Mental Health Parity and Addiction Equity Act (MHPAEA)

C. Newborns' and Mothers' Health Protection Act (Newborns' Act)

D. Consolidated Omnibus Budget Reconciliation Act (COBRA)

(*See answers next page.*)

38. A) Collaboration

This is an example of collaboration: working with individuals of other professions to maintain a climate of mutual respect and shared values to improve quality and safety of patient care. The term *advocacy* refers to the process of supporting a cause or proposal. The term *diversity* refers to factors that vary, such as race, culture, spirituality, ethnicity, socioeconomic status, age, lifestyle, and values. Reflective learning involves recurrent, thoughtful, personal self-assessment and analysis of strengths and weaknesses for improvement.

39. C) Office for Civil Rights

Within the U.S. Department of Health and Human Services, the Office for Civil Rights enforces HIPAA. The Office of the Surgeon General oversees the U.S. Public Health Service Commissioned Corps but does not enforce HIPAA. The practice protocols of each institution should be similar in regard to protecting patient health information as set forth by the Office for Civil Rights. OSHA is within the Department of Labor and works to ensure safe and healthy working conditions.

40. D) Consolidated Omnibus Budget Reconciliation Act (COBRA)

COBRA gives patients and their families who lose their health benefits the right to continue group health benefits provided by their group health plan for limited periods of time under certain circumstances, such as voluntary or involuntary job loss, reduction in hours worked, transition between jobs, death, divorce, and other life events. ERISA sets minimum standards for most voluntarily established retirement and health plans to provide protection for these individuals. This patient has not voluntarily retired, so ERISA would not be applicable. MHPAEA requires that health plans ensure that financial requirements applicable to mental health or substance use disorder are no more restrictive than those applied to other medical-surgical benefits. Although this patient has a history of anxiety, the patient is presenting with chest pain concerning for ST-elevation myocardial infarction. Because this patient is not presenting with a mental health concern, MHPAEA would not be applicable. The Newborns' Act protects postpartum patients and their newborns with regard to length of the hospital stay after childbirth. Because this patient does not have newborn children, it would not be applicable.

41. An AGACNP is approached by a patient visitor in the cafeteria. The visitor reports that they are the neighbor of a patient the AGACNP is caring for. The visitor asks how the patient is doing and poses specific questions regarding their laboratory and diagnostic test results. The patient is alert and oriented and has not consented to release information to this person. How should the AGACNP respond?

A. "The patient is doing much better; their laboratory results are much improved as of this morning."
B. "I appreciate your concern, but I am unable to disclose this information without the patient's consent."
C. "I'm sorry, but I need to get back to work now."
D. "Why don't you give the patient's mother a call? She's up to date on all the patient's information."

42. Which of the following is true regarding the benefits of the Consolidated Omnibus Budget Reconciliation Act (COBRA)?

A. Coverage under COBRA is the same as the individual had as an employee.
B. An individual must enroll within 30 days once employer-sponsored benefits end.
C. Dependents are not eligible for COBRA coverage.
D. COBRA is temporary and individuals can stay on it for up to 1 year.

43. A patient's protected health information was involved in a healthcare data breach. The Health Insurance Portability and Accountability Act (HIPAA) requires that the patient be informed based on the rule called:

A. Breach Notification
B. Privacy
C. Security
D. Enforcement

(*See answers next page.*)

41. B) "I appreciate your concern, but I am unable to disclose this information without the patient's consent."

The Health Insurance Portability and Accountability Act (HIPAA) Privacy Rule has been established to protect patient medical records and other identifiable health information. Validating the visitor's concern and acknowledging that the AGACNP needs to check with the patient prior to releasing information protects the patient and follows the guidelines of HIPAA. Disclosing patient information without discussing with the patient first releases protected health information. Additionally, telling the visitor to get information from the patient's family member without consulting the patient first compromises protected health information. Ignoring the visitor and putting them off is not appropriate; many people may not be aware of what constitutes protected health information, so education is important.

42. A) Coverage under COBRA is the same as the individual had as an employee.

COBRA gives patients who lose their health benefits, and their families, the right to continue group health benefits provided by their group health plan for limited periods of time under certain circumstances, such as voluntary or involuntary job loss, reduction in hours worked, transition between jobs, death, divorce, and other life events. COBRA coverage is the same as employee-sponsored benefits so the individual can see the same providers and receive the same benefits. COBRA includes coverage for dependents (i.e., spouse, children) even if the dependent does not sign up for COBRA coverage. COBRA allows individuals to avoid a lapse in coverage; they have up to 60 days to enroll once employer-sponsored benefits end. COBRA is temporary, but individuals can stay on for 18 to 36 months.

43. A) Breach Notification

The Breach Notification Rule requires HIPAA-covered entities to provide notification following a data breach of unsecured, protected health information. The Privacy Rule defines and limits the circumstances in which an individual's protected health information may be used or disclosed by HIPAA-covered entities. The Security Rule protects individuals' electronic personal health information that is created, received, used, or maintained by a covered entity. The Enforcement Rule provides standards for compliance, as well as investigations and penalties for violations.

44. Which of the following is not considered a covered entity under the Health Insurance Portability and Accountability Act (HIPAA)?

A. Written information by the physician in the medical record
B. Patient billing information stored in a dentist's office
C. Patient information stored in a health insurance company computer system
D. Life insurance company requests for patient medical records

45. While managing the care of a patient recently diagnosed with pancreatic cancer, the AGACNP works with the patient and their family to coordinate care with hospice care and home health nursing. This standard of care ensures the patient is comfortable and all needs are met by demonstrating:

A. Systems thinking
B. Ethics
C. Collaboration
D. Leadership

46. The holistic practice of participating in and improving organizational structures and processes to ensure optimal outcomes is known as:

A. Systems thinking
B. Ethics
C. Collaboration
D. Leadership

47. The practice of considering cost-effectiveness as it relates to treatment choices is an example of which AGACNP standard of professional performance?

A. Professional practice
B. Education
C. Resource utilization
D. Clinical inquiry

(*See answers next page.*)

44. D) Life insurance company requests for patient medical records

HIPAA rules apply to covered entities and business associates. Covered entities include healthcare providers (e.g., doctors, clinics, psychologists, dentists, chiropractors, nursing homes, pharmacies), health plans (e.g., company health insurance, government programs such as Medicare and Medicaid, military and veterans' healthcare programs), and healthcare clearinghouses (entities that process nonstandard health information they receive from another entity into a standard, which includes standard electronic format or data content). A life insurance company calling to request patient medical records would need consent from the patient prior to the release of information.

45. C) Collaboration

Collaboration centers on interaction and communication with the patient, family, and other members of the care team. Systems thinking is an AGACNP standard that focuses on engaging within organizational structures and systems to improve outcomes. Ethics is focused on applying moral principles toward patient care. Leadership focuses on the AGACNP's ability to guide and influence the care practice setting.

46. A) Systems thinking

Systems thinking is an AGACNP standard that focuses on engaging within organizational structures and systems to improve outcomes. Ethics is focused on applying moral principles toward patient care. Collaboration centers on interaction and communication with the patient, family, and other members of the care team. Leadership focuses on the AGACNP's ability to guide and influence the care practice setting.

47. C) Resource utilization

Resource utilization relates to implementing strategies to use resources efficiently in order to deliver optimal care. The professional practice competency involves an AGACNP's evaluation of their own practice as it relates to institutional and professional standards and regulations. Education relates to ongoing learning to maintain an understanding of current practices and guidelines. Clinical inquiry centers around participation in research and the advancement of evidence-based practice.

48. Which example best exemplifies ethical consideration when working with a patient in early stages of dementia?

A. Collaborating with family members to ensure that decisions regarding care are being made in the best interests of the patient

B. Maintaining respect for the patient's autonomy by including them in all decisions regarding care now and for the future

C. Including the social worker in conversations around choosing a medical proxy and durable power of attorney

D. Obtaining documentation from the patient that transfers decision-making to a caregiver or family member

49. The AGACNP examines an older adult patient and notes rhonchi in the right upper lobe of the lung as well as increased respiratory rate. Which standard of clinical practice does this address?

A. Advanced assessment

B. Differential diagnosis

C. Outcomes identification

D. Care planning and management

50. An AGACNP routinely assesses their own performance against accepted standards. With which standard of practice is this aligned?

A. Professional practice

B. Quality of practice

C. Resource utilization

D. Clinical inquiry

51. The AGACNP is planning to present a community educational offering to residents at an assisted living facility on the topic of nutrition in older adults. What type of learning style strategy will the AGACNP emphasize with this patient population?

A. Video

B. Self-study

C. Group activity

D. Lecture

(*See answers next page.*)

48. B) Maintaining respect for the patient's autonomy by including them in all decisions regarding care now and for the future

Ethics is focused on applying moral principles toward patient care, which includes respecting and promoting a patient's autonomy with regard to care decisions. While collaborating with the family and other members of the care team is appropriate, leaving the patient out of conversations regarding care is not the most ethical practice. Similarly, while it is appropriate to begin efforts to identify an individual who can make care decisions when the patient is no longer capable, that process should not exclude the patient from participating actively at this early stage.

49. A) Advanced assessment

The examination of the patient and the identification of normal versus abnormal findings is part of an advanced assessment. Differential diagnosis involves analysis of the gathered information to identify potential diagnoses. Outcomes identification focuses on establishing goals of care. Care planning and management center on interventions and collaboration that are necessary to achieve goals and optimal care.

50. A) Professional practice

The professional practice standard includes an AGACNP's evaluation of their own practice as it relates to institutional and professional standards and regulations. Quality of practice dictates that the AGACNP contribute to quality of care, but it does not involve self-assessment. Resource utilization relates to implementing strategies to use resources efficiently to deliver optimal care. Clinical inquiry centers around participation in research and advancement of evidence-based practice.

51. C) Group activity

Social learning by using group activities or games can help facilitate an older adult's reception to new learning by taking advantage of a collective group's convergence of past experiences and individualized strengths. Older adults may be impacted by visual or auditory deficits that may not be conducive to learning by formal lecture or use of visual aids. Older adults living in a community setting may not be receptive to learning alone or isolated with self-study.

52. The AGACNP evaluates an older adult patient and, based on symptoms and examination, documents that the patient has pneumonia versus exacerbation of chronic obstructive pulmonary disease. This documentation is an example of which standard of clinical practice?

A. Advanced assessment
B. Differential diagnosis
C. Outcomes identification
D. Care planning and management

53. The AGACNP is rounding on an older adult patient who just underwent emergency abdominal surgery for ruptured diverticulitis and has a new colostomy. The patient currently lives alone and has comorbidities of rheumatoid arthritis and glaucoma. Who will the AGACNP consult *first* in order to plan for the patient's discharge?

A. Occupational therapist
B. Wound, ostomy, and continence nurse
C. Rheumatologist
D. Physical therapist

54. An advanced practice registered nurse is asked by their manager to be a preceptor for a new AGACNP team member at a large extended care corporation. What about the new AGACNP will be *most* important for the preceptor to assess during the first few days of orientation?

A. Past work experience
B. Past educational training
C. Learning style preference
D. Patient assignments

55. The AGACNP is examining an older adult patient admitted from a nursing home to the emergency department with reports of acute pain in the left hip after a fall. The patient, who came by ambulance and is alone, is confused and disoriented but stable. An x-ray reveals a fractured left hip, and the AGACNP needs to admit the patient for surgery. Because there is no immediate family or other contact information available, what will the AGACNP do next?

A. Contact the nursing home to obtain assistance in locating next of kin or a person with durable power of attorney
B. Contact the on-call orthopedic surgeon about the patient and inform them of the need to locate a family member or durable power of attorney
C. Contact an on-duty colleague to witness the patient's signature in the room while the patient signs the consent form
D. Call the dispatcher of the transporting ambulance company to determine if they have any contact information available

(*See answers next page.*)

52. B) Differential diagnosis

This documentation is an example of differential diagnosis, in which analysis of the gathered information is used to identify potential diagnoses. Advanced assessment centers on the examination of the patient and the identification of normal versus abnormal findings. Outcomes identification focuses on establishing goals of care. Care planning and management center on interventions and collaboration that are necessary to achieve goals and optimal care.

53. B) Wound, ostomy, and continence nurse

The first consultation would be placed with the wound, ostomy, and continence nurse (WOCN) to ensure that this specialist evaluates the patient's needs and begins planning for their learning and discharge management plan with the new stoma. This interdisciplinary team member will be the most important professional to guide the AGACNP (and likely the social worker) in planning further discharge needs. Consultation with the occupational therapist and physical therapist may be more effective after the WOCN initially assesses and determines the patient's dexterity and potential mobility deficits pertaining to future, independent colostomy care. A rheumatologist would be consulted only for medical guidance and support for the patient's rheumatoid arthritis needs that present while hospitalized.

54. C) Learning style preference

The preceptor will evaluate the new AGACNP's individual learning style preferences in order to enhance the educational experience. By doing so, the preceptor can develop effective teaching strategies to strengthen the orientee's educational experience and ensure that the teaching approach is meaningful and receptive to the learner. Information regarding the AGACNP's work experience, educational training, and patient assignments is useful but not the priority for the preceptor when first developing an effective teaching plan.

55. A) Contact the nursing home to obtain assistance in locating next of kin or a person with durable power of attorney

The AGACNP's most accurate and immediate source of contact information will be the patient's nursing home staff since the patient is currently living there. Notifying the on-call orthopedic surgeon and not preparing the patient ahead of time with this information is not conducive to the patient's smooth hand-off between departments and will only cause delays. The patient is confused and cannot give reliable and informed consent; having another healthcare professional witness their signature will not solve the problem. The ambulance dispatcher is less likely than the nursing home to have contact information.

56. During an exceptionally busy and stressful time, the AGACNP allowed their advanced practice registered nurse license to lapse and become 5 days overdue. The AGACNP worked 2 of those 5 days, picking up on-call provider coverage as a per diem at a local long-term care acute care hospital (LTACH), without any adverse or eventful situations in patient care on those days. The AGACNP did not work at their full-time employer during that time. What next step will the AGACNP take?

A. Proceeding with renewing their license as quickly as possible
B. Notifying the LTACH director of nursing and state board of nursing to determine their policies
C. Resigning from the per diem LTACH AGACNP position
D. Notifying the full-time employer about seeing patients at the LTACH with an expired license

57. A patient with end-stage renal disease elects to discontinue dialysis. Four days later, the patient stops responding to outside stimuli and has a blood pressure of 66/32 mmHg, a pulse of 36 bpm, and a respiratory rate of 4 breaths/min. As-needed medications ordered include alprazolam (Xanax), 1 mg intravenously (IV) every 4 hours for agitation, and morphine sulfate, 2 mg IV every 2 hours for pain. Which scenario best demonstrates a double effect encounter?

A. The patient begins pulling at the IV tubing. Agitation continues 30 minutes after alprazolam (Xanax), 1 mg IV, is given, so the nurse contacts the ordering provider for additional options.
B. The nurse knows the patient must feel terrible and administers 2 mg morphine sulfate IV every 1 hour to ease the transition.
C. The patient becomes combative. The nurse administers lorazepam (Ativan), 2 mg IV, because the patient has not yet required a dose today.
D. The patient transitions into active dying and begins gasping respirations. This activity interferes with the roommate's sleep, so the nurse administers a dose of morphine sulfate.

(See answers next page.)

56. B) Notifying the LTACH director of nursing and state board of nursing to determine their policies

The AGACNP should be professionally transparent and notify the LTACH nursing administrator to determine what their policy and procedures are for this type of incident, as well as their state board of nursing representative. The AGACNP will then renew their license before returning to any patient care at either work location. Resigning or informing the full-time employer does not address the status of the license, which is the priority.

57. A) The patient begins pulling at the IV tubing. Agitation continues 30 minutes after alprazolam (Xanax), 1 mg IV, is given, so the nurse contacts the ordering provider for additional options.

The principle of double effect holds that a provider's actions are justified, even if an adverse outcome is possible, so long as the intent is for a good outcome and no other option is available with a lesser risk of a bad outcome. Administering IV alprazolam (Xanax) as ordered to an agitated patient could cause central nervous system depression; however, the intent implied is the alleviation of agitation and reduced risk of harm to self. If a patient cannot verbally communicate troubling symptoms, the nurse must assess nonverbal cues. It is inappropriate for the nurse to treat a patient's condition based on personal convictions. Nursing judgment is not a substitution for an order. While gasping respirations may indicate an air-hungry patient, the implied intent of morphine administration is to reduce the nuisance to the patient's roommate.

58. A patient hospitalized for failure to thrive has a body mass index of 15.5 on admission. The patient has oropharyngeal dysphagia related to advanced esophageal carcinoma and fails a swallow study. Advanced directives state no artificial nutrition and name the patient's spouse as a healthcare proxy. The AGACNP reviews options for artificial nutrition versus palliative care with the patient and their spouse. The patient, who is alert, oriented, and appropriate throughout the hospital stay, maintains declination of artificial nutrition. The following day, the patient's spouse pleads for a feeding tube. The AGACNP explains:

A. "I will request ethics and psychology consults to evaluate the patient's competency."

B. "As the healthcare proxy you have the final say. Can you sign the consent this afternoon?"

C. "When your spouse loses capacity, we will meet again and complete the consent at that time."

D. "Your spouse retains decision-making capacity. It is unethical to ignore treatment directives."

59. The AGACNP is getting ready to see a new patient in the urgent care clinic. The patient only speaks Croatian and is accompanied by a neighbor who is fluent in this same language. The AGACNP does not speak Croatian. What *next* step will the AGACNP take in this situation?

A. The AGACNP can ask the patient's neighbor if they speak English so that they can be an interpreter.

B. The AGACNP can notify their organization's language hotline for a medical interpreter.

C. The AGACNP can use an app as a language interpreter on their own smartphone as a translator.

D. The AGACNP can call the patient's family member and ask if they can interpret over the phone.

60. The AGACNP is presenting a poster at a national gerontology nursing conference. Which standard of professional performance does this exemplify?

A. Leadership

B. Resource utilization

C. Systems thinking

D. Beneficence

(*See answers next page.*)

58. D) "Your spouse retains decision-making capacity. It is unethical to ignore treatment directives."

The patient demonstrates competency to make decisions and is alert, oriented, and involved in daily activities. Additionally, the patient's declination of artificial feeding aligns with the advanced directives. While an interdisciplinary approach, in which the AGACNP consults with ethics and psychology, can be valuable in such situations, it does not devalue a competent patient's decision. A healthcare proxy may not overrule a competent patient's treatment directives. The healthcare proxy may not make treatment decisions unless the patient lacks decision-making capacity. Further, it is unethical for an AGACNP to make plans to diverge from a patient's treatment directives once that patient no longer has decision-making capacity.

59. B) The AGACNP can notify their organization's language hotline for a medical interpreter.

It is best practice to use trained, certified, medical translation services for interpreter assistance in healthcare. The majority of healthcare organizations have contracts with medical translation service vendors/companies. A neighbor, friend, or family member should not be utilized as it may violate confidentiality and/or the information may not be relayed in an assured, reliable fashion. The AGACNP should not use their personal phone nor any nonapproved translation app to substitute for professional medical translation as this could violate confidentiality and Health Insurance Portability and Accountability Act (HIPAA) regulations since these devices are not encrypted by the hospital's own malware protection and licensing technological authorizations.

60. A) Leadership

Speaking at a nursing conference exemplifies leadership, which focuses on the AGACNP's ability to guide and influence the care and practice setting. Resource utilization relates to implementing strategies to use resources efficiently to deliver optimal care. Systems thinking is an AGACNP competency that focuses on engaging within organizational structures and systems to improve outcomes. Beneficence is one's obligation to act in the best interest of the patient.

61. The AGACNP is evaluating a new patient with type 2 diabetes and a non-healing left foot ulcer. The patient is transferring from another provider, and past medical records indicate that the patient's most recent arterial doppler demonstrated partial occlusion of the left femoral artery. When developing a treatment plan for the patient, what specialist will the AGACNP consult *first*?

A. Vascular specialist
B. Endocrinologist
C. Dietitian
D. Orthotist

62. A 70-year-old female patient arrives at urgent care for complaints of lower abdominal pain with new-onset vaginal bleeding. An accompanying visitor is introduced by the patient as her partner, and they join her in the exam room. The AGACNP initially greets the patient and partner and states that the plan is to perform a pelvic exam. Before proceeding further, what question is essential for the AGACNP to ask the patient?

A. "Are you currently sexually active?"
B. "When was your last pelvic exam/Pap smear?"
C. "Do you want your partner present during the exam?"
D. "At what age did you stop having your menstrual cycle?"

63. The AGACNP has been asked to lead a unit-wide committee to develop an evidence-based initiative to decrease hospital-acquired pressure injuries. Members of the team have been assigned and include multi-disciplinary healthcare professionals. To prepare for the "kick-off" and initial team meeting, what will the AGACNP plan to do *first*?

A. Collect data regarding the unit's trends in pressure injury occurrences
B. Notify the hospital institutional review board (IRB) of an impending study
C. Order brochures on pressure injury prevention from the National Pressure Injury Advisory Panel
D. Arrange a meeting during the week of the quarterly pressure injury incidence/prevalence audit

(*See answers next page.*)

61. A) Vascular specialist

Perfusion concerns demonstrated on the arterial doppler report of the patient's left femoral artery along with a nonhealing wound requires further evaluation by a vascular specialist. The vascular specialist is key to this patient's care in determining the need to revascularize the extremity in hopes of healing the foot wound. Since there is evidence of arterial occlusion, the endocrinologist, dietitian, and orthotist can be consulted *after* the vascular specialist.

62. C) "Do you want your partner present during the exam?"

It is important to ensure that the patient's privacy and comfort are addressed prior to the physical exam. Since this exam involves a sensitive anatomical location, it is even more vital to make certain that the patient's modesty is respected. To obtain the patient's medical history, it is necessary to ask the patient about their sexual activity, their last pelvic exam/Pap smear, and when their menstrual cycle stopped, but these questions should not be asked until the patient gives permission for others to be present during the interview.

63. A) Collect data regarding the unit's trends in pressure injury occurrences

Collecting objective data and preparing to share and evaluate this information with the team should be an initial plan for this committee leader. This will assist with developing a strategy and goals as it will stimulate clinical inquiry in order to provide informed decision-making and practice. At this early phase of planning, it is not yet necessary to notify the institutional review board (IRB) of the impending study, order brochures on pressure injury prevention, or arrange the meeting date.

64. The AGACNP is rounding on a patient who is on hospice care with a diagnosis of end-stage Alzheimer disease. The patient's adult daughter is present at bedside. This is the AGACNP's first encounter with the daughter, and the AGACNP notices she has been crying. Which response is *most* appropriate?

A. Immediately walk toward the daughter and give her a hug
B. Acknowledge the daughter's sadness by saying, "This must be very difficult for you"
C. Quickly excuse oneself and leave the room to provide privacy
D. Stand quietly in the back of the room to avoid disturbing the daughter

65. The AGACNP is leading a team of colleagues for a hospital-wide quality initiative project focusing on reducing catheter associated urinary tract infections. At yesterday's committee meeting, two of the members became argumentative regarding differing opinions on an implementation plan. The conflict subsided, but now the AGACNP would like to follow up with these individuals to facilitate smoother collaboration in the future. What is the *most* appropriate next step for the AGACNP?

A. Arrange a separate, in-person meeting with both members (including the AGACNP serving as the facilitator) to discuss a resolution in an open, but constructive fashion
B. Send an email to both members that includes reminders of the committee charter's stipulations on behavioral expectations
C. Meet with each member, their unit manager, and recommend/delegate disciplinary action to this manager
D. Do not pursue the issue any further to avoid embarrassment or risk of the member quitting the committee

66. The AGACNP is working in the emergency department and would like to develop a method to "check on" the health, well-being, and follow-up status of patients discharged from the hospital 48 to 72 hours prior. Considering the generational characteristics of older patients, what is the *most* important factor the AGACNP will need to consider when developing a format for this communication?

A. Cultural differences
B. Religious beliefs
C. Transportation
D. Sensory deficits

(*See answers next page.*)

64. B) Acknowledge the daughter's sadness by saying, "This must be very difficult for you"

Acknowledging the daughter's sadness by offering empathy is the most appropriate response as it does not minimize her impending loss. Since this is the first time the AGACNP has met the daughter, it would not be professionally appropriate to provide physical contact with a hug, especially without permission. Leaving the daughter immediately after entering the room or standing "out of the way" does not convey emotional support.

65. A) Arrange a separate, in-person meeting with both members (including the AGACNP serving as the facilitator) to discuss a resolution in an open, but constructive fashion

As the leader, the AGACNP should call a separate meeting with the two members and act as a facilitator to oversee a cordial, respectful, and constructive discussion on the situation to resolve differences and come to a professional agreement. Sending an email, meeting with their unit manager to delegate disciplinary action, and avoiding the issue are not effective methods that will improve future communication and collaborative efforts.

66. D) Sensory deficits

When considering potential obstacles to participating in their own care, it is important to be mindful of sensory deficits that can occur in this patient population. Thus, designing tools that may have a larger print or that can be clearly audible are examples of improving communication delivery. Although other factors such as cultural differences, religious beliefs, and transportation are important, the first priority for this particular age group is to focus on how the communication will be received.

67. An AGACNP has been appointed to lead a small team on their unit that will focus on alternative methods to off-load patients' heels from the bed to prevent pressure injuries. The AGACNP is fairly new to the organization and does not personally know all of the key stakeholders involved in this project. What is the best route for the AGACNP to take to communicate information about the project?

A. Monthly employee email reminders and updates
B. The organization's quarterly electronic newsletter
C. Posted notes in the staff breakrooms and cafeteria areas
D. Sending a survey to review what the members prefer

68. The AGACNP is providing ostomy care instructions to a patient who had a colon resection with an end-colostomy placement. Which behavior by the patient *best* indicates comprehension of teaching?

A. The patient maintains eye contact and nods their head appropriately.
B. The patient takes notes and asks to have an educational brochure.
C. The patient relays the information back to the AGACNP in their own words.
D. The patient responds "yes" when asked if they understand the instructions.

69. An AGACNP is new to an organization and would like to learn more about how speech therapy collaborates with the team regarding patient swallowing studies as well as other speech-related pathology needs. What would be an effective approach for the AGACNP to gain more knowledge regarding this ancillary service?

A. Ask her manager for the departmental manual
B. Ask to speak with a patient who is under speech therapy's care
C. Attend next month's speech therapy staff meeting
D. Ask to shadow a speech therapist for a day

70. The AGACNP is rounding on a patient who is terminal and has just agreed to hospice care. When they walk into the patient's room, they notice that the patient is alone, crying, and holding a rosary, crucifix, and Bible in their hand. What will be the *best* approach for the AGACNP to take next?

A. Ask the patient if they should leave and come back later
B. Tell the patient that they understand how they are feeling
C. Ask the patient if they can call the hospital chaplain for them
D. Ask the patient if they need anything for pain or anxiety

(*See answers next page.*)

67. D) Sending a survey to review what the members prefer

Since the AGACNP is new to the organization and not very familiar with all of the team members, it is best if they send out an initial survey to poll the members to determine preferences for communication. While email reminders and updates, quarterly electronic newsletters, and posted notes in public areas are also potential routes of communication that the AGACNP can take, given the number of multiple communication platforms that exist, a survey may help the AGACNP narrow down which one is being utilized the most by team members.

68. C) The patient relays the information back to the AGACNP in their own words.

A positive indication that the patient is comprehending information provided to them is hearing the patient relay the information back to the AGACNP in their own words, which is called "teach-back." While eye contact and nodding, note-taking and asking for brochures, and responding in the affirmative are positive steps, teach-back is the only way the AGACNP can validate that the patient has full understanding of the information being relayed to them.

69. D) Ask to shadow a speech therapist for a day

Interprofessional competency assists in mutual respect, shared values, and increased teamwork. For a new professional employee, it would benefit the AGACNP to shadow a speech therapist for a day or two to gain a greater appreciation for the team's input on overall patient care. Reading the departmental manual, speaking with a patient in speech therapy care, or attending a staff meeting are not effective ways to develop a collaborative practice.

70. C) Ask the patient if they can call the hospital chaplain for them

The patient is end-of-life and is demonstrating profound sadness. Some patients report that prayer provides assurance, comfort, and inner strength for them. Offering to call the hospital chaplain may aid in additional spiritual support for the patient. Leaving the patient and returning later does not build empathy. Expressing understanding for their feelings is neither empathetic nor authentic. Asking them if they need something for pain or anxiety does not address the patient's emotions and actions.

71. The AGACNP is new to an organization. Their manager wants them to feel welcomed and a part of the team. What would be the *best* approach for the manager to take in order to promote team building?

A. Plan a staff luncheon to welcome the AGACNP and also invite interdisciplinary colleagues as guests
B. Include the AGACNP's name in the quarterly hospital newsletter
C. Send out a mass email that announces the new hire
D. Inform the AGACNP to set up one-on-one meetings with as many staff members as possible

72. The AGACNP is providing teaching to a patient with testicular cancer who underwent a retroperitoneal lymph node dissection and will be discharged tomorrow. Which statement by the patient indicates understanding of a low-fat diet for management of a chyle leak?

A. "I understand what to eat."
B. "I can eat vegetables with butter."
C. "I need to use fat-free milk products."
D. "I will just have my spouse take care of it."

73. When preparing discharge for a trauma survivor, the AGACNP will be sure to include information based on the patient's:

A. Diversity
B. Socioeconomic status
C. Resiliency
D. Spiritual needs

74. A home health AGACNP is seeing a patient for their annual physical exam. The patient has a history of depression and was hospitalized 3 years ago for a previous suicide attempt. Which component of their socioeconomic health history would be the greatest risk factor for suicide?

A. History of alcohol and substance use
B. Level of education
C. Long work hours
D. Large family

(*See answers next page.*)

71. A) Plan a staff luncheon to welcome the AGACNP and also invite interdisciplinary colleagues as guests

The best response to promote team building for a new employee is to plan a luncheon to welcome them and include other colleagues so that they can all be introduced; it also enhances the AGACNP's perception of feeling included. Including the AGACNP's name in the newsletter or a mass email announcement of their hiring is not personal and will not help them feel part of the team. Setting up a one-on-one meeting with as many staff members as possible, while personal, is not realistic.

72. C) "I need to use fat-free milk products."

Positive indication that the patient is comprehending information provided to them is their restating specific descriptors of a fat-free diet, that is, "fat-free milk products." Simply saying they understand does not give evidence that they understand how to follow a low-fat diet. Saying they can eat vegetables with butter is contraindicated with a low-fat diet. The AGACNP cannot discharge a patient without confirming the capability of a family member, such as their wife, to follow the instructions for a low-fat diet.

73. C) Resiliency

The term *resiliency* refers to the adaptability of an individual in the face of adversity, including trauma and stress. The AGACNP will include education information geared toward the patient's ability to care for themselves based on their resiliency. If the patient shows impaired levels of resiliency, educational information will include steps needed to improve this state. Diversity is an understanding that each individual is unique and different, and while it may play a role in an individual's ability to adapt, it is not specific to trauma survivorship and discharge education. Socioeconomic status and spiritual needs are areas of concern for all patients, but not when planning educational information for discharge of the trauma survivor.

74. A) History of alcohol and substance use

A history of alcohol and substance use is a risk factor for suicide due to the ability of alcohol and illicit drugs to decrease inhibitions and affect ability to think clearly. An individual's level of education is not a characteristic indicator of risk for suicide. Working long hours and coming from or living in a large family are not typically considered risk factors.

75. Although evidence-based guidelines are essential in selecting appropriate therapy, treatment must also consider:

A. Convenience of available treatment options from the perspective of the healthcare organization
B. Patient-specific factors such as allergies, medication interactions, and disease-specific contraindications
C. Discussion of upfront cost of treatment options with the patient
D. Not deviating from a selected treatment plan or therapy for any reason

76. What does it mean to apply deductive reasoning?

A. Using observations and information collected about a particular phenomenon either to confirm or to refute the theory suspected
B. Recognizing a particular pattern by observation and determining a theory or idea about a particular phenomenon or subject matter
C. Understanding sensitivity and specificity
D. Formulating a firm clinical diagnosis

77. In which manner would the AGACNP define scope of practice?

A. Legal boundaries of the license held by the practitioner including procedures, actions, and processes contained within the role for which the practitioner has specified education and training
B. Documents describing the boundaries of all AGACNPs across all recognized specialties, regardless of specificity of education and training or licensure of patient population
C. Authoritative statements that describe level of care or performance by the nursing professional
D. Area of expertise that gives the AGACNP competencies of expected behavior without legal binding or jurisdiction

(*See answers next page.*)

75. B) Patient-specific factors such as allergies, medication interactions, and disease-specific contraindications

Consideration of patient-specific factors such as allergies, medication interactions, and disease-specific contraindications should be considered when selecting appropriate therapy for a patient. Convenience of treatment options would be considered from a patient's perspective but should have no relevance when the AGACNP is selecting an appropriate treatment therapy. Cost of treatment would not be discussed before considering all pertinent patient-specific factors. Deviation from a treatment plan may, at times, be appropriate and determined by a number of factors in a patient's case.

76. A) Using observations and information collected about a particular phenomenon either to confirm or to refute the theory suspected

Deductive reasoning begins with generalizations, either observed or from information collected, and moves toward specific predictions about the theory. The process of inductive reasoning involves noting particular details about a phenomenon or subject matter, recognizing a pattern, then developing a theory about that phenomenon. The terms *sensitivity* and *specificity* refer to the ability of measurement to detect those who have a condition (i.e., a true positive). Forming a clinical diagnosis uses both inductive and deductive reasoning, depending largely on the provider's experience level and expertise in gathering key clinical information.

77. A) Legal boundaries of the license held by the practitioner including procedures, actions, and processes contained within the role for which the practitioner has specified education and training

Scope of practice defines boundaries held by the practitioner, including procedures, actions, and processes contained within the practitioner role. Scope of practice is specific to the education, training, licensure, and certification needed to practice, including the recognition of specialty-specific populations and practice requirements for such. One scope of practice for all specialties would not define safe practice, nor would it delineate functions within each specific role. Competencies and behavior expectations are outlined in professional standards of the AGACNP role, rather than defining legal boundaries defined by education and training under scope of practice. Authoritative statements describing level of care and performance are professional standards, not scope of practice.

78. Which type of collaboration is recognized as best practice for delivery of optimal quality care that meets the needs of acute and critically ill patients?

A. Consortium collaboration
B. Discussion among critical care practitioners
C. Elite circle communication
D. Multidisciplinary collaboration

79. The AGACNP demonstrates appropriate scope of practice by:

A. Assessing critically ill patients and relaying that information to the provider for diagnosis
B. Ordering diagnostic studies only under the direction of the attending physician
C. Formulating nursing diagnoses for suspected problems
D. Independently formulating a differential diagnosis

80. What action will the AGACNP take *first* to address a reported concern of an unsafe work environment?

A. Discussing policy and procedures for reporting with unit staff
B. Establishing a team-building activity to repair unit rapport
C. Discussing the reported concern with team members and documenting all findings
D. Conducting an evaluation of safety issues to date

81. Which component of AGACNP competencies fits the established standards of practice?

A. Practicing beyond regulatory constraints if in the best interests of the patient
B. Avoiding political activity to maintain a focus on clinical care
C. Advocating for legislation and policies that promote health and improve care delivery
D. Working to remove organizational barriers that are not consistent with personal values and beliefs

(*See answers next page.*)

78. D) Multidisciplinary collaboration

Multidisciplinary collaboration is essential to optimize patient outcomes, especially in the acute and critical care settings. Research shows that collaboration among the multidisciplinary team promotes quality improvement and decreases morbidity and mortality. A consortium is a private group of participants that make care and ethical decisions, but it may lack a multidisciplinary perspective. Expanding information sharing beyond interdepartmental collaboration is best practice and is supported in a multitude of quality improvement studies. Elite circle communication is not an effective multidisciplinary collaborative effort. Communication regarding patient care should encompass a variety of perspectives across the care continuum; a small or "elite" circle involves subjective decision-making and does not support best-practice guidelines.

79. D) Independently formulating a differential diagnosis

The AGACNP's scope of practice recognizes the completion of formal education preparing the practitioner to independently perform, order, interpret, and provide interventions for the individualized patient population, including formulation of a differential diagnosis. Ordering and interpreting diagnostic studies are also key components of the AGACNP role. Formulating a nursing diagnosis is not an advanced practice skill.

80. C) Discussing the reported concern with team members and documenting all findings

Formally documenting the concern and discussing with appropriate team members helps to directly address the concern as well as to capture important data that can be retrieved and reviewed. Discussing reporting policy and procedures does not formally address the concern of the employee. A team building activity may help morale and encourage sharing of ideas, but it does not address the underlying concern of an unsafe work environment. Conducting an evaluation on safety issues to date may be needed, but this would take place after discussion with team members has occurred.

81. C) Advocating for legislation and policies that promote health and improve care delivery

Advocating for legislation and policies that promote health and improve care delivery is a component of established standards of practice. Practicing beyond regulatory constraints demonstrates practice outside the defined AGACNP scope. Limiting participation in legislation and policies that improve health outcomes and delivery of care would negatively impact practice standards and patient outcomes. Removal of organizational barriers to achieve optimal patient care rather than to promote personal values and beliefs should be prioritized and is consistent with established practice standards.

82. The AGACNP displays ethical practice by:

A. Encouraging a patient's family member to refrain from sharing thoughts that can impact the patient's decision process until a more appropriate time

B. Informing extended family and support members of a patient's worsening state

C. Providing counseling for critically ill patients

D. Demonstrating nonjudgmental and nondiscriminatory attitudes and behaviors toward patients and families

83. After analyzing assessment data for a patient transported to the emergency department for shortness of breath, the AGACNP notices a deterioration in the patient's condition. Which action will the AGACNP take first?

A. Ordering chest x-ray and respiratory therapy

B. Interviewing caregivers for history of present illness and current treatments

C. Evaluating the need for pharmacological and therapeutic interventions appropriate to care

D. Performing a pertinent problem-focused exam according to the patient's immediate needs

84. The AGACNP evaluates an older adult patient with confusion, dizziness, and difficulty voiding and attempts to determine whether the patient is suffering from dehydration or from a urinary tract infection. This is an example of which clinical practice standard?

A. Differential diagnosis

B. Care planning

C. Outcomes identification

D. Diagnosis

85. Which gene is associated with the development of late-onset Alzheimer disease?

A. *BRCA*

B. *APOE-e4*

C. *KRAS*

D. *RET*

(*See answers next page.*)

82. D) Demonstrating nonjudgmental and nondiscriminatory attitudes and behaviors toward patients and families

Demonstration of nonjudgmental and nondiscriminatory attitudes and behaviors is an example of ethical practice. Asking the patient or family member to keep thoughts to themselves rather than encouraging open discussion does not demonstrate ethical practice and may impede the relationship with the patient. Providing information to extended family members and support systems is considered a breach of confidentiality unless prior permission has been given, and providing counseling is not within the scope of practice for the AGACNP.

83. C) Evaluating the need for pharmacological and therapeutic interventions appropriate to care

A change in patient condition warrants an immediate assessment for any pharmacological and/or therapeutic interventions that can address the change (e.g., supplemental oxygen). A problem-focused physical examination would be conducted when appropriate—that is, after necessary interventions—and would gather critical information related to potential causes or immediate concerns. Ordering chest x-rays or respiratory therapy and interviewing family members or caregivers are steps that would be taken once the immediate need is addressed.

84. A) Differential diagnosis

Differential diagnosis is the process of considering the range of disorders that could explain the patient's condition with the goal of arriving at a final diagnosis. Care planning involves establishing and documenting a program of clinical care that will meet the patient's individual needs. Outcomes identification focuses on establishing goals of care. The term *diagnosis* refers to the underlying disorder that has been identified after the differential diagnosis has been established and subsequent testing has yielded results for analysis.

85. B) *APOE-e4*

APOE-e4 is a susceptibility gene that is associated with (but not indicative of) late-onset Alzheimer disease. *BRCA, KRAS,* and *RET* are genes that are associated with certain cancer types.

86. A decrease in physiologic reserve that results in an increased risk of health problems is called:

A. Dementia
B. Frailty
C. Delirium
D. Exercise tolerance

87. Which statement is *most* accurate regarding an older individual's decision-making capacity?

A. The Montreal Cognitive Assessment (MoCA) is the only approved test to determine capacity
B. Decision-making capacity depends on the decision in question
C. Decision-making capacity remains consistent over time
D. If necessary, a surrogate decision-maker may be designated by the health-care provider

88. Which statement most accurately describes the significance of the *APOE-e4* allele?

A. The presence of two copies guarantees that the individual will develop Alzheimer disease.
B. The absence of any copies guarantees that the individual will not develop Alzheimer disease.
C. Genetic testing for *APOE-e4* is recommended for all individuals older than 50 years.
D. The presence of *APOE-e4* increases an individual's risk for developing Alzheimer disease.

89. Which class of medication is particularly likely to cause delirium in older individuals?

A. Proton pump inhibitor
B. Insulin
C. Anticholinergic
D. Selective serotonin reuptake inhibitor (SSRI)

90. What tool can assess delirium in an older adult patient?

A. Confusion Assessment Method (CAM)
B. Patient Health Questionnaire-2 (PHQ-2)
C. Patient Health Questionnaire-9 (PHQ-9)
D. Montreal Cognitive Assessment (MoCA)

(*See answers next page.*)

86. B) Frailty

The term *frailty* refers to the loss of physiologic reserve that can lead to multisystem issues. It is a prognostic indicator of poor health outcomes. Dementia is a condition involving progressive loss of cognitive function. Delirium is an acute change in cognition. Exercise tolerance (or lack thereof) may be a component of frailty.

87. B) Decision-making capacity depends on the decision in question

Decision-making capacity depends on the complexity of the decision at hand. The MoCA can assess cognitive function, but it is not the only approved test. Decision-making capacity can vary over time. A surrogate decision-maker is designated by the patient, not the healthcare provider.

88. D) The presence of *APOE-e4* increases an individual's risk for developing Alzheimer disease.

The presence of the *APOE-e4* allele increases one's risk of developing Alzheimer disease. However, two copies do not guarantee that one will develop the disease, and an individual can develop Alzheimer disease despite a lack of the *APOE-e4* allele. Genetic testing is not widely recommended.

89. C) Anticholinergic

There are several classes of medications that can cause delirium, including anticholinergic drugs. Proton pump inhibitors, insulin, and SSRIs are not likely to induce delirium.

90. A) Confusion Assessment Method (CAM)

CAM is an instrument that can be used at the bedside to assess delirium. PHQ-2 and PHQ-9 are instruments used to screen for depression. The MoCA is best used to assess cognitive impairment.

91. The AGACNP sees an older adult patient with a history of falls. What behavioral intervention does the AGACNP recommend as *most* effective in reducing falls?

A. Minimizing environmental hazards
B. Exercising regularly
C. Using assistive devices
D. Supplementing with vitamin D

92. A patient with dementia is demonstrating disruptive behavior. What strategy should the AGACNP employ in managing this patient?

A. Confronting the patient when they are disruptive
B. Keeping a log that describes the behavior and events leading up to it
C. Ordering antianxiety medication to calm the patient
D. Providing a variable schedule to prevent the patient from becoming bored

93. An older male patient reports urinary urgency and leakage over the past 6 months. The AGACNP suspects that the most likely cause is:

A. Urinary tract infection (UTI)
B. Stool impaction
C. Benign prostatic hyperplasia
D. Overhydration

94. An older patient asks the AGACNP about vitamin D supplementation to decrease fall risk. What is the AGACNP's *best* response?

A. "Vitamin D strengthens bones and is therefore beneficial in decreasing risk of falls."
B. "There is a benefit to vitamin D supplementation, but only with very high doses."
C. "Vitamin D supplementation is not recommended for community-dwelling older adults."
D. "Only postmenopausal women have been found to see a reduced fall risk with vitamin D."

(*See answers next page.*)

91. B) Exercising regularly

Regular exercise has most consistently shown effectiveness in reducing fall risk. Minimizing environmental hazards and using assistive devices are beneficial but have not shown the same degree of effectiveness as exercising regularly. Vitamin D supplementation is a pharmacologic intervention, not a behavioral intervention.

92. B) Keeping a log that describes the behavior and events leading up to it

When a patient with dementia exhibits disruptive behavior, it is best to keep a log to identify patterns. It is better to distract, not confront, the patient. Nonpharmacologic interventions are always preferred. It is best to keep the patient's routine structured and predictable.

93. C) Benign prostatic hyperplasia

Benign prostatic hyperplasia is the most common cause of detrusor overactivity (urge incontinence) in older male patients. UTI, stool impaction, and overhydration are all potential causes but are less common chronic causes.

94. C) "Vitamin D supplementation is not recommended for community-dwelling older adults."

The U.S. Preventive Services Task Force recommends against vitamin D supplementation for fall prevention in adults residing in the community. High-dose vitamin D supplementation has been shown to increase falls.

95. The AGACNP is evaluating an older adult patient with dementia who presents with involuntary weight loss. What intervention is appropriate?

A. Percutaneous endoscopic gastrostomy (PEG) insertion
B. Megestrol acetate administration
C. Hand feeding of the patient
D. Prednisone administration

96. Which older adult patient would the AGACNP diagnose with involuntary weight loss?

A. 120-lb woman with a loss of 3 lbs over the past month
B. 150-lb man with a loss of 6 lbs over the past 6 months
C. 160-lb woman with a loss 8 lbs over the past 6 months
D. 200-lb man with a loss of 9 lbs over the past 12 months

97. The AGACNP examines a patient with a nonblanchable maroon discoloration on intact skin of the sacrum that has been present for 6 months. How does the AGACNP define this pressure injury?

A. Stage 1
B. Stage 2
C. Stage 3
D. Deep tissue

98. The AGACNP is assessing an older adult hospitalized patient with dementia who has experienced recent weight loss. What intervention would be contraindicated for this patient?

A. Assisted hand feeding
B. Oral nutritional supplements
C. Sodium-containing flavor enhancers
D. Megestrol acetate administration

99. The AGACNP is assessing an older adult patient in the hospital who is at high risk for pressure injury. What should the AGACNP order to reduce the risk of development of a pressure injury in this patient?

A. Low–air loss mattress
B. Gel dressing
C. Strict bed rest
D. Low-protein diet

(*See answers next page.*)

95. C) Hand feeding of the patient

It is recommended that individuals with dementia who have weight loss be assisted with hand feeding. Although PEG insertion or administration of megestrol acetate or prednisone may be indicated for weight gain in specific populations, they are not recommended for weight maintenance in older adults.

96. C) 160-lb woman with a loss 8 lbs over the past 6 months

Involuntary weight loss in community-dwelling older adults is defined as unintentional and unexplained loss of 5% of body weight within 6 months or a loss of 10% body weight within 1 year. A 160-lb patient who has lost 8 lbs in 6 months has lost 5% of their body weight within that span. The other patients have lost less than 5% of their body weight.

97. D) Deep tissue

A deep tissue injury is characterized by an area of nonblanchable purple, maroon, or dark-red discoloration of intact skin. Stage 1 injury is characterized by nonblanchable erythema of intact skin, stage 2 by partial-thickness skin loss with exposed dermis, and stage 3 by full-thickness skin loss.

98. D) Megestrol acetate administration

Megestrol acetate is not indicated as an appetite stimulant for older adult patients because it has not been shown to be effective and is associated with numerous side effects. Assisted hand feeding, oral nutritional supplements, and sodium-containing flavor enhancers can be helpful in weight maintenance for patients with dementia.

99. A) Low–air loss mattress

Specialized mattresses, such as low–air loss mattresses, can reduce the risk of pressure injury. A gel dressing may be indicated to treat a pressure injury, but it does not play a role in prevention. Strict bed rest and a low-protein diet would increase, not decrease, the risk of developing a pressure injury.

100. The AGACNP examines a patient with a pressure injury covered by black eschar. What stage does the AGACNP assign to this pressure injury?

A. Stage 1
B. Stage 2
C. Stage 3
D. Unstageable

101. An older adult patient is experiencing nausea and vomiting secondary to partial gastric outlet obstruction. What medication should the AGACNP prescribe?

A. Diphenhydramine (Benadryl)
B. Lorazepam (Ativan)
C. Senna glycoside (Senokot)
D. Metoclopramide (Reglan)

102. The AGACNP is evaluating a patient with a stage 2 sacral pressure injury. What intervention is contraindicated for the treatment of this patient?

A. Polyurethane film dressing
B. Maintenance of a dry wound bed
C. Low–air loss mattress
D. Frequent repositioning

103. The AGACNP is seeing a patient for urinary incontinence secondary to detrusor overactivity. What does the AGACNP recommend as *first-line* treatment?

A. Bladder training
B. Tolterodine (Detrol)
C. Oxybutynin (Oxytrol)
D. Onabotulinum toxin A (Botox)

104. The AGACNP is discussing medication adherence with an older patient. What strategy should the AGACNP use to improve adherence?

A. Asking the patient to bring all medications to each provider visit
B. Encouraging the patient to use multiple pharmacies to fill medications
C. Changing the medication dosing schedule frequently
D. Keeping the medications in their original bottles

(*See answers next page.*)

100. D) Unstageable

A pressure injury that is obscured by eschar or other slough is considered unstageable. Stage 1 injury is characterized by nonblanchable erythema of intact skin, stage 2 by partial-thickness skin loss with exposed dermis, and stage 3 by full-thickness skin loss.

101. D) Metoclopramide (Reglan)

Metoclopramide (Reglan) and other prokinetic agents are indicated for nausea and vomiting secondary to partial gastric outlet obstruction. Diphenhydramine (Benadryl) is indicated for nausea secondary to vestibular apparatus disturbance. Lorazepam (Ativan) is indicated for anticipatory nausea. Senna glycoside (Senokot) is indicated for nausea secondary to constipation.

102. B) Maintenance of a dry wound bed

Treatment of pressure injury depends on maintaining a moist, not dry, wound bed. Polyurethane film dressings, a low–air loss mattress, and frequent repositioning are interventions that are indicated for the treatment of pressure injuries.

103. A) Bladder training

Bladder training, among other behavioral strategies, is the first-line treatment for detrusor overactivity. Tolterodine (Detrol), oxybutynin (Oxytrol), and injection of onabotulinum toxin A (Botox) are pharmacologic interventions that may be used if behavioral interventions are ineffective.

104. A) Asking the patient to bring all medications to each provider visit

Asking patients to bring all medications to each visit for review helps to ensure adherence and reinforces the reasons for taking each medication. It is best to use one pharmacy only and to keep the medication dosing schedule consistent and simple. Using a pillbox, rather than keeping each medication in its original bottle, can also be helpful to ensure adherence.

105. The AGACNP is evaluating a patient with a nonhealing sacral pressure injury. The area is foul smelling, but the patient is exhibiting no signs of systemic infection. What intervention is most appropriate?

A. Topical silver sulfadiazine
B. Oral clindamycin
C. Intravenous clindamycin
D. Superficial wound culture

106. An older adult patient exhibits sudden urinary urgency and leakage as well as suprapubic discomfort. What should the AGACNP do first?

A. Order urinalysis and cystoscopy
B. Educate patient on bladder training
C. Prescribe oxybutynin (Oxytrol)
D. Insert a Foley catheter

107. Which of the following diagnoses should be reported to the Centers for Disease Control and Prevention (CDC)?

A. Hand, foot, and mouth disease
B. Lyme disease
C. Lung cancer
D. Rheumatoid arthritis

108. The AGACNP is using the CAGE questionnaire while performing a health history. Under which level of disease prevention does this fall?

A. Primary
B. Secondary
C. Tertiary
D. Quaternary

109. A researcher performed a study, and an AGACNP wants to evaluate if they are able to obtain the same results under the same experimental conditions. What concept of empirical research is the AGACNP testing?

A. Controlled observation
B. Reliability
C. Validity
D. Confounds

(*See answers next page.*)

105. A) Topical silver sulfadiazine

A patient who has a suspected infected pressure injury without systemic infection should be treated with a topical agent such as silver sulfadiazine. Oral or parenteral antibiotics are indicated only if there is a systemic infection present, and the choice of therapy depends on tissue culture. A superficial wound culture is not indicated if an infection is localized.

106. A) Order urinalysis and cystoscopy

Sudden urge incontinence and detrusor overactivity should raise concern for the possibility of bladder stones or tumors and should be evaluated with a urinalysis and cystoscopy. Bladder training and oxybutynin (Oxytrol) are interventions for urinary incontinence, but if the incontinence occurs acutely, then the priority is identifying the underlying cause. Insertion of a Foley catheter is not indicated for urinary leakage and urgency.

107. B) Lyme disease

Lyme disease requires mandatory reporting to the CDC. The CDC maintains a reportable disease list, which is upgraded and revised as necessary and reissued on July 1 of each year. Each state also maintains its own reportable disease list. Diagnosis of hand, foot, and mouth disease; lung cancer; or rheumatoid arthritis does not require reporting to the CDC.

108. B) Secondary

Secondary prevention is the level of screening that identifies diseases in the earliest stages, before the onset of signs and symptoms. Primary prevention is intervening before health effects occur; vaccinations are an example of primary prevention. Tertiary prevention is treating the disease after diagnosis to prevent or mitigate its effects. Quaternary prevention involves protecting patients from excessive medical interventions.

109. B) Reliability

The term *reliability* refers to repeatability or consistency; the outcome of data collection should lead to the same conclusions if the data collection is replicated. Reliability also describes the precision of measuring instruments. The term *controlled observation* refers to the precision of conditions under which data are collected. The term *validity* refers to whether empirical research is appropriate, meaningful, and useful; tests are valid if they measure the characteristics they were intended to measure. Confounds are other explanations of results—variables that may be operating in conjunction with the manipulated variable that make it impossible to determine if the differences in the dependent variable are due to manipulation, the confound, or a combination of the two.

110. An AGACNP receives a year-end bonus from the hospital system if their department is able to meet or exceed key metrics such as liberating (extubating) patients in less time than the national average. The hospital system's bonus incentive is likely aligned with what system of payment?

A. Value-based purchasing
B. Retrospective payment
C. Fee for service
D. Prospective payment

111. The AGACNP is noting a high mortality in patients being admitted with septic shock across the hospital system. Which would be the most effective process to try to improve this situation?

A. Implementing the goals of *Healthy People 2030* in the hospital system's ICUs and emergency departments
B. Forming an interdisciplinary team to help incorporate the bundles recommended in the Surviving Sepsis Campaign throughout the hospital system
C. Becoming a spokesperson to advocate for broader Medicare and Medicaid coverage for patients
D. Beginning to document incident reports for each casualty associated with sepsis

112. Which of the following statements about Medicare is true?

A. Eligibility for Medicare is not impacted by the patient's income.
B. Medicare is jointly administered by state and federal governments.
C. Only patients age 65 years and older qualify for Medicare coverage.
D. AGACNPs are reimbursed at 100% of physician fee schedule when billing independently at an outpatient office.

(*See answers next page.*)

110. A) Value-based purchasing

Value-based purchasing, or pay-for-performance, was developed to resolve the issue of linking payment of services to quality and performance. Under this system, providers receive a higher rate of reimbursement for improved outcomes and cost-effective care. Fee-for-service involves payment for service provided, regardless of outcome. A retrospective payment system is a type of fee-for-service payment in which providers bill for actual costs of services provided. In a prospective payment system, payments are made according to fixed, predetermined rates, regardless of provider cost.

111. B) Forming an interdisciplinary team to help incorporate the bundles recommended in the Surviving Sepsis Campaign throughout the hospital system

The Surviving Sepsis Campaign is a global initiative to bring together professional organizations in reducing mortality from sepsis. The use of its recommended bundles has an effect on outcome beyond implementing the individual elements alone. The bundles are distilled from evidence-based practice guidelines. *Healthy People 2030* aims to prevent disease and promote health; its focus is on keeping people safe and healthy. It does not specifically aim to address mortality in sepsis, nor is it designed for the acute care setting. There is no association between broader insurance coverage and decreased sepsis mortality. While determining and prioritizing areas of potential improvement is important, and data collection and analysis would be helpful in analyzing specific trends in the hospital system's treatment of patients with sepsis, this information does not need to be collected through incidence reports.

112. A) Eligibility for Medicare is not impacted by the patient's income.

Income level does not impact eligibility for Medicare. Those age 65 years and older who are eligible for Social Security are automatically enrolled in Medicare, and individuals younger than 65 years may also qualify for coverage if they are affected by disability, end-stage renal disease, or amyotrophic lateral sclerosis. Medicare is a federal program; Medicaid is a joint federal and state program that provides additional coverage for those who meet income requirements. AGACNP reimbursement under Medicare is at 85% of the physician fee schedule when billing independently at an outpatient office.

Part II

Practice Exams and Answers With Rationales

Practice Exam 1

1. A patient presents to the emergency department with reports of cough, shortness of breath, green sputum production, and fever. With consideration of cost efficiency, which radiologic examination of the chest does the AGACNP order first?

   A. MRI
   B. CT
   C. CT with angiography
   D. X-ray

2. Which diagnostic study is most cost-effective for diagnosing deep vein thrombosis (DVT) in the leg?

   A. X-ray
   B. D-dimer
   C. Lung perfusion study
   D. Venous Doppler ultrasound

3. An older adult patient presents to the office for their yearly physical examination. The AGACNP reviews their electronic medical record and notes a history of elevated blood pressure readings. Which systolic and diastolic blood pressure range is categorized as stage II hypertension according to the American College of Cardiology/American Heart Association?

   A. Systolic blood pressure <120 mmHg and diastolic blood pressure <80 mmHg
   B. Systolic blood pressure 130 to 139 mmHg or diastolic blood pressure 80 to 90 mmHg
   C. Systolic blood pressure 120 to 129 mmHg and diastolic blood pressure <80 mmHg
   D. Systolic blood pressure ≥140 mmHg or diastolic blood pressure ≥90 mmHg

4. An older adult patient presents with triglycerides of 180 mg/dL, fasting glucose of 162 mg/dL, and hypertension. Which diagnosis does the AGACNP suspect?

   A. Metabolic syndrome
   B. Myocardial hibernation
   C. Obesity
   D. Coronary artery disease

5. The AGACNP is educating their patient on the importance of lipid control post-myocardial infarction. The patient is on maximum statin therapy, and the most recent laboratory studies report a low-density lipoprotein (LDL) level of 100 mg/dL. Which action does the AGACNP take next?

   A. Encourages diet and lifestyle modification
   B. Rechecks lipid profile in 6 months
   C. Starts omega-3 fatty acid supplementation
   D. Prescribes a cholesterol absorption inhibitor

6. An older adult patient reports intermittent chest pain that occurs with activity and is relieved with rest. Which diagnostic tool should the AGACNP order first?

   A. EKG
   B. Echocardiogram
   C. Cardiac stress test
   D. Cardiac angiogram

7. The AGACNP suspects that an older adult patient may have primary hypothyroidism. Which lab test should the AGACNP order first?

   A. Free T4
   B. Free T3
   C. Thyroglobulin
   D. Thyroid-stimulating hormone

8. An older adult patient has an elevated thyroid-stimulating hormone (TSH) level and a normal free T4 level. The AGACNP diagnoses this as:

   A. Hypothyroidism
   B. Hyperthyroidism
   C. Subclinical hypothyroidism
   D. Autoimmune thyroiditis

9. An older adult patient presents with suspected brain metastases. Which imaging modality is best at diagnosing a brain tumor?

A. CT scan of the head
B. MRI of the brain
C. EEG
D. PET scan

10. The AGACNP is conducting a psychiatric evaluation on an older adult patient. Which patient characteristic is most concerning for suicide risk?

A. Female sex assigned at birth
B. Involvement in church group
C. Close relationship with children
D. History of generalized anxiety disorder

11. A patient reports episodes of mania that alternate with depression. The AGACNP suspects which diagnosis?

A. Major depressive disorder
B. Bipolar I disorder
C. Bipolar II disorder
D. Hypothyroidism

12. Which test should be ordered as part of an initial asthma evaluation?

A. Arterial blood gas
B. Spirometry
C. Bronchial provocation testing
D. Chest x-ray

13. Which statement is *true* regarding changes in vision with age?

A. Older adults are at decreased risk of narrow-angle glaucoma.
B. Older adults have decreased lacrimal secretions.
C. Visual acuity begins to decline after age 30 years.
D. Older adults are more light sensitive because pupil size increases with age.

14. The AGACNP is prescribing bisacodyl (Dulcolax) for an older adult with constipation. Which advisory should be included in this education?

A. "This medication is an osmotic laxative."
B. "Bisacodyl typically requires 12 to 24 hours to take effect."
C. "You may experience abdominal cramping."
D. "You should take the medication daily."

15. The AGACNP is seeing an older adult patient with hearing loss. Which communication technique is best?

A. Using a high-tone voice
B. Speaking loudly
C. Speaking slowly
D. Talking to a family member to relay information

16. The AGACNP is educating an older adult patient on how to use a cane. What statement does the AGACNP include in this education?

A. "The cane should be used on your stronger side."
B. "The cane should reach the height of your hip."
C. "The cane should be moved in unison with the stronger leg."
D. "A cane is more effective than a walker in preventing falls."

17. An older adult patient reports recent leakage of urine when sneezing. The AGACNP diagnoses this as which type of incontinence?

A. Stress
B. Urge
C. Overflow
D. Functional

18. The AGACNP is evaluating a patient with transient urinary incontinence. Which medication does the AGACNP suspect as a likely contributor?

A. Pantoprazole (Protonix)
B. Famotidine (Pepcid)
C. Furosemide (Lasix)
D. Fluoxetine (Prozac)

19. An acute, fluctuating course of cognitive impairment is called:

A. Dementia
B. Alzheimer's disease
C. Delirium
D. Cerebrovascular accident

20. The AGACNP examines a patient with a pressure injury and notes partial-thickness skin loss and exposed dermis. What stage does the AGACNP assign to this pressure injury?

A. 1
B. 2
C. 3
D. 4

21. The AGACNP assesses a patient who has had multiple falls due to postural hypotension after starting furosemide (Lasix). What is the most appropriate initial intervention?

A. Ordering a medical alert system
B. Referring the patient to physical therapy
C. Assessing the feasibility of discontinuing the drug
D. Educating the patient on sleep hygiene

22. The AGACNP is rounding on an 85-year-old patient in the ICU who was admitted a short time ago from a nursing home. The patient's record indicates acute respiratory distress syndrome, body mass index of 17, and stage 1 pressure injuries on the bilateral heels upon admission. The patient's spouse, who is at the bedside, turns to the AGACNP and states, "You gave him bedsores!" The AGACNP responds by:

A. Stating that the record shows that the patient developed the sores at the nursing home
B. Saying, "Your spouse is at higher risk because of their status. I will order some heel-relief splints."
C. Replying, "I'm sure this is a stressful time for you. Is there anything we can do to make you more comfortable?"
D. Remaining quiet and allow the spouse to vent their feelings during this stressful time

23. The AGACNP asks an older adult patient whether they are experiencing hearing impairment. When the patient answers "No," what is the *most* appropriate next step?

A. Inquiring again at the next visit
B. Asking the patient's family
C. Referring the patient to audiometry
D. Conducting a whispered voice test

24. The AGACNP, who is a manager of a large outpatient clinic that specializes in senior care, is notified by a staff member that one of the providers who reports to them was seen apparently smoking marijuana in their car during a lunch break. What is the *priority* next step that this manager will take?

A. Locating the person who witnessed the alleged event and interviewing them for more details
B. Taking no action because there is no way to know if the person who made the allegation is correct
C. Asking the provider to meet at the end of their shift to discuss the issue
D. Asking Human Resources to assist with guidance on how to proceed with this allegation

25. The AGACNP is in the emergency department examining an 85-year-old patient who is accompanied by her adult son. The patient is silent while the son, who states that he lives with the patient, reports that the patient missed her footing and fell down a set of stairs. The son continues to answer all of the AGACNP's questions while the patient remains silent and seemingly avoids eye contact. On assessment, the AGACNP observes that the injuries do not seem consistent with the reported accident and notes what appears to be a thermal burn. What action does the AGACNP take next?

A. Telling the son, "These injuries don't appear consistent with what you described. Could you explain the accident to me again?"
B. Telling the son, "The exam may require your mother to disrobe. Could you leave the room briefly until she can dress again?"
C. Telling the son, "I need to ask your mother about these injuries in private. Could you leave the room for a few minutes?"
D. Asking the patient, "Did you really fall down the stairs?"

26. The AGACNP is instructing other members of the practice on screening older adult patients for signs of frailty. What sign would the AGACNP include in the instruction?

A. Decreased gait speed
B. Increased body mass index
C. Hearing loss
D. Forgetfulness

27. An AGACNP is rounding on a patient who was just placed on hospice and has a do-not-resuscitate order. Several family members are gathered at the bedside and are arguing in loud whispers that are clearly audible in the hallway. The patient is actively dying, exhibits labored breathing, and has their eyes closed. What response by the AGACNP is appropriate?

A. "Could you have this discussion some other time?"
B. "Your argument is disturbing other patients."
C. "Your loved one may be able to hear you."
D. "We can hear you out in the hallway."

28. What behavior is required of an AGACNP to demonstrate good leadership skills?

A. Exhibits the greatest clinical knowledge on the team
B. Provides patient care that is free from errors
C. Possesses effective communication skills
D. Never takes a sick day

29. While rounding in the hospital, the AGACNP notices that an older adult patient has fallen out of bed and is confused and combative, believing they are at home. After caring for the patient, the AGACNP notifies the patient's adult child, who demands that a 1:1 sitter be assigned to stay with the patient at all times. How can the AGACNP best respond given that there is a staffing shortage at the hospital?

A. "I'm sorry, but we aren't able to accommodate this request."
B. "Unfortunately, we don't have the staff to do what you have asked."
C. "Let me speak to the nurse manager and see what we can do."
D. "I will see if I can locate someone to sit with your parent for the rest of the day."

30. The AGACNP is preparing a continuing nursing education presentation for a group of healthcare professionals on the topic of providing an effective telehealth patient visit. What teaching-learning format will most effectively deliver this type of content?

A. Lecture
B. Self-learning module
C. Group discussion
D. Role-play

31. The AGACNP is evaluating an 81-year-old patient who lives alone in their home. The patient has stopped driving but is mobile and is able to take short walks in the neighborhood without assistance. Other than some mild forgetfulness, the patient does not exhibit any signs or symptoms of confusion and is able to provide self-care. The patient has a body mass index (BMI) of 17.5 and has limited financial resources for groceries. What will the best strategy be for the AGACNP regarding meal planning?

A. Provide the patient with information regarding the nearest community food kitchen
B. Provide information on stretching their food budget
C. Help them sign up for a free meal delivery service through the local senior center
D. Teach the patient about the importance of good nutrition and the risk of a low BMI

32. The AGACNP is asked by their manager to give peer-review feedback for the scheduled performance review of a work colleague with whom the AGACNP is friendly. The AGACNP has occasionally witnessed the colleague performing shortcuts that are not considered best practice techniques in patient care, although the AGACNP is not aware of any impact on patient outcomes. What action is best for the AGACNP to take?

A. Provide feedback but avoid mentioning the shortcuts. It seems unlikely that patient harm will occur.
B. Ask the manager to be excused from providing feedback. The friendly relationship makes it difficult to remain objective.
C. Provide feedback, including mention of the shortcuts. Mention that no patient harm was identified.
D. Ask the manager for a delay in providing feedback. Ask the colleague to avoid making shortcuts so the feedback will not have to mention them.

33. The AGACNP recognizes that which feature is an important component of collaboration with the healthcare team?

A. Being friends with the team members
B. Letting each member's input carry equal weight
C. Deferring to senior members
D. Being willing to listen to others' viewpoints

34. A patient recently underwent coronary angiography and asks the AGACNP to explain the findings of "significant stenosis." The AGACNP's best response is:

A. "At least half of your coronary arteries had blockages."
B. "You had a major heart attack."
C. "At least one of your major arteries or its branches was at least 75% blocked."
D. "Your femoral artery is hardened, which made it difficult to assess your coronary vessels."

35. The ultimate goal of promoting health literacy is to:

A. Allow patients to attain and act on health information in an informed way
B. Provide health information to patients in their primary language
C. Accommodate cultural needs in the communication of health information
D. Convey health information in ways that are easy to understand

36. The AGACNP is providing education to a patient with newly diagnosed left ventricular hypertrophy (LVH). Which of the following would the AGACNP state?

A. "Your LVH is not hereditary, so your children should be unaffected."
B. "It is important to control your blood pressure to avoid worsening your LVH."
C. "Patients with LVH should avoid aerobic activity and exercise."
D. "LVH is a normal variant and does not require any treatment."

37. A patient presents with unintentional weight loss and loose stools that the patient describes as "foul." The AGACNP orders gastrointestinal testing focusing on the:

A. Stomach
B. Small intestine
C. Large intestine
D. Liver

38. Which lab results are consistent with diabetic ketoacidosis (DKA)?

A. Glucose 240 mg/dL, bicarbonate 14 mEq/L, pH 7.2
B. Glucose 305 mg/dL, bicarbonate 19 mEq/L, pH 7.3
C. Glucose 180 mg/dL, bicarbonate 20 mEq/L, pH 7.5
D. Glucose 305 mg/dL, bicarbonate 14 mEq/L, pH 7.1

39. When evaluating for pancreatitis, which lab testing will the AGACNP order to confirm diagnosis?

A. Cholinesterase
B. Uric acid
C. Bile acids
D. Amylase

40. The AGACNP is seeing a patient with pyelonephritis. What would prompt the AGACNP to order imaging?

A. Dysuria
B. Urinary urgency
C. Patient's request
D. Fever for 4 days

41. What pathogen is the *most* common cause of community-acquired urinary tract infections (UTI)?

A. *Staphylococcus saprophyticus*
B. *Escherichia coli*
C. *Klebsiella pneumoniae*
D. *Proteus mirabilis*

42. The AGACNP is caring for an older adult patient who has reported itching skin after being exposed to poison ivy. Which medication would the AGACNP *avoid* in the patient's treatment plan for mild pruritis?

A. Diphenhydramine (Benadryl)
B. Loratadine (Claritin)
C. Hydrocortisone 1% topical cream
D. Topical pramoxine/calamine

43. The major limiting factors for the use of aminoglycoside antibiotics include:

A. Increased glomerular filtration rate
B. Visual toxicity
C. Nephrotoxicity
D. Creatinine reduction

44. Diffuse application of topical glucocorticoids can lead to:

A. Increase in adrenal production
B. Adrenal suppression
C. Extensive burns to skin
D. Decreased peripheral perfusion

45. The AGACNP working in endocrinology considers PICO while formulating the following clinical question when practicing best-evidence medicine: "Among patients with type 2 diabetes mellitus, is metformin 500 mg once daily more effective than glipizide 2.5 mg once daily in controlling blood glucoses?" Which of the following is the intervention being considered?

A. Patients with type 2 diabetes mellitus
B. Metformin 500 mg once daily
C. Glipizide 2.5 mg once daily
D. Blood glucoses

46. Evidence-based practice involves the care of patients using the best available research to guide clinical decision-making. One of the basic elements of evidence-based medicine is:

A. Relying on expert opinion
B. Reviewing historical data to understand what has been tried in the past
C. Applying the best available research medicine, combined with clinical expertise and patient preference
D. Formulating broad clinical questions

47. When formulating a clinical question regarding the effectiveness of an intervention, which of the following components should be considered (commonly referred to as PICO)?

A. Patient population
B. Internal validity
C. Chance
D. Obstacles

48. Which of the following describes the correct hierarchy of categories of evidence from highest to lowest?

A. Expert opinion, case-controlled studies, meta-analysis of randomized controlled trials

B. Meta-analysis of randomized controlled trials, expert opinion, qualitative studies

C. Systematic reviews, descriptive studies, randomized controlled trials

D. Meta-analysis of randomized controlled trials, case-controlled studies, expert opinion

49. An AGACNP is working on a research study to determine if nicotine inhalers assist with smoking reduction. Failure to blind relevant study participants to group assignment in a randomized trial could lead to which of the following?

A. Chance

B. Bias

C. Indirect evidence

D. Low statistical power

50. An AGACNP is conducting a literature review on the treatment strategies for a stroke patient with cardiovascular disease. Which of the following databases would be the *least* appropriate to use to find evidence-based data?

A. Wikipedia

B. PubMed

C. Cumulative Index for Nursing and Allied Health Literature (CINAHL)

D. Cochrane databases

51. Results from a randomized clinical trial found that stringent blood glucose control led to better outcomes in patients with diabetes mellitus. The AGACNP is able to generalize the findings from a study's sample to the larger population based on which component of the study?

A. Internal validity

B. Sensitivity

C. External validity

D. Specificity

52. A patient who is healthy with no past medical history undergoes secondary prevention screening for cervical cancer. The pap smear is negative for the detection of cancerous cells. This diagnostic test can be described as having:

A. Specificity
B. Sensitivity
C. False negative
D. Positive predictive value

53. A patient with syphilis has a rapid plasma regain test that is positive. The performance of this diagnostic test can be described as having:

A. Negative predictive value
B. Specificity
C. False positive
D. Sensitivity

54. The number of new cases of colon cancer per 100,000 people per year is an example of which of the following epidemiological terms?

A. Odds ratio
B. Incidence
C. Relative risk
D. Prevalence

55. Which of the following is true regarding confidence intervals?

A. They can be used to directly infer how confident one should be in a result.
B. A larger confidence interval implies a more precise range of values.
C. It is a fixed-point estimate that can be reflected to the entire population.
D. They can be interpreted as a range of believable values that is likely to include the true value.

56. The AGACNP is evaluating a research study and notes that the *p*-value is <0.05. Which of the following is true regarding the *p*-value?

A. It is the probability that the result of the study is true.
B. It can be used to directly infer how confident one should be in a result.
C. It is a measure of the effect of chance within a study.
D. A higher *p*-value indicates stronger evidence in support of the hypothesis.

57. An AGACNP is participating in a research project on a new cancer drug. The null hypothesis is that the drug does not affect the growth of cancer cells. During the experimental phase, cancer cell growth has stopped after application of the drug. The AGACNP rejects the null hypothesis. However, later testing discovers that another factor has contributed to impeding growth rather than solely administration of the drug. This is an example of:

A. Type I error
B. Type II error
C. Insufficient power
D. Poor reliability

58. A large number of nurses are followed over time to assess for certain diseases, such as colon cancer, to provide an estimate of the risk of a particular disease for this population. Dietary intake is assessed, and the risk of colon cancer in those with high and low intake of fiber can be evaluated to determine if fiber is a risk factor (or a protective factor) for colon cancer. This is an example of which type of study design?

A. Case-control study
B. Randomized controlled trial
C. Cohort study
D. Systematic review

59. Which of the following is the most common measurement to assess interobserver agreement when assessing reliability?

A. Standard deviation
B. Kappa statistic
C. Confidence interval
D. Level of significance

60. A study design is assessing the role of dietary fiber in colon cancer. A group of patients with colon cancer are compared with controls without colon cancer. The fiber intake of the two groups is compared. This is an example of which type of study design?

A. Randomized controlled trial
B. Cohort study
C. Systematic review
D. Case-control study

61. Why are clinical practice guidelines important for the AGACNP to incorporate into practice?

A. They are widely agreed upon between professional organizations.
B. Most guidelines are based on clinical expertise and quality improvement projects.
C. They rely on systematic reviews and include cost-effective approaches to patient care.
D. Recommendations for the same topic can be found in multiple guidelines.

62. The AGACNP is participating in a research design that is evaluating blood glucose stability in patients with diabetes mellitus. The study participants are randomized into treatment groups to test blood glucoses of patients with diabetes mellitus who use implanted insulin pumps against the blood glucoses of patients with diabetes who receive multiple insulin injections. This is an example of which type of study design?

A. Randomized controlled trial
B. Systematic review
C. Cohort study
D. Case-control study

63. A patient presents with acute changes in memory impairment. During the head-to-toe physical assessment, the AGACNP asks the patient to take the Mini-Mental State Examination. To ensure consistency with the results, the AGACNP asks the patient to complete the same exam during their follow-up appointment. A similar score is obtained. This is an example of assessment of which type of reliability?

A. Inter-observer reliability
B. Internal consistency
C. Intra-observer reliability
D. Test-retest reliability

64. A trauma patient presents to the emergency department after a motor vehicle crash. The patient was found to be in acute respiratory distress with agonal breathing, a low oxygen saturation, and extremely abnormal arterial blood gas. The patient arrived alone with no identification, and no family has been identified. What is the next best step for the AGACNP?

A. Continue to work with social work to identify a family member who could consent for the patient
B. Use all noninvasive respiratory interventions until the durable power of attorney can be consulted
C. Proceed with endotracheal intubation as delay would pose risk of serious, imminent harm to the patient
D. Ask another AGACNP to consent with you as this is an emergency exception to informed consent

65. The AGACNP is obtaining a consent for a patient to receive blood products that may be needed postoperatively. For the consent from the patient to be valid, which of the following is true?

A. Medical information regarding the decision can be relayed to the patient's family member.
B. The patient must have the mental ability to understand and make decisions about medical treatments.
C. The consent form can be obtained after the unit of blood products is ordered.
D. Technical medical knowledge and a complete list of all the risks are essential to ensure the patient receives all the information.

66. A patient admitted to the ICU with septic shock has been comatose and deemed incompetent to make decisions regarding their medical care. Of the following, who would be responsible to direct this patient's care?

A. The patient's next of kin
B. Any close living family member
C. The patient's spouse
D. The patient's durable power of attorney for healthcare

67. The justification for informed consent is based on upholding which ethical principal?

A. Respect for autonomy
B. Nonmaleficence
C. Beneficence
D. Justice

68. The AGACNP obtains informed consent from the patient for a nonurgent procedure that is within their scope of practice and that they have the credentials and privileges to perform. The patient has been receiving opioid pain medication preoperatively and seemed very drowsy during their conversation. The AGACNP assumes that the patient does not have any questions and drifts off to sleep after signing the consent form. The AGACNP continues planning for the procedure. Did the AGACNP obtain informed consent?

A. Yes, the informed consent discussion and its documentation were completed by the provider who will be performing the procedure—in this case the AGACNP.

B. Yes, the AGACNP communicated with the patient regarding the medical procedure to be performed and obtained permission to perform the intervention.

C. No, the AGACNP should have obtained consent from the patient's surrogate decision-maker because the was too lethargic.

D. No, the AGACNP provided the pertinent medical information, but they did not ensure that the patient had adequately understood the information.

69. The AGACNP is considering a clinical trial for a patient with leukemia, which may help slow disease progression but may also cause troublesome and possibly debilitating side effects. This decision takes into consideration which ethical principle?

A. Fidelity

B. Nonmaleficence

C. Beneficence

D. Justice

70. A patient has been managed on supportive care in the ICU for necrotizing pancreatitis for weeks. The patient has suffered from acute respiratory failure and has been unable to be weaned from the ventilator. Continuous dialysis has been necessary for the patient's kidney failure. The patient's durable power of attorney for healthcare has been making decisions for this patient and has been pressing to continue aggressive care. The AGACNP on the ICU team explains that any further intervention would likely cause harmful side effects and minimal, if any, potential benefits or prolongation of life. This conflict regarding overly aggressive end-of-life treatment relates to which type of futility?

A. Physiologic

B. Quantitative

C. Imminent demise

D. Qualitative

71. Which of the following establishes the ethical standard for the AGACNP and a guide to use in ethical analysis and decision-making?

A. Institutional protocols
B. Clinical practice guidelines
C. American Nurses Association Code of Ethics
D. State nurse practice acts

72. In the event the patient loses decisional capacity, which of the following is a signed legal document authorizing another person to make medical decisions on the patient's behalf?

A. Durable power of attorney for healthcare
B. Living will
C. Physician Orders for Life-Sustaining Treatment (POLST)
D. Instructional directive

73. What is the most common type of skin cancer?

A. Basal cell carcinoma
B. Squamous cell carcinoma
C. Malignant melanoma
D. Kaposi sarcoma

74. When caring for patients, it is important for the AGACNP to participate in advance care planning because:

A. All patients should have an advance directive to delineate preferences for future medical care.
B. It ensures patients receive medical care consistent with their values and preferences.
C. It helps patients with terminal diseases come to terms with their disease.
D. It provides the identification of the healthcare proxy.

75. A patient in the neurological ICU is being treated for subdural hematoma posttraumatic fall. Which clinical manifestation suggests expansion of the bleed?

A. Hypotension
B. Tachycardia
C. Decreased respiratory rate
D. Fever

76. The AGACNP is evaluating an older adult patient in the hospital who has new-onset urinary incontinence. The AGACNP suspects which *most common* cause of urinary incontinence in hospitalized patients?

A. Urinary tract infection
B. Delirium
C. Atrophic urethritis
D. Restricted mobility

77. Which is an example of a nonopioid adjuvant analgesic?

A. Amitriptyline
B. Acetaminophen (Tylenol)
C. Aspirin
D. Haloperidol (Haldol)

78. When an AGACNP fails to meet their licensing state's requirements, this is an example of which of the following?

A. Deception
B. Fraud
C. Unprofessional conduct
D. Violation of Health Insurance Portability and Accountability Act (HIPAA)

79. The AGACNP has been providing education to a patient with type 1 diabetes. Which of the following statements by the patient would indicate that the AGACNP's teaching has been effective?

A. "As long as I don't need glasses, I won't worry about going blind."
B. "I know that I need to have my eyes checked every year."
C. "I will see my primary care physician if I experience eye pain."
D. "I will see my eye doctor when my vision gets blurry."

80. A 50-year-old patient presents with breathing difficulty after working in a factory setting for the last 25 years. The patient states a belief that being exposed to chemicals at work has created their health issues. The AGACNP knows that determining occupational exposure in the workplace is difficult because of:

A. Possible inaccuracy of occupational disease reporting
B. Confidential information within company records
C. Length of time between exposure and disease development
D. Unreliable documentation of time at work

81. What is the main goal of tertiary prevention?

A. Slowing or stopping disease progression
B. Detecting and treating disease in an early stage
C. Screening for presence of disease
D. Educating to prevent disease from occurring

82. A 65-year-old patient has been recently diagnosed with osteoarthritis. The AGACNP has explained that the goals for managing osteoarthritis include controlling pain, maximizing functional independence and mobility, minimizing disability, and preserving quality of life. The patient explains that their first choice would be to use complementary therapies to control the condition and asks which therapies are most effective in treating osteoarthritis. What would be the most appropriate response by the AGACNP?

A. "I would be happy to discuss treatment options available to you. Complementary therapies such as acupressure have shown promise when used with standard medical therapy for osteoarthritis."
B. "It would be inadvisable to use complementary therapies to treat such a serious condition."
C. "I am unfamiliar with the available complementary therapies for osteoarthritis and prefer to discuss more mainstream treatments such as medication and physical therapy to manage your condition."
D. "Complementary therapies should be considered only if surgical interventions are not successful."

83. An 85-year-old patient is newly diagnosed with colon cancer, and surgery is indicated. The patient is mentally alert but refuses to give consent for the procedure. The AGACNP responds by:

A. Respecting the patient's wishes
B. Insisting that the patient listen a surgeon's advice
C. Ordering a psychiatric consult
D. Contacting the family so they can persuade the patient to have surgery

84. Evidence-based practice is important in healthcare because it involves the provider's clinical expertise, the patient, and:

A. Medication orders
B. Traditional beliefs
C. Historical ideas
D. Current research

85. AGACNPs at times may need to use the therapeutic privilege. This privilege involves the right of a healthcare professional to:

A. Use mental health therapy to treat their patients
B. Have free access to mental health therapy
C. Withhold some truths from patients if they believe complete honesty could be harmful
D. Not be legally responsible for what a patient may do after receiving bad news

86. Behavior change is one of the most effective ways to improve patient outcomes. What is the best way to promote personal behavior change in patients?

A. Stressing compliance with a treatment plan
B. Discussing options and letting the patient decide
C. Writing an order for a treatment plan
D. Sending the patient for mental health services

87. Access to neighborhood transportation is an example of which of the following health determinants?

A. Physical
B. Social
C. Biological
D. Behavioral

88. The AGACNP is performing a visual examination and observes that the patient is unable to turn both eyes in the same direction simultaneously. The AGACNP identifies the abnormal assessment findings as:

A. Disconjugate gaze
B. Conjugate gaze
C. Mydriasis
D. Nystagmus

89. An AGACNP participates in a hospital-based quality improvement project by performing chart reviews of colleagues to ensure certain protocols are met. What is this process an example of?

A. Peer review
B. Standard auditing
C. Hospital policy
D. Risk analysis

90. Which type of shock is caused by large loss of blood or fluids and is characterized by confusion, anxiety, and pallor?

A. Cardiogenic
B. Septic
C. Hypovolemic
D. Distributive

91. The AGACNP is educating a community group on the signs of opioid overdose. Which side effect is most commonly associated with this type of overdose?

A. Respiratory depression
B. Hypertension
C. Tachycardia
D. Fever

92. The AGACNP is counseling a patient with cystic fibrosis on reproductive considerations. Which statement by the AGACNP accurately describes the risk of the patient passing the disease on?

A. "Cystic fibrosis is a nongenetic disease, so you don't have anything to worry about."
B. "Cystic fibrosis skips a generation, so you don't need to worry about passing it on."
C. "Both parents must be carriers of the gene in order for the child to inherit the disease."
D. "Only one parent has to be a carrier of the gene in order for the child to inherit the disease."

93. The AGACNP is reviewing echocardiogram results with a patient. The AGACNP informs the patient that the normal range for left ventricular ejection fraction (LVEF) is:

A. 15% to 35%
B. 35% to 55%
C. 55% to 75%
D. 75% to 95%

94. A patient presents to the emergency department with thyroid storm. What medication should the AGACNP order during the initial treatment period?

A. Propranolol (Inderal)
B. Levothyroxine (Synthroid)
C. Vancomycin (Vancocin)
D. Albuterol (Proventil)

95. The AGACNP is calculating the cardiac output for a patient whose stroke volume is 80 mL and heart rate is 75 beats/min. What is the cardiac output for this patient in L/min?

A. 1.55
B. 5
C. 6
D. 8

96. A patient presents to the emergency department with suspected acute adrenal insufficiency. What should the AGACNP order as an initial treatment?

A. Beta-blockers
B. Corticosteroids
C. Insulin
D. Antibiotics

97. A patient asks the AGACNP why she gets urinary tract infections (UTIs) while her husband has never experienced one. How does the AGACNP respond?

A. "Your hygiene practices must not be as thorough as your husband's hygiene practices."
B. "The daily calcium supplements you take put you at higher risk for UTIs."
C. "Urine produced by women is less acidic and therefore promotes bacterial growth."
D. "The length and location of the male urethra helps protect against UTIs."

98. A patient who was discharged from the hospital 1 week ago now presents with severe, watery diarrhea over the past 2 days. After obtaining a stool culture, the AGACNP should treat the patient empirically for suspected *Clostridioides difficile* (*C. difficile*) with which medication?

A. Loperamide (Diamode)
B. Diphenoxylate/atropine (Lomotil)
C. Metronidazole (Flagyl)
D. Cephalexin (Keflex)

99. The AGACNP is seeing a patient with type 2 diabetes mellitus who has been experiencing recurrent urinary tract infections (UTIs). What educational point related to UTIs is important to include in this patient's care plan?

A. It is important to keep glucose levels well-controlled.
B. It is not necessary to obtain a urine culture before starting treatment.
C. Treatment is not indicated unless fever or hematuria is present.
D. Douching will decrease the risk of developing UTIs.

100. The AGACNP diagnoses a patient with otitis media with effusion (OME). The patient inquires about receiving a prescription for antibiotics. The AGACNP's best response is:

A. "I will prescribe ciprofloxacin for a one-week course."
B. "OME is not due to a bacterial infection, so it does not require antibiotics."
C. "OME requires antibiotics only if it is accompanied by fever."
D. "A culture is necessary prior to prescribing any antibiotic treatment."

101. The AGACNP sees a male patient with dysuria and a temperature of 101.2°F (38.4°C). On examination, the patient reports tenderness upon palpation of the right renal angle. What is the AGACNP's top differential diagnosis?

A. Prostatitis
B. Renal carcinoma
C. Pyelonephritis
D. Urinary tract infection

102. The AGACNP is evaluating the complete blood count with differential results of a patient experiencing an acute allergic reaction. What value would the AGACNP expect to see increased?

A. Neutrophils
B. Eosinophils
C. Monocytes
D. Platelets

103. Which endocrine disorder can cause myxedema crisis?

A. Adrenal insufficiency
B. Hypothyroidism
C. Hyperthyroidism
D. Acromegaly

104. The AGACNP is assessing a patient of Native American descent. Physical examination reveals a bluish discoloration of the sacral area. The patient reports that they have had this discoloration since birth. The AGACNP identifies this discoloration as a(n):

A. Deep tissue injury
B. Unstageable pressure ulcer
C. Slate gray nevus
D. Keloid scar

105. The AGACNP is reviewing the medication list for a patient with thyrotoxicosis. Which medication does the AGACNP identify as a potential cause of this condition?

A. Metoprolol (Lopressor)
B. Amiodarone (Cordarone)
C. Acetaminophen (Tylenol)
D. Omeprazole (Prilosec)

106. The AGACNP is seeing a patient post hospitalization as follow-up for a cerebral vascular accident. An MRI report shows a left temporal lobe territory infarct. The AGACNP anticipates which deficits on the clinic exam considering the territory of infarct?

A. Visual field defects
B. Personality changes accompanied by impulsive behavior
C. Expressive or receptive language deficits
D. Ataxia, dysmetria, and astereognosis

107. The AGACNP is assessing an older adult patient with a past medical history of hypertension, dyslipidemia, and uncontrolled type 2 diabetes mellitus. During the assessment, the AGACNP notes that the patient is able to detect vibration on the lower extremities only at the level of the upper shin and has no great toe proprioception. The AGACNP knows that the patient has disease of what part of the central nervous system?

A. Spinothalamic tract
B. Posterior column lateral meniscus tract
C. Cerebellum
D. Corticospinal tract

108. An adult patient complains of several episodes of severe lacerating pain that shoots up the right cheek and is precipitated by drinking cold liquids or chewing. These episodes begin suddenly and spontaneously after a few seconds, with several episodes per day. The patient denies any trauma, facial weakness, or difficulty swallowing. The patient has stopped drinking cold liquids because of the pain. Which of the following is the most likely diagnosis?

A. Trigeminal neuralgia
B. Cluster headache
C. Acute sinusitis
D. Sinus headache

109. Which of the following findings would prompt the AGACNP to listen to transmitted sound, such as egophony and bronchophony?

A. Bronchial breath sounds in most areas of the lungs
B. Vesicular breath sounds in most areas of the lungs
C. Bronchial breath sounds in trachea area
D. Bronchovesicular breath sound between scapulae

110. When grading muscle strength on a scale from 0 to 5, what does a grade of four indicate?

A. Active range of motion (ROM) against gravity with full resistance
B. Active ROM against gravity with some resistance
C. Active ROM with gravity
D. Active ROM with gravity eliminated

111. An older adult patient presents with an itchy rash on the head, especially in the nasolabial folds and eyelids, behind the ears, and on the scalp. The patient reports that sweating seems to make symptoms worse. On exam, the AGACNP notes plaques on the eyelids, on the nasolabial folds, behind the ears, and on the scalp that appear oily with some flaking and scaling. The AGACNP knows that findings are most consistent with what condition?

A. Seborrheic dermatitis
B. Rosacea
C. Atopic dermatitis
D. Contact dermatitis

112. The AGACNP adjusts warfarin (Coumadin) to target an international normalized ratio (INR) within what range for a patient with nonvalvular atrial fibrillation?

A. 2.0 to 3.0
B. 2.0 to 3.5
C. 2.5 to 3.0
D. 2.5 to 3.5

113. Sulfamethoxazole-trimethoprim (SMZ-TMP) is a sulfonamide antibiotic that may contribute to a potassium imbalance. The AGACNP knows:

A. To avoid use in patients taking angiotensin-converting enzyme if possible
B. To reduce the dose by 50% in a patient with chronic liver disease
C. That this antibiotic will treat streptococcal pharyngitis
D. That drug clearance is unchanged in chronic kidney disease (CKD)

114. The AGACNP is ready to discharge a patient who is hospitalized for acute graft-versus-host disease (GVHD). The patient weighs 67 kg and takes cyclosporine 3 mg/kg/day intravenously (IV). How many 100-mg capsules of cyclosporine per day will the AGACNP prescribe to transition the patient to oral therapy?

A. 3
B. 4
C. 2
D. 6

115. Management of a thyroid storm includes blunting the action of the sympathetic nervous system with an agent, such as propranolol, and blocking the formation and release of thyroid hormone with another agent, such as:

A. Liothyronine
B. Methimazole
C. Mycophenolate
D. Hydrocortisone

116. A patient presents 4 weeks after a total thyroidectomy with sluggishness, weight gain, and edema and is so drowsy and confused that their accompanying family member must provide the patient's past medical history. The patient did not fill medication prescriptions after the surgery, which included levothyroxine (Synthoid). Vital signs today reveal heart rate of 58 beats/min, blood pressure of 114/90 mmHg, oral temperature of 96.2°F (35.7°C), and normal arterial oxygen saturation (SaO_2). A cardiac workup is negative for an acute process. The toxicology screen is negative. The basic metabolic panel reveals a serum sodium of 128 mEq/L (135–145 mEq/L), cortisol of 6 mcg/dL (6–23 mcg/dL), thyroid-stimulating hormone (TSH) of 32 mIU/L (0.5–5 mIU/L), and free T4 of 0.2 ng/dL (0.8–1.8 ng/dL). The chest x-ray is notable for pulmonary congestion and cardiomegaly. What is the AGACNP's most likely differential diagnosis?

A. Encephalitis
B. Angioedema
C. Anaphylaxis
D. Myxedema

117. To treat emergent hyperkalemia in a patient with diabetes who is euglycemic, the AGACNP chooses 50 g intravenous (IV) dextrose and:

A. Albuterol via nebulizer treatment
B. Regular insulin given IV
C. Sodium polystyrene sulfonate
D. Metoprolol given IV

118. What hearing test is performed by placing a tuning fork on the mastoid bone and then in front of the ear canal?

A. Weber
B. Rinne
C. Whisper
D. Audiogram

119. Which condition is an indication for negative-pressure wound therapy (NPWT)?

A. Infected diabetic foot ulcer
B. Dehisced surgical wound
C. Pressure injury covered in eschar
D. Arterial ulcer

120. A patient presents with a suspected asthma exacerbation. What test would the AGACNP order to evaluate the degree of airflow obstruction for this patient?

A. Arterial blood gas
B. Bronchial provocation testing
C. Spirometry
D. Chest x-ray

121. What is the smallest variation in peak expiratory flow (PEF) value that suggests inadequate control of asthma?

A. 5%
B. 10%
C. 20%
D. 50%

122. What test would the AGACNP order to determine if a patient with asthma is eligible for anti-interleukin-5 therapy?

A. Spirometry
B. Arterial blood gas
C. Chest x-ray
D. Absolute eosinophil count

123. A patient with asthma has a peak expiratory flow (PEF) of 180 L/min. The AGACNP interprets this value as:

A. Normal airflow
B. Mild airflow obstruction
C. Moderate airflow obstruction
D. Severe airflow obstruction

124. What is the most common cause of community-acquired pneumonia?

A. Viruses
B. *Streptococcus pneumoniae*
C. *Legionella pneumophila*
D. *Pseudomonas aeruginosa*

125. The AGACNP would expect what lab abnormality in a patient with bronchitis-predominant chronic obstructive pulmonary disease (COPD)?

A. Elevated hemoglobin
B. Decreased hematocrit
C. Elevated creatinine
D. Decreased platelet count

126. Which patient would the AGACNP diagnose as having hospital-acquired pneumonia (HAP)?

A. 72-year-old patient who was admitted to the hospital 24 hours ago and now has fever and leukocytosis
B. 51-year-old patient who presents to the emergency department with leukocytosis, fever, and parenchymal opacities on chest CT
C. 48-year-old patient who was intubated 3 days ago and now has purulent sputum and leukocytosis
D. 60-year-old patient who was admitted to the hospital 5 days ago and now has fever, purulent sputum, and parenchymal opacities on chest CT

127. A patient presents with a new, unexplained right-sided pleural effusion on chest x-ray. What is the *best* next step in the diagnostic workup?

A. Chest CT
B. Echocardiogram
C. Bronchoalveolar lavage
D. Thoracentesis

128. What lab abnormality is expected in acute pancreatitis?

A. Decreased lipase
B. Elevated amylase
C. Hypokalemia
D. Hyperkalemia

129. What value on arterial blood gas constitutes respiratory failure?

A. Partial pressure of carbon dioxide (pCO_2) 45 mmHg
B. Partial pressure of oxygen (pO_2) 64 mmHg
C. pCO_2 55 mmHg
D. pO_2 70 mmHg

130. The AGACNP is evaluating a patient with alcohol-induced hepatic injury. What lab pattern would the AGACNP expect to see?

A. Aspartate aminotransferase (AST) 160, alanine transaminase (ALT) 70
B. AST 900, ALT 850
C. AST 50, ALT 120
D. AST 20, ALT 33

131. The AGACNP is evaluating a patient with suspected hepatocellular jaundice. What lab value would the AGACNP expect to be decreased?

A. Direct bilirubin
B. Indirect bilirubin
C. Serum albumin
D. Prothrombin time

132. The AGACNP evaluates a patient with suspected mitral valve regurgitation. What diagnostic study is the best to confirm this diagnosis?

A. Echocardiogram
B. EKG
C. Chest CT
D. Cardiac catheterization

133. An older adult patient reports clear rhinorrhea triggered by cold air and perfume. Which will the AGACNP choose as the initial treatment?

A. Fluticasone (Flovent)
B. Loratadine (Claritin)
C. Fexofenadine (Allegra)
D. Amoxicillin and clavulanate acid (Augmentin)

134. An older adult patient reports rhinorrhea for 1 week with no other associated symptoms. The AGACNP notes erythematous nasal mucosa and clear nasal discharge. What is the AGACNP's differential diagnosis?

A. Viral rhinitis
B. Vasomotor rhinitis
C. Bacterial pneumonia
D. Viral pneumonia

135. An adult patient reports sore throat and fever over the past 4 days. Examination reveals exudative tonsillopharyngitis and tender anterior cervical adenopathy. Which is the AGACNP's priority differential diagnosis?

A. Squamous cell carcinoma
B. Oral candidiasis
C. Group A beta-hemolytic streptococcal infection
D. Hairy leukoplakia

136. A new patient is seen in the AGACNP's clinic for complaints of a nagging cough that has been going on for the "last few months." The 63-year-old patient has a medical history of asthma, hypertension, hyperlipidemia, chronic gastroesophageal reflux disease, and current 1- to 2-pack per day smoking history of over 35 years. They describe their cough as productive, consisting of white or yellow sputum. The patient states that they use their spouse's albuterol (Ventolin) inhaler "once in a while" with only mild relief and have not been to the doctor "for some time." They also report that they experience wheezing on occasion and shortness of breath with exertion. Based on this presentation, the AGACNP suspects emphysema. The AGACNP will perform an exam that will indicate elevated right-sided heart pressures. What is this exam called?

A. Jugular venous examination
B. Lincoln sign
C. Ankle-brachial index test
D. Cullen's sign

137. Which screening tool would be ordered to determine metastasis when a patient's repeat prostate-specific antigen (PSA) is 11.8 ng/mL?

A. Digital rectal examination
B. 4Kscore PSA testing
C. Transrectal ultrasonography (US)
D. CT of abdomen and pelvis

138. A patient presents to the ED after sustaining a head injury. The patient's Glasgow Coma Scale (GCS) score is 8. How would the AGACNP classify the severity of the patient's head injury based on their GCS scoring?

A. No injury
B. Mild
C. Moderate
D. Severe

139. The AGACNP is ordering an insulin infusion and fluid replacement for a patient with diabetic ketoacidosis. What rule does the AGACNP need to remember when caring for a patient with fluid deficit concerns?

A. Insulin therapy should start simultaneously with fluid deficit correction.
B. Insulin therapy should start first and then fluid replacement 2 hours later.
C. Insulin therapy should start first and then fluid replacement 4 hours later.
D. Fluid replacement is initiated only if the patient has clinical signs of dehydration.

140. The AGACNP is caring for a patient in the emergency department who is alert and oriented but speaks limited English. They were transported this morning after an automobile crash with a fracture of the femur. The patient is awaiting orthopedic evaluation and is currently stable. No family members are present, and the AGACNP, who speaks only English, is waiting for the interpreter. What is the *best* method to evaluate the patient's current pain level?

A. Visual analog scale
B. Numeric rating scale
C. Interpreter
D. Vital signs

141. The AGACNP has just diagnosed a patient with *Heliobacter pylori* (*H. pylori*). The first-line recommended treatment regimen to treat this pathogen is a combination of:

A. Amoxicillin (Amoxil), ciprofloxacin (Cipro), and cimetidine (Tagamet)
B. Amoxicillin (Amoxil), rabeprazole sodium (Aciphex), and clarithromycin (Biaxin)
C. Amoxicillin (Amoxil), metoclopramide (Reglan), and cimetidine (Tagamet)
D. Amoxicillin (Amoxil), ciprofloxacin (Cipro), and sulfamethoxazole-trimethoprim (Bactrim)

142. The AGACNP rounds on the burn unit and examines a patient with a second-degree burn. The AGACNP notes that the wound is primarily covered with eschar and prescribes which topical antimicrobial agent?

A. Silver sulfadiazine 1% cream (Silvadene)
B. Mafenide acetate 10% cream (Sulfamylon)
C. Silver nitrate 0.5% in water
D. Triamcinolone 0.025% (Cinolar)

143. The AGACNP knows that a full-thickness pressure injury with tunneling and visible subcutaneous fat is an injury at which stage?

A. Stage 1
B. Stage 3
C. Stage 4
D. Unstageable

144. A patient presents to the emergency department after sustaining a chemical burn from lye while making homemade soap. The AGACNP's initial intervention reflects the understanding that neutralizing chemical burns with another chemical-based solution is contraindicated due to the risk for:

A. Tissue-damaging heat production
B. Chemical adherence to the skin
C. Crystallization within the dermis
D. Loss of motor function

145. The AGACNP is evaluating a patient in the ED who reports a new-onset complaint of "not being able to sit still." The patient is alert and oriented. Their medical history is significant for schizophrenia, and the patient reports that their psychiatrist changed their medication to fluphenazine (Modecate) 1 week ago. The patient is standing and pacing and appears restless and anxious. Based on these initial presenting symptoms, the AGACNP suspects which diagnosis?

A. Akathisia
B. Dystonia
C. Akinesia
D. Parkinson's disease

146. The AGACNP sees a patient with back pain caused by disk herniation. The AGACNP knows that this pain is classified as:

A. Mechanical
B. Visceral
C. Neuropathic
D. Nonmechanical

147. An alert and awake patient is transported to the ED by ambulance with a diagnosis of attempted suicide. The report from emergency medical services states that the patient was found "early enough" and was still conscious in their car within a closed garage with the motor running and a suicide note on the seat. In acute carbon monoxide poisoning with this origin and description, what other signs, symptoms, or findings should the AGACNP look for?

A. Irregular heart rate
B. Low blood glucose
C. Smoke inhalation
D. Rectal bleeding

148. The AGACNP is seeing a patient in the clinic with a chief complaint of unilateral hand pain. The patient reports nocturnal hand numbness, dropping of objects, and difficulty with twisting lids off jars. The AGACNP has the patient perform forced flexion of the wrist and notes reproduction of symptoms. The AGACNP will confirm the suspected diagnosis by ordering what gold standard of diagnostics for the suspected diagnosis?

A. Electromyogram
B. Nerve conduction test
C. Ultrasound of wrist
D. Two-view radiographs

149. A normal finding on a digital rectal prostate exam is best described as:

A. Reported tenderness on palpation
B. Prostate approximately 5 cm wide
C. Smooth surface of the prostate
D. Nodule noted on palpation

150. Which of the following statements is *true* regarding active immunity?

A. It can be obtained with an injection of immunoglobulin.
B. It is short, lasting for about 3 months.
C. It provides immediate protection against disease.
D. It takes 2 to 4 weeks for the body to develop immunity.

151. A limitation of the Fracture Risk Assessment Tool (FRAX) is:

A. Measurement of bone mineral density (BMD) at femoral neck only
B. Score adjustment for chronic prednisone dosing up to 10 mg only
C. Measurement of BMD of wrist and vertebral spine only
D. Inclusion of recent hip but not vertebral fracture in the calculation

152. The AGACNP is called to the ICU to evaluate a postoperative patient who underwent a wound debridement of the right groin. The patient has been undergoing negative-pressure wound therapy, and three canisters have been filled with bloody output over the past 2 hours. The AGACNP's first intervention is to:

A. Order blood
B. Assess vital signs
C. Order a complete blood count
D. Contact the surgeon

153. The patient reports to the AGACNP: "I had my last tetanus shot about 12 years ago." The AGACNP explains that tetanus booster should be administered every:

A. 1 year
B. 5 years
C. 10 years
D. Season

154. A patient presents to the emergency department with stroke-like symptoms. CT of the head shows no evidence of hemorrhage; however, MRI reveals occlusion of the middle cerebral artery. Which condition noted in the patient's electronic medical record contraindicates the use of tissue plasminogen activator (tPA)?

A. Gastrointestinal bleed 2 years previously
B. Cerebral vascular accident 6 months previously
C. Appendectomy 10 days previously
D. History of hypertension stage 1

155. The AGACNP is educating a group of nursing students on management of acute cerebral vascular accident. Per treatment guidelines, how many hours after onset of symptoms is a patient a candidate for tissue plasminogen activator (tPA)?

A. 3
B. 6
C. 9
D. 12

156. Which modifiable risk factor is most commonly associated with chronic obstructive pulmonary disease (COPD)?

A. Alcohol consumption
B. Secondhand smoke exposure
C. Environmental pollutant exposure
D. Cigarette smoking

157. The AGACNP is educating a patient with a fasting blood glucose of 105 mg/dL on interventions associated with delaying or preventing the development of type 2 diabetes mellitus (DM). Which statement by the patient indicates that they understand?

A. "If I focus on diet and exercise, I may delay or prevent progression to diabetes."
B. "I am going to get diabetes no matter what I do."
C. "I should start a metformin (Glucophage) regimen now."
D. "As long as I exercise, I can continue to eat however I want."

158. While reviewing the health history of an adult patient, the AGACNP notes hypertension and hyperlipidemia but no other significant history. How often should this patient have their lipid profile checked?

A. Every 6 months
B. Yearly
C. Every 2 years
D. Every 5 years

159. The AGACNP is caring for an older adult patient who has recently been diagnosed with type 2 diabetes mellitus. The patient has numerous comorbidities, poor functional status, and a limited life expectancy. Which target hemoglobin A1C (HbA1C) level is appropriate for this patient?

A. 6.5%
B. 7.0%
C. 7.5%
D. 8.0%

160. How many months after the initial dose of the herpes zoster vaccine will the AGACNP recommend that a 75-year-old patient who is immunocompetent receive their second dose?

A. 1
B. 2 to 6
C. 12
D. 24

161. Review of a 60-year-old patient's electronic medical record shows that the patient has had three consecutive negative Pap smears. The AGACNP will recommend that the patient discontinue testing at what age?

A. 60 years
B. 65 years
C. 70 years
D. 75 years

162. Through which age is the human papillomavirus (HPV) vaccine most effective?

A. 18 years
B. 26 years
C. 30 years
D. 40 years

163. A patient has been diagnosed with uncomplicated gonorrhea. The chlamydia test is negative. The AGACNP prescribes ceftriaxone (Recophin) 500 mg:

A. Intramuscularly once
B. Orally once daily for 7 days
C. Orally twice daily for 7 days
D. Orally once daily for 14 days

164. A patient with a history of coronary artery disease has been prescribed ibuprofen (Motrin) for management of osteoarthritis. The AGACNP understands that this drug carries a boxed warning because:

A. The patient's bleeding risk decreases due to platelet aggregation.
B. The patient is at risk for elevated blood sugar levels.
C. There is an increased risk of a cardiovascular thrombotic event.
D. Studies do not support use of nonsteroidal anti-inflammatory drugs (NSAIDs) for osteoarthritis.

165. Which treatment regimen will the AGACNP prescribe for a patient diagnosed with chlamydia?

A. Azithromycin (Zithromax) 1 g orally once daily for 7 days
B. Doxycycline (Doxycin) 100 mg orally twice daily for 7 days
C. Doxycycline (Doxycin) 100 mg orally once daily for 14 days
D. Levofloxacin (Levaquin) 500 mg orally once daily for 14 days

166. Which vaccine is contraindicated in patients with symptomatic HIV?

A. Varicella
B. Tetanus
C. Hepatitis B
D. Pneumococcal

167. A young adult is brought to the emergency department after ingesting a bottle of alprazolam (Xanax) 45 minutes before arrival. The patient has decreased level of consciousness and is having periods of extended apnea. The AGACNP will prioritize which intervention?

A. Administering flumazenil (Romazicon)
B. Preparing for endotracheal intubation
C. Administering charcoal
D. Obtaining baseline laboratory studies

168. Which treatment is in accordance with first-line therapy guidelines for a patient diagnosed with uncomplicated acute cystitis?

A. Sulfamethoxazole/trimethoprim (Bactrim) 160/800 mg orally every 12 hours for 3 days
B. Ciprofloxacin (Cipro) 250 mg orally every 12 hours for 3 days
C. Levofloxacin (Levaquin) 250 mg orally every 24 hours for 3 days
D. Cephalexin (Keflex) 500 mg orally every 6 to 12 hours for 7 days

169. How would the AGACNP describe red blood cells (RBCs) in patients with folic acid deficiency?

A. Macrocytic, normochromic
B. Microcytic, hypochromic
C. Hemolytic
D. Normocytic, normochromic

170. A male patient has been diagnosed with acute epididymitis secondary to chlamydia. What treatment regimen will the AGACNP prescribe?

A. Ceftriaxone (Rocephin) 500 mg intramuscularly once plus doxycycline (Doxycin) 100 mg orally twice a day for 10 days
B. Ceftriazone (Rocephin) 250 mg intramuscularly once
C. Levofloxacin (Levaquin) 500 mg orally once per day for 10 days
D. Ofloxacin (Floxin) 300 mg orally twice a day for 10 days

171. The AGACNP is following an established patient in primary care who completed their first round of chemotherapy for stage IIIA colon cancer last week at an outpatient infusion center. Today, the patient's hemoglobin level is 8.3 g/dL. Based on this finding, what medication will the AGACNP prescribe for this patient?

A. Fondaparinux (Arixtra)
B. Gefitinib (Iressa)
C. Ondansetron (Zofran)
D. Epoetin alfa (Procrit)

172. Reagent strip testing for nitrites to detect urinary tract infections has:

A. High sensitivity, high specificity
B. High sensitivity, low specificity
C. Low sensitivity, high specificity
D. Low sensitivity, low specificity

173. A patient with a history of recurrent sinus and pulmonary infections as well as a recent diagnosis of rheumatoid arthritis presents to a clinic. Which laboratory value will the AGACNP treat as most important?

A. Immunoglobulin A (IgA)
B. Complete blood count (CBC)
C. Erythrocyte sedimentation rate (ESR)
D. C-reactive protein (CRP)

174. A patient comes to the urgent care clinic for complaints of an "unusual" vaginal discharge, dysuria, and pain in the lower abdomen. The AGACNP performs a pelvic examination and notes that the vaginal discharge is purulent and yellow-green in color. The cervix is friable with positive cervical motion tenderness. What diagnosis does the AGACNP suspect?

A. Vaginal yeast infection
B. Urinary tract infection
C. Gonorrhea
D. Cervical cancer

175. The AGACNP educates a patient's family that the best way to reduce the risk of infection is to:

A. Wear a face mask
B. Wash hands often
C. Cook all vegetables
D. Take prophylactic antibiotics

5

Practice Exam 1 Answers

1. D) X-ray

The patient is presenting with signs and symptoms of pneumonia. The most efficient and cost-effective radiologic exam indicated for this differential diagnosis is a chest x-ray. An MRI of the chest would provide advanced images of all chest structures and is often indicated if an abnormality has been identified on a lower level of radiologic imaging. A CT scan of the chest adequately diagnoses pneumonia, but it is not the most efficient test due to radiation exposure, time, and cost. A chest CT scan with angiography is indicated for patients suspected to have a pulmonary embolism, not pneumonia.

2. D) Venous Doppler ultrasound

Venous Doppler ultrasounds are the least invasive and most cost-efficient diagnostic study for diagnosing DVT. An x-ray shows only the bony structures of the leg and is unable to assess for DVT. D-dimer is a laboratory study that assesses for the presence of fibrin degradation in the blood and is not specific to DVT. Lung perfusion studies assess for pulmonary embolism, not DVT.

3. D) Systolic blood pressure ≥140 mmHg or diastolic blood pressure ≥90 mmHg

The ACC and AHA classify a systolic blood pressure of ≥140 mmHg or a diastolic blood pressure of ≥90 mmHg as stage II hypertension. A systolic blood pressure of <120 mmHg and a diastolic blood pressure of <80 mmHg is considered normal. A systolic blood pressure of 120 to 129 mmHg and a diastolic blood pressure of <80 mmHg is considered elevated, and a systolic blood pressure of 130 to 139 mmHg or a diastolic blood pressure of 80 to 90 mmHg is categorized as stage I hypertension.

4. A) Metabolic syndrome

Metabolic syndrome is a cluster of conditions that increase one's risk for stroke, diabetes, and heart disease. The diagnosis is made if the patient exhibits at least three of the following conditions: triglycerides 150 mg/dL or higher; abdominal obesity; high-density lipoprotein less than 40 mg/dL in men or less than 50 mg/dL in women; fasting glucose 110 mg/dL or greater; and hypertension. Myocardial hibernation is a condition in which parts of the heart are underperfused. Coronary artery disease is a potential consequence of metabolic syndrome but is not reflected itself by this patient.

5. D) Prescribes a cholesterol absorption inhibitor

Patients with a documented history of coronary artery disease should have a goal LDL of less than 70 mg/dL. The next appropriate intervention would be to prescribe a cholesterol absorption inhibitor such as ezetimibe (Zetia). Encouraging diet and lifestyle modification is a complementary intervention but is not sufficient to prevent the progression of cardiovascular disease. Starting an omega-3 fatty acid supplement would also be helpful, but data does not indicate this intervention alone would adequately reduce LDL levels to the goal.

6. C) Cardiac stress test

The patient is eliciting symptoms consistent with angina. A cardiac stress test is a noninvasive test that can help in diagnosing and determining the severity of angina. EKG and echocardiogram can diagnose other cardiac issues but will usually be normal with angina. A cardiac angiogram may be indicated if angina is present, but it would not be the best diagnostic exam at this point.

7. D) Thyroid-stimulating hormone

Thyroid-stimulating hormone is the best and most sensitive screening test for primary hypothyroidism with an increased value indicating hypothyroidism. Free T4 and free T3 may be decreased with hypothyroidism but should not be used as an initial screening tool. Thyroglobulin may be increased in thyroid cancer.

8. C) Subclinical hypothyroidism

Subclinical hypothyroidism is characterized by an elevated TSH and a normal free T4 level. It is common in older adults. Hypothyroidism is typically characterized by an elevated TSH and a low free T4 level. Hyperthyroidism is typically characterized by a low TSH and a high free T4 level. Autoimmune thyroiditis can present as either hyperthyroidism or hypothyroidism.

9. B) MRI of the brain

An MRI of the brain with gadolinium is the best imaging test to identify brain lesions clearly. A CT of the head is less sensitive at identifying smaller tumors. EEG is used to detect seizure activity. A PET scan of the brain may be helpful in certain clinical scenarios but is typically not the best imaging modality for diagnosis of brain tumors.

10. D) History of generalized anxiety disorder

A psychiatric comorbidity such as anxiety increases one's risk for a suicide attempt. Female sex assigned at birth and having close ties (e.g., to family, to church) are considered suicide-inhibiting factors.

11. B) Bipolar I disorder

Bipolar I disorder is characterized by mood shifts of manic episodes alternating with depressive episodes. Major depressive disorder and bipolar II disorder do not include manic episodes. Hypothyroidism may cause some changes in mood but would typically not cause mania.

12. B) Spirometry

Spirometry helps to identify reversible versus irreversible airflow obstruction by testing expiratory volume before and after bronchodilator use. It should be done as part of asthma evaluation. Arterial blood gas testing and chest x-ray are typically normal with asthma. Bronchial provocation testing should be done only if spirometry is not diagnostic.

13. B) Older adults have decreased lacrimal secretions.

Older adults experience a reduction in lacrimal secretions, which leads to dry eyes. Older adults are at increased risk of narrow-angle glaucoma. Visual acuity begins to decline after age 40 years, not 30 years. Pupil size decreases with increasing age, so older adults tend to require increased lighting to perform tasks such as reading.

14. C) "You may experience abdominal cramping."

The patient should be counseled that bisacodyl (Dulcolax) may cause abdominal cramping because it works by stimulating colonic contractions. It is a stimulant, not an osmotic, laxative, and typically takes 6 to 8 hours to take effect. It should be used as a rescue agent, and daily use should be avoided.

15. C) Speaking slowly

Speaking in a slow-paced, low-tone voice helps patients with hearing loss understand more clearly. Speaking more loudly or quickly or in a high-tone voice can distort words, making it more difficult for the individual to understand. Speaking to the patient, rather than to the family, is always preferable.

16. A) "The cane should be used on your stronger side."

A cane is most effective when being used on an individual's stronger side. The height should reach the wrist when the arm is held straight down, not the hip. The patient should move the cane in unison with the weaker leg and hold the cane in place when moving the stronger leg. Canes are not necessarily more effective than walkers in preventing falls; proper equipment selection depends on the individual's needs.

17. A) Stress

Incontinence or leakage of urine that occurs with straining, such as sneezing, is considered stress incontinence. Urge incontinence is characterized by urgency and the inability to hold urine in the bladder. Overflow incontinence involves leakage that occurs due to the inability to completely empty the bladder. Functional incontinence results from a physical or mental impairment that prevents the individual from reaching bathroom facilities in time.

18. C) Furosemide (Lasix)

Furosemide (Lasix) and other diuretics are among the most common medications that cause transient urinary incontinence. Pantoprazole (Protonix), famotidine (Pepcid), and fluoxetine (Prozac) are not typically agents that cause this issue.

19. C) Delirium

Delirium is an acute, variable course of cognitive impairment. It is distinguished from dementia or Alzheimer's disease, which involve a gradual, progressive course of cognitive impairment. A cerebrovascular accident may cause cognitive impairment but is not, in itself, defined as such.

20. B) 2

A pressure injury with partial-thickness skin loss and exposed dermis is considered stage 2. Stage 1 is characterized by nonblanchable erythema of intact skin, stage 3 by full-thickness skin loss, and stage 4 by full-thickness skin and tissue loss.

21. C) Assessing the feasibility of discontinuing the drug

Medication use is a common, significant cause of falls and should be discontinued (as feasible) if it is found to be impacting patient safety. If discontinuation is not feasible, the AGACNP should explore other options. Ordering a medical alert system is most beneficial for patients who have difficulty getting up after falling. Physical therapy is most beneficial for patients who are experiencing strength and balance issues. Sleep hygiene will not address risks related to postural hypotension.

22. B) Saying, "Your spouse is at higher risk because of their status. I will order some heel-relief splints."

Because the patient's spouse is expressing verbal concerns about the patient's pressure injuries, this is a good time to educate the spouse about the patient's condition and describe the risk factors for pressure injury development. The AGACNP can also assure the spouse that staff will immediately address the injury by ordering off-loading devices. While it may eventually be appropriate to indicate that the injury was present upon admission, assigning blame elsewhere as a first response does not address the spouse's concern or emotional needs, and the AGACNP has no way to know for sure when and where the injuries occurred. While acknowledging the spouse's emotions is valid, limiting the response to that acknowledgment fails to address the specific concern the spouse expressed and may be seen as patronizing. Similarly, remaining silent is nontherapeutic and nonresponsive and may allow the spouse's stress to escalate.

23. D) Conducting a whispered voice test

Older adult patients should be asked if they are experiencing hearing impairment. If they answer no, they should still be screened with a whispered voice test rather than simply asked again at the next visit. Asking the patient's family may be beneficial, but it is not the most appropriate next step. Referral to audiometry should take place if the patient answers affirmatively or if they fail the whispered voice test.

24. D) Asking Human Resources to assist with guidance on how to proceed with this allegation

The manager has received a claim of behavior that may negatively impact patient care and that is illegal at the federal level. The manager will contact the Human Resources department for guidance on how to proceed. If an investigation is required, including interviewing the person who witnessed the alleged event, Human Resources should coordinate it. Failing to take any action on the report is inappropriate; if the allegation is true, the provider's behavior may place patients at risk. Meeting with the provider prior to coordinating with Human Resources is inappropriate and unwise.

25. B) Telling the son, "The exam may require your mother to disrobe. Could you leave the room briefly until she can dress again?"

The AGACNP should consider the possibility of abuse and try to interview the patient in private to assess further and to inquire about the patient's safety. By keeping the focus on the exam and asking the son to leave "briefly," the AGACNP may be able to speak with the patient alone without rousing the son's suspicion. Telling the son that the injuries are inconsistent with his description may increase his suspicion—if abuse truly is occurring—and decrease the likelihood he will leave the patient alone with the AGACNP. Emphasizing the need to hear directly from the patient may have a similar effect. Asking the patient in the son's presence is unlikely to be helpful; the patient already appears to be unwilling to speak while the son is present. Additionally, asking, "Did you really fall down the stairs?" is accusatory, which may be counterproductive if abuse is taking place and unfair to the son if it is not.

26. A) Decreased gait speed

Slower or decreased ambulation or gait speed is one indicator of frailty, along with unintentional weight loss (not increased body mass index), muscle weakness, fatigue, and low physical activity. Hearing loss and forgetfulness are frequently associated with normal aging and are not signs of frailty.

27. C) "Your loved one may be able to hear you."

In order to ease tensions and redirect the family back to the patient's present condition, it would be best to point out that the patient may still be able to hear. Asking the family to continue the argument at another time, or stating that the argument is audible in the hallway, may come across as condescending or lecturing, and it fails to place the focus on the patient. It may be true that the family is disturbing other patients, but focusing initially on their own family member may be more effective.

28. C) Possesses effective communication skills

Having effective and professional communication skills that encourage collaboration and team-building is a positive attribute of a good leader. An AGACNP with emotional intelligence who is approachable, respectful, and instrumental in conflict resolution exhibits the characteristics of a good leader. Effective leadership does not necessarily require being the best clinical performer on the team. Therefore, exhibiting the greatest degree of clinical knowledge is not required; similarly, while providing care that is completely free from errors is ideal (and is certainly the goal), it is not necessarily representative of leadership ability. Never taking a sick day does not depict leadership; in fact, reporting to work while ill could be considered irresponsible.

29. C) "Let me speak to the nurse manager and see what we can do."

As a healthcare professional, the AGACNP is viewed as a clinical leader and therefore is expected to conduct themselves as a positive role model while communicating to all stakeholders using empathy, understanding, and respect. Although it may be easy to initially dismiss this family member's unrealistic request, the AGACNP needs to maintain a calm, reassuring manner and attempt to find a way to solve the underlying problem (e.g., using volunteers from the family, assigning a low-height bed, placing protective floor mats). Although it is true that the hospital cannot assign staff to sit with the patient full-time, merely stating that does not address the family member's legitimate concern about their parent or the impression that the AGACNP takes the patient's health and safety seriously. On the other hand, immediately agreeing to the sitter request is unrealistic and risks offending the family member when the AGACNP inevitably has to break that commitment.

30. D) Role-play

Since this is an educational presentation addressing the effective delivery of a telehealth patient visit, participants can engage actively in the learning by using the equipment and engaging in role-play to practice the visits. Verbal lecturing, self-learning modules, or group discussion may not be as beneficial as the hands-on, kinesthetic learning approach.

31. C) Help them sign up for a free meal delivery service through the local senior center

Setting the patient up with a free community meal delivery service for seniors and the homebound population is the best approach at this time. Unless the nearest food kitchen is very close to the patient, expecting them to use the facility is unreasonable; the patient no longer drives, and although they walk short distances, they should not be expected to walk longer distances while carrying food items. A patient with this financial situation is likely already stretching their food budget; the meal delivery service provides nutrition without additional financial sacrifice. While it may be appropriate to teach the patient about the importance of nutrition and a healthy BMI—if the patient is not already aware—this education would not address the patient's need for adequate nutrition on a regular basis.

32. C) Provide feedback, including mention of the shortcuts. Mention that no patient harm was identified.

Providing honest, fair, and objective feedback as a peer reviewer is the ethical approach because patient advocacy is one of the primary values for a healthcare professional to adhere to. Avoiding mention of the shortcuts—either by omitting it from feedback or by asking to be excused from providing feedback—fails to advocate for the patient and to provide the best care. It also may leave the colleague unaware of their performance deficiency and, therefore, unable to correct it. If the AGACNP wishes to speak to the colleague about avoiding shortcuts and maintaining best practices, delaying that conversation until a scheduled performance review is inappropriate.

33. D) Being willing to listen to others' viewpoints

The willingness to listen to others' viewpoints is an important component of collaborating with the professional healthcare team as it can increase and clarify communication and understanding. Openness to other suggestions and feedback is crucial. Friendly relationships are not necessary; cordial, professional relationships are. It is unlikely that input from each team member should carry equal weight; different areas of expertise and scopes of practice mean that certain team members will have greater say depending on the situation. Although seniority may carry some weight in team dynamics, it is not appropriate to automatically defer to senior members, particularly when doing so would reduce the effectiveness or appropriateness of care or planning.

34. C) "At least one of your major arteries or its branches was at least 75% blocked."

Stenosis in blood vessels refers to narrowing of the lumen due to fatty or calcium deposits, and significant stenosis refers to narrowing of at least 75% of a major artery or its branches. It does not mean half of the coronary arteries are blocked, nor does it imply a major heart attack. It also does not refer to femoral artery hardening.

35. A) Allow patients to attain and act on health information in an informed way

Health literacy is the patient's ability to obtain, communicate, process, and understand health information with the ultimate goal of equipping them to effectively use that information to make appropriate health decisions. Providing information in the patient's primary language (e.g., through qualified interpreters), accounting for culture-specific needs in communication, and communicating using language that is easy to understand are ways in which the healthcare community can contribute to health literacy, but none is the primary goal.

36. B) "It is important to control your blood pressure to avoid worsening your LVH."

The most common cause of LVH is hypertension, and it is therefore important to maintain good blood pressure control to prevent worsening of the condition. It is genetically hereditary. It is not a normal variant. The AGACNP should encourage aerobic activity rather than discourage it.

37. B) Small intestine

The small intestine is responsible for breaking down fats into fatty acids and monoglycerides. Fat malabsorption manifests as unintentional weight loss as well as steatorrhea that is often described as "foul" or particularly smelly. The stomach and large intestine are responsible for digestion and absorption of other nutrients and substances. The liver plays a role in digestion but does not break down fats.

38. D) Glucose 305 mg/dL, bicarbonate 14 mEq/L, pH 7.1

DKA typically presents with a glucose level >300 mg/dL, acidosis (pH <7.3), and a low bicarbonate level (<18 mEq/L).

39. D) Amylase

Amylase is an enzyme present in the saliva and pancreas that breaks down starch into disaccharides. In pancreatitis, this enzyme is elevated and would be a strong indicator to use in confirming diagnosis. Uric acid is present in the stomach and helps break down food. It would be increased with a diagnosis of gout. Bile is produced by the liver and plays a role in other aspects of digestion. Cholinesterase would be a test used to determine nervous system dysfunction.

40. D) Fever for 4 days

While most cases of pyelonephritis do not require radiographic workup, fever lasting more than 72 hours warrants imaging, preferably with a CT scan. Urinary urgency and dysuria are typical symptoms of pyelonephritis and would not prompt the nurse to order imaging. Patient request for imaging should not necessarily prompt an order but rather patient education.

41. B) *Escherichia coli*

Escherichia coli accounts for 75% to 90% of community-acquired UTI cases. *Staphylococcus saprophyticus* causes approximately 10% to 15% of cases. *Klebsiella pneumonia* and *Proteus mirabilis* are more rare pathogens seen in UTIs.

42. A) Diphenhydramine (Benadryl)

Antihistamines such as diphenhydramine (Benadryl) are associated with sedation, which may increase in the older adult population. This can increase risk for falls. Extended use, although unlikely in this scenario, can contribute to cognitive deterioration. Second-generation antihistamines such as loratadine may be a safer option. Topical creams and lotions such as pramoxine/calamine are beneficial over-the-counter options with little side effect profile.

43. C) Nephrotoxicity

Nephrotoxicity is a major limiting factor with the use of aminoglycoside antibiotics. Nephrotoxicity is estimated to occur in nearly 30% of acutely ill patients, notably with a baseline serum creatinine of 0.5 mg/dL. Nephrotoxicity is associated with a reduction in glomerular filtration rate, increased serum creatinine, and increased urea nitrogen. Although ototoxicity is another limiting factor, visual toxicity is much less likely.

44. B) Adrenal suppression

The diffuse application of topical glucocorticoid preparations can lead to adrenal suppression due to absorption of high fluorinated steroid concentrations. Absorption leads to suppression of the hypothalamus-pituitary-adrenal axis, causing inefficient production of cortisol. Diffuse application will not lead to an increase in adrenal production. Although irritation may be present with excessive use, extensive burns to the skin are not likely with diffuse application of a glucocorticoid. Topical glucocorticoid use does not cause an increase in peripheral perfusion.

45. B) Metformin 500 mg once daily

When formulating a clinical question, PICO is often used to evaluate the effectiveness of an intervention. PICO refers to the following: the relevant patient *p*opulation, the *i*ntervention being considered, the *c*omparison intervention or patient population, and the *o*utcomes of interest. In this case, the patient population is patients with type 2 diabetes mellitus. When formulating the PICO question, it is essential to specify the intervention being considered, which in this case is treatment with metformin. The dose, timing, and duration of treatment should be considered. The comparison can be a placebo, usual care, or other treatment, which in this case is treatment with glipizide. The outcome of a clinical question, in this case blood glucoses, should be well-defined, measurable, reliable, and sensitive to change, and should assess clinically relevant aspects of a patient's health.

46. C) Applying the best available research medicine, combined with clinical expertise and patient preference

Evidence-based practice involves the use of current best practice to facilitate decision-making about patient care. The basic elements are formulating specific clinical questions, finding the best available evidence that is relevant and current, assessing the validity of the evidence (including internal and external validity), and applying the evidence in practice, in combination with clinical expertise and patient preferences.

47. A) Patient population

A well-developed PICO question helps the AGACNP search for focused evidence. When formulating questions regarding the effectiveness of an intervention, the following four components should be considered: *p*atient population, *i*ntervention, *c*omparison, and *o*utcomes (PICO). Validity (including internal and external validity) is important to consider when AGACNPs assess and evaluate research articles that are important to their practice. Internal validity considers whether the results of clinical research are correct for the patients studied. Bias and chance can threaten internal validity. Chance is random error, common in all observations. While obstacles are inevitable and may make research difficult, it should not interfere with moving forward with the clinical research study.

48. D) Meta-analysis of randomized controlled trials, case-controlled studies, expert opinion

Meta-analysis of randomized controlled trials and systematic reviews are the two highest levels of evidence, followed by randomized controlled trials, then controlled trials without randomization, cohort studies, case-controlled and cross-sectional studies, descriptive and qualitative studies, and then expert opinion.

49. B) Bias

Bias includes any systematic error that can produce a misleading impression of a true effect. While randomized controlled trials are conducted with the consideration of reducing all potential sources of bias, there is a potential for a low risk of bias, and flaws can produce biased results. A potential source of bias is failure to blind relevant individuals (including study participants, clinicians, data collectors, outcome adjudicators, and data analysts) to group assignment. Chance is random error, common in all observations. Indirect evidence occurs when a study involves a somewhat different population than is of interest to the researcher. Even though it does not apply to the population being studied, it can still help inform medical decision-making. A lower statistical power can be seen when fewer subjects are used than needed to detect a true effect.

50. A) Wikipedia

Keeping current with evidence-based practice is not feasible without a reliable source. Many resources are available online, but just because a source is online and easily accessible does not mean it is evidence based. Wikipedia entries can have major omissions and have been deemed inadequate to use for evidence-based practice. Medical articles can be accessed by a multitude of other databases; for example, with the use of PubMed, CINAHL, Ovid, Medical Literature Analysis and Retrieval System online, and UpToDate.

51. C) External validity

External validity refers to whether the study can be applied to patients outside of the study, particularly the specific patient (or population) being considered. Internal validity refers to whether the results of the clinical research are correct for the patients studied. Sensitivity refers to the number of patients who have the disease screen or test positive for the disease (true positives). Specificity refers to those who do not have the disease and screen or test negative for the disease (true negative).

52. A) Specificity

Specificity refers to those who do not have the disease and screen or test negative for the disease (true negative). A test with high specificity will rarely identify patients as having a disease when they do not (i.e., few false-positive results). Sensitivity refers to the number of patients who have the disease who screen or test positive for the disease (true positives). A test with high sensitivity will not miss many patients who have the disease (i.e., few false-negative results). The positive predictive value of a test represents the likelihood that a patient with a positive test has the disease; the negative predictive value represents the likelihood that a patient who has a negative test is free of the disease. A false negative (i.e., negative predictive value) would occur if the patient truly has the condition and the result from the screening test is negative.

53. D) Sensitivity

Sensitivity refers to the number of patients who have the disease who screen or test positive for the disease (true positives). A test with high sensitivity will not miss many patients who have the disease (i.e., few false-negative results). Specificity refers to those who do not have the disease and screen or test negative for the disease (true negative). A test with high specificity will rarely identify patients as having a disease when they do not (i.e., few false-positive results). The positive predictive value of a test represents the likelihood that a patient with a positive test has the disease; the negative predictive value represents the likelihood that a patient who has a negative test is free of the disease. A false positive (i.e., positive predictive value) would occur if the patients does not have the condition and the result from the screening test is positive.

54. B) Incidence

Incidence represents the number of new events that have occurred in a specific time interval. It describes the frequency with which a disease or disorder appears in a particular population or area at a given time. Prevalence refers to the number of individuals with a given disease at a given point in time. This involves the proportion of a population that is affected by a disease or disorder at a particular time. The relative risk is often done in a cohort study and can be calculated by dividing the incidence of exposed individuals by the incidence of unexposed individuals. The odds ratio is used in case-control studies and refers to the odds that an individual with a specific condition has been exposed to a risk factor.

55. D) They can be interpreted as a range of believable values that is likely to include the true value.

Confidence intervals are a way to show the range of reasonable and likely values after statistics are performed on gathered data. Confidence intervals and *p*-values cannot be used to directly infer how confident one should be in a result. Often, confidence intervals are interpreted as representing a range of believable values. It provides a degree of assurance or confidence that the interval actually contains the true value. A small confidence interval implies a very precise range of values. A single value from a sample population may not reflect the true value from the entire population. As such, a confidence interval is helpful to provide a range that is likely to include the true value. The confidence intervals are calculated based upon the number of observations and the standard deviation of the data.

56. C) It is a measure of the effect of chance within a study.

Statistical testing is performed on results once data is gathered from the study to assess the likelihood that a certain result would have occurred given some assumptions about the population being studied. A *p*-value is the statistical test that is a measure of the effect of chance within a study. It is not the probability that the result of the study is true or correct. Instead, it is the likelihood that if the null hypothesis were true, and if the results were not affected by bias, then one would see a result as extreme or even bigger than that seen in the study. A confidence interval is used to show the range of values that could be considered reasonably likely after statistical analysis is performed on gathered data. Confidence intervals and *p*-values cannot be used to directly infer how confident one should be in a result. Often, a *p*-value of 0.05 and a confidence interval of 95% is often the conventional cutoff point to decide if a study had statistically significant results. Regardless, a smaller *p*-value is in favor of stronger evidence compared to those with a *p*-value closer to or above 0.05.

57. A) Type I error

A type I error is incorrectly concluding that there is a statistically significant difference in a data set; the probably of making a type I error is known as alpha. This leads to a decision to reject the null hypothesis, when in fact likely random chance or variations that occurred within the sample led to a mistaken conclusion that there was an effect. A type II error is incorrectly concluding that there was no statistically significant difference in a dataset; random chance leads to a mistaken conclusion that there was no effect. Power refers to the ability of a study to detect a true difference; it is the statistical probably of avoiding a type II error. Often, negative findings may reflect that the study was underpowered to detect a difference. Whenever a study finds no statistically significant difference, there is concern as to if there was adequate power. It is necessary to look at the confidence intervals and see whether clinically important values exist within the range. Since this study found a significant difference due to a type I error, there is little concern for insufficient power as this often reflects a type II error. Reliability refers to the consistency of a measurement or the degree to which repeated measurements fall closely to each other. Since this study was only completed once, it is difficult to interpret the reliability.

58. C) Cohort study

This is an example of a cohort study because there is a clearly identified group of people to be studied. The cohort uses a group of individuals who are alike in many ways (nurses) but differ by a certain characteristic (dietary intake). A cohort study often moves forward to observing the outcome of interest, even if the data is collected retrospectively over time. A case-control study starts with the outcome of interest and moves backward to the exposure. This is particularly useful for uncommon diseases in which a very large cohort would be required to accumulate enough cases for analysis. A randomized controlled trial includes experimental manipulation of variables using randomization and a control group to test the effects of an intervention or experiment. A systematic review is a comprehensive summary of all available evidence that meets certain eligibility criteria to address a specific clinical question or range of questions.

59. B) Kappa statistic

The kappa statistic is the most common measurement for assessing interobserver agreement. The value for perfect agreement is 1.0; the value is 0 if expected by chance alone. Standard deviation measures the variability of data around the mean; it provides information on how much variability can be expected among individuals within a population. Confidence intervals are a way to show the range of reasonable and likely values after statistics are performed on gathered data. It provides a degree of assurance or confidence that the interval actually contains the true value. The level of significance is the probability level of which the results of statistical analysis are judged to indicate a statistically significant difference between groups.

60. D) Case-control study

A case-control study moves backward to the exposure, starting with the outcome of interest. Patients with a disease are identified and compared with controls for exposures to a risk factor. This is particularly useful for uncommon diseases in which a very large cohort would be required to accumulate enough cases for analysis. A randomized controlled trial includes experimental manipulation of variables using randomization and a control group to test the effects of an intervention or experiment. A systematic review is a comprehensive summary of all available evidence that meets certain eligibility criteria to address a specific clinical question or range of questions. The cohort study uses a group of individuals who are alike in many ways but differ by a certain characteristic. A cohort study often moves forward to observing the outcome of interest, even if the data is collected retrospectively over time.

61. C) They rely on systematic reviews and include cost-effective approaches to patient care.

Clinical practice guidelines are developed as a decision-making aid to caregivers. They represent a combination of systematic reviews, original research, clinical expertise, and patient preferences. This comprehensive synthesis of the best available evidence provides guidelines that the practitioner can consider when making cost-effective approaches to patient care. However, the quality of published guidelines can vary and may differ based on each sponsored professional organization. Additionally, multiple guidelines on the same topic can make contradictory recommendations and discrepancies exist from major organizations. Guidelines cannot also be expected to account for the uniqueness of each patient and their illness. Standards have been set forth for guideline development and include that they rely on systematic reviews, grade the quality of available evidence, grade the strength of recommendations, and make an explicit connection between evidence and recommendations. The AGACNP should incorporate the useful recommendations provided by the experts in guidelines and incorporate them into the care of each individual patient.

62. A) Randomized controlled trial

A randomized controlled trial includes experimental manipulation of variables using randomization and a control group to test the effects of an intervention or experiment. In this case, the patients who use insulin pumps are the active group and are tested against the control group who are the patients receiving multiple insulin injections. Study subjects are randomly allocated into the different treatment groups, and all groups are followed to observe the effect of the various treatments. A systematic review is a comprehensive summary of all available evidence that meets certain eligibility criteria to address a specific clinical question or range of questions. The cohort study uses a group of individuals who are alike in many ways but differ by a certain characteristic. A cohort study often moves forward to observing the outcome of interest, even if the data is collected retrospectively over time. A case-control study moves backward to the exposure, starting with the outcome of interest. Patients with a disease are identified and compared with controls for exposures to a risk factor.

63. D) Test-retest reliability

Reliability is the consistency of a measurement or the degree to which repeated measurements of a relatively stable notion fall closely to each other. There are several different types of reliability, such as inter- and intra-observer (rater) reliability, test–retest reliability, and internal consistency. Test–retest reliability is consistency of the same scores by the same person on two or more separate occasions, as noted in this case. Initial scores are compared with those obtained after taking the same test after a certain period of time. Internal consistency is a function of the number of items and their covariation and is often estimated by the Cronbach's alpha coefficient. It is used to assess the consistency of results across items within a test. Inter-observer reliability refers to the consistency of data recorded by two or more raters, measuring the same subjects over a single trial. Intra-observer reliability refers to the consistency of the data recorded by one rater over several trials (best determined when multiple trials are administered over a short period of time).

64. C) Proceed with endotracheal intubation as delay would post risk of serious, imminent harm to the patient

When emergent, lifesaving procedures are required (e.g., endotracheal intubation in the setting of acute hypoxic respiratory failure), the courts have recognized a doctrine of implied consent. This means that the clinical providers may assume that the patient would consent based on the assumption that no reasonable person would refuse the procedure in the circumstances. This emergency exception to the requirement for informed consent is used when delaying the procedure or treatment intervention in order to obtain informed consent would pose a risk of serious, imminent harm (e.g., death, serious disability). This patient is presenting with acute hypoxic respiratory failure, and delaying intubation could cause serious harm. In some states, two-physician consent may be obtained in certain situations in which emergent intervention is needed or the patient does not have the capacity to consent, and no family member or durable power of attorney has been identified or is able to consent. However, this is unlikely within the scope of the AGACNP in most areas.

65. B) The patient must have the mental ability to understand and make decisions about medical treatments.

In order for consent to be valid, the patient must be competent and have the mental ability to understand problems and make decisions about accepting or rejecting medical treatments. No intervention can be performed without the patient's consent, which must be both voluntary and knowing. Therefore, the blood products should not be ordered and prepared for administration before consent is obtained. When obtaining consent from a patient, the AGACNP should use comprehensible language. An exhaustive list of every possible thing that may go wrong is unnecessary; a personal transmission of truly relevant data is warranted. The information presented should be what the patient needs to know in order to make a truly educated decision. The AGACNP has a responsibility to provide adequate information to the patient, not the family member, so that they are able to process the information and make appropriate decisions.

66. D) The patient's durable power of attorney for healthcare

Comatose or incompetent patients lack adequate decision-making capacity to make informed consent decisions. When patients are comatose or otherwise incompetent, living wills may provide some elements of the patient's wishes, and durable powers of attorney will name surrogate decision-makers who can direct care. If surrogate decision-makers have not been chosen by the patient in advance, laws may vary as to who may serve as the patient's healthcare proxy. In general, the order is the spouse, adult children, parents, siblings, and other relatives.

67. A) Respect for autonomy

Obtaining informed consent from patients respects their right to determine what happens to their bodies (i.e., respect for autonomy). Respecting autonomy upholds that the patient has a right to participate in medical decision-making. Beneficence mandates that clinicians act in the best interest of their patients. Nonmaleficence is the duty to do no harm. Justice requires that all people be treated well and fairly, and that health resources be used equitably.

68. D) No, the AGACNP provided the pertinent medical information, but they did not ensure that the patient had adequately understood the information.

Obtaining informed consent is a communicative process that involves certain steps, rather than obtaining a signed consent document. Before obtaining consent, the AGACNP needs to ensure that the patient has decision-making capacity. In this case, the patient does not have a clear mental state after receiving pain medication. Decision-making abilities involve understanding, expressing a choice, appreciation, and reasoning. Since the patient is lethargic, the AGACNP cannot assume that the patient does not have any questions nor that the patient understood all of the information. Obtaining informed consent involves providing pertinent medical information about the proposed treatment and the reasonable alternatives, ensuring that the patient has adequately understood the information, and deliberating with the patient and then obtaining permission to perform the intervention. In some areas, inadequate disclosure of the risks and obtaining consent when the patient does not have a clear mental state adds up to no consent at all; thus, a claim for battery may be made, even if the procedure is a success. While it is true that the informed consent discussion and its documentation should be done by the provider performing the procedure, this patient does not have the capacity to consent in the current state. Unless the procedure is an emergency, efforts should be made to identify and correct any reversible causes of impairment, particularly in hospitalized patients with impaired capacity due to medications or delirium. Because this procedure is nonurgent, treatment of the underlying causes may restore decision-making capacity of the patient.

69. B) Nonmaleficence

The principle of nonmaleficence is to first do no harm and, if necessary, inflict the least harm possible to reach a beneficial outcome. While there may be some hope with this clinical trial, the benefits must be weighed against the risks; harmful side effects are considerations and part of the ethical decision-making process in healthcare. Harm, while unintentional, can often accompany life-saving treatment. Fidelity is the duty to remain faithful and keep commitment to the patient. Beneficence mandates that clinicians act in the best interest of their patients. Justice requires that all people be treated well and fairly, and that health resources be used equitably.

70. D) Qualitative

Qualitative futility occurs when the quality of benefit an intervention will produce is extremely poor. If an intervention may prolong survival even the slightest amount, with minimal suffering and an improvement in quality of life, futility may be debated. However, if an intervention could cause intense pain and suffering while offering only a brief extension in length of life, it would be considered futile. Qualitative futility is subjective and requires individuals to make judgment calls on what quality means for that patient. Quantitative futility focuses on the numeric probably of achieving the intended goal. This involves using published data on medical outcomes in addition to clinical expertise to determine a probably of survival after a given treatment. Physiological futility describes medical interventions that could not result in a physiological goal (e.g., using an antimicrobial that is resistant to a patient's bacterial infection). Imminent demise futility relays that the underlying condition is terminal in the short term and cannot be reserved or impacted by treatment.

71. C) American Nurses Association Code of Ethics

The American Nurses Association has established the Code of Ethics for Nurses, which establishes the ethical standard for the profession and provides a guide for nurses to use in ethical analysis and decision-making. This nonnegotiable code has been the foundation to nursing theory and practice. All nurses are expected to adhere to and embrace the values, moral norms, and ideals set forth by the code of ethics. It includes ethical values, obligations, duties, and professional ideas and is an expression of nursing's own understanding of its commitment to society. Institutional protocols, clinical practice guidelines, and state nurse practice acts may guide the scope and standards of practice, but the code of ethics provides the ethical standard for nursing practice.

72. A) Durable power of attorney for healthcare

The durable power of attorney for healthcare is a signed legal document authorizing another person to make medical decisions on the patient's behalf if they lose decision-making capacity. A living will is a document summarizing a person's preferences for future medical care. POLST relays what specific care should be administered or withheld for a specific patient (e.g., cardiopulmonary resuscitation, certain medical interventions), as directed by a physician. Because they are medical orders, they are signed by a physician and considered portable. The instructional directive advance care plan is rarely used and is not a sanctioned document in the United States.

73. A) Basal cell carcinoma

Basal cell carcinoma is the most commonly occurring skin cancer, and the incidence increases with age. It most often affects light-skinned people, but the risk for this form of cancer is increased in all persons who have repeated exposure. The lesions are often found on the head and neck in areas of hair growth. Squamous cell carcinoma, the second most common skin cancer, is nonspecific to skin pigmentation and occurs on sun-exposed areas. Malignant melanoma is a form of skin cancer that affects light-skinned individuals with a history of repeated exposure. Unlike the other two forms of skin cancer, this type often metastasizes and is associated with a high mortality rate if left untreated. Kaposi sarcoma are cancerous lesions that grow on the skin, lymph nodes, and mucous membranes of the mouth and the gastrointestinal tract. This cancer is commonly associated with patients who are immune compromised.

74. B) It ensures patients receive medical care consistent with their values and preferences.

Advance care planning is a multistage process that supports patients at any stage of health in understanding and sharing their personal values, life goals, and preferences regarding current and future medical care. While the timing and nature may vary for each patient, the discussion should be appropriately timed, integrated into routine care, and readdressed every time a patient's medical condition changes. The advance care planning discussion provides communication between patients, families, and other decision-makers and their healthcare providers. Thus, it is best accomplished when taking into consideration the patient's culture. Advance care planning is appropriate for all patients, whether they are healthy, have chronic illness, or have an advanced life-threatening terminal illness. While the discussion may include the completion of an advance directive and identification of a healthcare proxy, that should not be the primary intent. Rather, the goal is to ensure that patients receive care that is aligned with their values.

75. C) Decreased respiratory rate

A decrease in respiratory rate is a clinical indication that intracranial pressure (ICP) is increasing, a common complication associated with subdural hematomas. This change, along with bradycardia and increased blood pressure (hypertension), make up Cushing triad, an indication of elevated ICP. Fever does not result from elevated ICP.

76. B) Delirium

Delirium is the most common cause of urinary incontinence among hospitalized patients. Urinary tract infections, atrophic urethritis, and restricted mobility can also contribute to urinary incontinence but are not the most common causes.

77. A) Amitriptyline

Amitriptyline, a tricyclic antidepressant, is an example of a nonopioid adjuvant analgesic clinically shown to help alleviate pain when used in conjunction with traditional opioid pain relievers. Acetaminophen and aspirin, both over-the-counter nonopioid analgesics, do not increase the effectiveness of opioids when used concurrently. Haloperidol (Haldol), an antipsychotic, is not indicated for adjuvant analgesia.

78. C) Unprofessional conduct

Unprofessional conduct has occurred when state requirements have not been met. Fraud is the intent to deceive, and deception is the act of deceiving. Failing to meet state licensing requirements is not a violation of the HIPAA.

79. B) "I know that I need to have my eyes checked every year."

Diabetic retinopathy, a type of diabetic eye disease, is the leading cause of new cases of blindness in working-age adults in the United States. However, many people with diabetes, especially in minority populations, do not have yearly eye exams. Annual eye exams can help prevent vision loss by finding diabetic retinopathy early, when it is usually easier to treat. Seeing a healthcare provider only when vision problems are noticed is not the recommended action to help treat diabetic retinopathy in its early stages.

80. C) Length of time between exposure and disease development

Although work-related illnesses and injuries may be easily identified by known precipitants, some may only become apparent after a prolonged period of exposure. At that point, it may be difficult to determine the true cause of illness.

81. A) Slowing or stopping disease progression

Tertiary prevention manages disease post diagnosis to slow or stop its progression. Patient education to help prevent disease is an example of primary prevention, and screening to detect disease in its early stages is an example of secondary prevention.

82. A) "I would be happy to discuss treatment options available to you. Complementary therapies such as acupressure have shown promise when used with standard medical therapy for osteoarthritis."

Proposing shared decision-making in treatment, such as by offering education on the patient's first choice of treatment, is the most appropriate response by the AGACNP. Complementary therapy may be used alongside conventional treatment for many patient conditions, and it is inappropriate for the nurse to dismiss the patient's desire for complementary therapy or to suggest that it be used only as a last resort.

83. A) Respecting the patient's wishes

Patients have the right to self-determination, which means that they have the right to make their own decisions about treatment and relief of pain. This also includes the patient's right to not receive treatment at all.

84. D) Current research

Evidence-based practice involves the patient, the provider's clinician expertise, and current research.

85. C) Withhold some truths from patients if they believe complete honesty could be harmful

A healthcare provider may withhold information about a patient's diagnosis or treatment if disclosing it could pose a serious psychological threat to the patient.

86. B) Discussing options and letting the patient decide

The most effective way to promote behavior change is by emphasizing patient ownership and allowing the patient to decide among options. The AGACNP can also promote behavior change by partnering with patients; identifying small steps; scheduling frequent follow-up visits to cheer successes, problem solve, or both; and showing caring and concern for patients.

87. B) Social

Social determinants of health are conditions in the environments where people are born, live, learn, work, play, worship, and age. Social determinants of health affect a wide range of health, functioning, and quality-of-life outcomes and risks. Access to reliable public transportation is an example of a social determinant of health that may affect quality of life.

88. A) Disconjugate gaze

A disconjugate gaze involves a misalignment of the eyes and the inability to move both eyes in the same direction simultaneously. Nystagmus is the abnormal eye movement of one or both eyes characterized by rhythmic jerking movements. Conjugate gaze describes appropriate extraocular movements and is a normal exam finding. Mydriasis is the dilation of the pupil.

89. A) Peer review

The American Nurses Association (ANA) defines nursing peer-review as a process for evaluating the care provided by an individual according to accepted standards. Further, the ANA proposes that nurses with similar rank and clinical expertise should conduct these evaluations.

90. C) Hypovolemic

The symptoms described suggest hypovolemic shock. Cardiogenic, septic, and distributive shock are not caused by large loss of blood or fluids.

91. A) Respiratory depression

Respiratory depression is a common adverse effect associated with overdose of opioids. These patients are often hypotensive and bradycardic rather than hypertensive and tachycardic. Fever is an unrelated clinical finding.

92. C) "Both parents must be carriers of the gene in order for the child to inherit the disease."

Cystic fibrosis is an autosomal-recessive disease that requires both parents be carriers of the gene in order for the child to inherit the disease. The disease does not skip generations.

93. C) 55% to 75%

LVEF is the percentage of end-diastolic blood volume that is ejected during systole. The normal range is 55% to 75%. 15% to 35%, and 35% to 55% would be considered low, whereas 75% to 95% would be considered unusually high.

94. A) Propranolol (Inderal)

Thyroid storm results from uncontrolled hyperthyroidism. The mainstay of treatment is beta-blockers such as propranolol (Inderal) to control heart rate and symptoms. Levothyroxine (Synthroid) would only exacerbate the syndrome. Vancomycin (Vancocin) would be used for infection, and albuterol (Proventil) would be used for dyspnea and wheezing.

95. C) 6

Cardiac output is the volume of blood the heart is able to pump per minute. It is calculated by multiplying stroke volume by heart rate. Therefore, 80 × 75 = 6,000 mL/min or 6 L/min.

96. B) Corticosteroids

Acute adrenal insufficiency is a life-threatening condition that should be treated with corticosteroids even before a diagnosis is confirmed. Beta-blockers are indicated for cardiac conditions and hyperthyroidism. Insulin would be used for hyperglycemia. Antibiotics are the mainstay of treatment for infections.

97. D) "The length and location of the male urethra helps protect against UTIs."

Male patients tend to get far fewer UTIs than female patient due to the increased length of the urethra and its separation from the anus. In addition, secretions from the prostate inhibit bacterial growth. It would not be appropriate or correct for the AGACNP to make assumptions about the patient's hygiene. Calcium supplements do not directly increase risk of UTIs. Urine produced by female patients is not less acidic.

98. C) Metronidazole (Flagyl)

C. difficile should be treated empirically with metronidazole (Flagyl). Loperamide (Diamode) and diphenoxylate/atropine (Lomotil) should be used in other types of diarrhea but not in cases of suspected *C. difficile.* Cephalexin (Keflex) is not an antibiotic indicated for this type of infectious diarrhea.

99. A) It is important to keep glucose levels well-controlled.

Diabetes and uncontrolled hyperglycemia increase the risk of UTIs, and the patient should be encouraged to maintain good control over glucose levels. Urine cultures should be obtained in patients with recurrent UTIs to assess resistance prior to selecting an antibiotic. Treatment is indicated regardless of fever or hematuria. Douching is discouraged as it disrupts normal, healthy flora.

100. B) "OME is not due to a bacterial infection, so it does not require antibiotics."

OME is typically caused by eustachian tube dysfunction or a viral infection and will therefore not be responsive to antibiotics. Prescribing ciprofloxacin (Cetraxal) and obtaining a culture are inappropriate. The presence or lack of fever is not relevant.

101. C) Pyelonephritis

Findings of fever, dysuria, and renal angle tenderness indicate the presence of pyelonephritis. Renal angle tenderness is not typically seen with prostatitis. Fever is typically not a presenting symptom of renal carcinoma. While urinary tract infection may have led to the pyelonephritis, the renal angle tenderness differentiates this condition as pyelonephritis.

102. B) Eosinophils

Eosinophils make up 1% to 3% of white blood cells and play a role in responding to allergic reactions. Neutrophils and monocytes respond to infectious organisms. Platelet count would be elevated in the presence of infection, cancer, some inflammatory diseases, and some anemias.

103. B) Hypothyroidism

Myxedema crisis is a life-threatening condition that occurs from severe hypothyroidism and manifests in a variety of ways, including impaired cognition, hyponatremia, and hypothermia. It is not caused by adrenal insufficiency, hyperthyroidism, or acromegaly.

104. C) Slate gray nevus

Slate gray nevus are painless bluish discolorations most frequently found in Native American, African American, Asian American, and Mexican American patients. Deep tissue injuries and unstageable pressure ulcers may appear bluish in nature but would not have been present since birth. Keloid scars are thick, rope-like scars that form most commonly after trauma.

105. B) Amiodarone (Cordarone)

Amiodarone (Cordarone) use is a common cause of thyrotoxicosis because the drug contains a high amount of iodine, which can trigger thyrotoxicosis. Metoprolol (Lopressor), acetaminophen (Tylenol), and omeprazole (Prilosec) are not known to affect thyroid function.

106. C) Expressive or receptive language deficits

The temporal lobe is responsible for auditory processing, including understanding the spoken word and speech formation; therefore, it would be anticipated to see deficits with infarction to this area. The parietal lobe controls vision, and the cerebellum is responsible for balance and coordination.

107. B) Posterior column lateral meniscus tract

In the posterior column system, the peripheral large fibers projection of the dorsal root ganglia transmits the sensation of vibration, proprioception, kinesthesia, fine touch from the skin, and joint receptors to the dorsal root ganglia. The spinothalamic tract is responsible for sensation of pain and temperature. The cerebellum controls balance and coordination. The corticospinal tract is responsible for voluntary movement in the trunk and limbs.

108. A) Trigeminal neuralgia

Trigeminal neuralgia is characterized by severe lacerating pain that travels through the divisions of the trigeminal nerve, including the maxillary, occipital, and mandibular division known as V1, V2, and V3, respectively; trigeminal pain is often incited by hot or cold temperatures to the divisions. Sinus headaches and sinusitis do not cause pain in the division of the trigeminal nerve, and cluster headaches cause severe pain behind the eye unilaterally.

109. A) Bronchial breath sounds in most areas of the lungs
Bronchial breath sounds in most areas of the lungs are an abnormal finding indicative of lung pathology with consolidation of tissue. Vesicular breath sounds would be indicative of healthy lung tissue, and bronchial breath sounds over the trachea are a normal finding, as are bronchovesicular breath sounds between the scapulae.

110. B) Active ROM against gravity with some resistance
Muscle strength is graded on a 0 to 5 scale. Grade 4 is defined as active ROM against gravity with some resistance. Active motion against gravity with full resistance with no evidence of muscle fatigue is a 5. Active ROM with only gravity is graded as a 3, and active ROM with gravity eliminated is graded as a 2.

111. A) Seborrheic dermatitis
Seborrheic dermatitis is characterized by bilateral symmetrical erythematous patches on the cheeks, eyebrows, and scalp and may have a greasy appearance. Rosacea most commonly affects the cheeks, causing blushing or flushing, and is exacerbated by extreme temperature. Atopic dermatitis is characterized by erythema scaling, dry skin, and intense itching. Contact dermatitis has erythema papules and vesicles with transudate crusting, not plaques or flaking skin.

112. A) 2.0 to 3.0
Warfarin (Coumadin) is an anticoagulant whose effects can be measured using the INR, which is a standardized ratio of prothrombin times. An INR between 2.0 and 3.0 is therapeutic for nonvalvular atrial fibrillation. While 2.5 is within the therapeutic range for nonvalvular atrial fibrillation, the narrow range of 2.5 to 3.0 may exclude many normal values. An INR above 3.0 is supratherapeutic in nonvalvular atrial fibrillation and risks adverse effects due to bleeding. The INR range of 2.5 and 3.5 is generally accepted for patients who have a mechanical heart valve, or at the prescriber's discretion, but it does increase the risk for bleeding events in patients without a mechanical valve.

113. A) To avoid use in patients taking angiotensin-converting enzyme if possible
SMZ-TMP may increase serum potassium. In CKD, coadministration of SMX-TMP with other agents that potentially increase potassium may exaggerate this response and lead to dangerously elevated potassium levels. Unless there is severe liver disease, a dose adjustment of SMZ-TMP for patients with chronic liver disease is not recommended. Using SMZ-TMP to treat streptococcal pharyngitis should be avoided because *Streptococcus pyogenes* is commonly accepted to be resistant to the drug. SMZ-TMP is cleared primarily by the kidneys and should be administered in CKD.

114. D) 6

The oral dose of cyclosporine should be three times the IV dose because it is poorly absorbed by the gastrointestinal tract. A patient weighing 67 kg who is taking 3 mg cyclosporine per day IV would be taking approximately 201 mg/day of cyclosporine. To transition to oral therapy, this dose needs to be multiplied by 3, which is 603 mg, or approximately 600 mg. Oral doses of cyclosporine lower than 600 mg daily would be subtherapeutic and risk recurrence of GVHD in this patient.

115. B) Methimazole

Methimazole is a thioamide that prevents further synthesis of thyroid hormone by interfering with the oxidation of iodine in the thyroid. It does not alter thyroid hormone already circulating, so it is often used in combination with medications like beta-blockers. Liothyronine is a synthetic thyroid hormone and would exacerbate a thyroid storm. Mycophenolate is an immunosuppressant, and hydrocortisone is a corticosteroid. Neither drug alters the formation of new thyroid hormone or circulating thyroid hormone.

116. D) Myxedema

Myxedema is a severe manifestation of hypothyroidism and often leads to hemodynamic instability and myxedema coma. This patient progressively declined as the hypothyroidism advanced without the exogenous source of thyroid hormone, levothyroxine (Synthroid). Encephalitis would have indications of acute neurologic inflammation or infection beyond sluggishness and confusion. The patient is afebrile with a normal complete blood, which does not completely exclude encephalitis, but it is not a leading differential given the patient's other values. While angioedema also produces profound edema, the onset is typically not insidious, and symptoms of angioedema are not as systemically vague. There is no indication that the patient has airway compromise or the hemodynamic instability that anaphylaxis often produces.

117. B) Regular insulin given IV

Insulin stimulates the uptake of potassium, which lowers the serum potassium. It is given alongside IV dextrose to avoid or minimize hypoglycemia. This can be used in a patient with or without diabetes; the dose of IV dextrose is titrated accordingly. Albuterol also reduces serum potassium, but it interacts with numerous medications and has no role to use alongside dextrose. Sodium polystyrene sulfonate also lowers potassium, but reports of intestinal necrosis are a concern, and other therapies are preferable. Beta-blockers like metoprolol can increase serum potassium on rare occasions.

118. B) Rinne

The Rinne test is performed by placing a tuning fork on the mastoid bone and then in front of the ear canal. It can help differentiate conductive and sensorineural hearing loss. The Weber test is performed by placing a tuning fork on the forehead or front teeth. The Whisper test involves testing a patient's hearing at different voice levels. An audiogram is a formal study in which patients are asked to identify the presence of sounds emitted at different decibel levels.

119. B) Dehisced surgical wound

NPWT has been approved by the U.S. Food and Drug Administration to manage the output of a wound or closed surgical incision to facilitate healing. NPWT is approved to help treat a myriad of conditions including partial-thickness burns, dehisced surgical wounds, pressure injuries, abdominal wounds, diabetic foot ulcers, trauma wounds, and flaps and grafts. Ischemic wounds, such as arterial ulcer, and infected wounds, such as an infected diabetic foot ulcer, are relative contraindications to use. Although NPWT is indicated as a treatment for pressure injuries, the wound must be free of eschar or necrotic tissue. The presence of eschar interferes with NPWT delivery.

120. C) Spirometry

Spirometry testing would be done when a patient presents with possible asthma exacerbation. Arterial blood gas is often normal in mild asthma exacerbations. Bronchial provocation testing may be used if spirometry is equivocal. A chest x-ray would not show the degree of airflow obstruction.

121. C) 20%

PEF values may vary from day to evening or from day to day. A change in PEF of 20% or more is suggestive of inadequate asthma control and warrants a change in therapy. A change of 5% or 10% may be expected. A change of 50% PEF is significant and may warrant further workup.

122. D) Absolute eosinophil count

Anti-interleukin-5 therapy is a treatment used to manage eosinophilic airway disease. Patients with allergen-related asthma and elevated eosinophil count may benefit from this therapy. Spirometry, arterial blood gas, and chest x-rays may be indicated in the workup of a patient with asthma but would not help determine the appropriateness of this therapy.

123. D) Severe airflow obstruction

A PEF of less than 200 L/min is considered severe airflow obstruction. Normal airflow in an adult ranges from 400 to 700 L/min. Mild and moderate airflow obstruction would fall between 200 and 400 L/min.

124. B) *Streptococcus pneumoniae*

Streptococcus pneumoniae is the most common pathogen responsible for community-acquired pneumonia. Viruses, *Legionella pneumophila*, and *Pseudomonas aeruginosa* can also cause community-acquired pneumonia but are not as common.

125. A) Elevated hemoglobin

Patients with bronchitis-predominant COPD typically have elevated hemoglobin due to compensation for chronic hypoxia. The hematocrit is more likely to be increased, not decreased, in these patients. The creatinine level and platelet count are not typically affected in patients with COPD.

126. D) 60-year-old patient who was admitted to the hospital 5 days ago and now has fever, purulent sputum, and parenchymal opacities on chest CT

HAP is defined as pneumonia that develops more than 48 hours after hospital admission and meets the following criteria: new or worsening parenchymal opacities on chest imaging, plus at least two of the following: fever, leukocytosis, or purulent sputum. A patient who was admitted to the hospital 24 hours ago or who presents to the emergency department with an infection already present would not meet the criteria for HAP. A patient who does not have evidence of opacities on chest imaging would also not be considered to have HAP.

127. D) Thoracentesis

A new pleural effusion with no clear cause warrants a diagnostic thoracentesis for pleural fluid analysis. Chest CT is not necessary because the chest x-ray has already established the presence of an effusion. An echocardiogram may be done to assess for congestive heart failure but would not be the best next step. Bronchoalveolar lavage is typically used for lung sampling in other clinical scenarios.

128. B) Elevated amylase

Amylase levels are elevated in the majority of acute pancreatitis cases. Lipase is typically elevated in cases of pancreatitis as well. White blood cell count, serum lactate dehydrogenase, and aspartate aminotransferase are often elevated, and hypocalcemia may be noted. Potassium levels are typically not affected.

129. C) pCO_2 55 mmHg

Respiratory failure occurs from abnormal oxygenation or ventilation resulting in organ dysfunction. A pO_2 under 60 mmHg or a pCO_2 over 50 mmHg on arterial blood gas meets the criteria for respiratory failure. A pCO_2 of 45 mmHg, pO_2 of 64 mmHg, or pO_2 of 70 mmHg would not constitute respiratory failure.

130. A) Aspartate aminotransferase (AST) 160, alanine transaminase (ALT) 70

A patient with alcohol-induced hepatic injury typically has mildly elevated liver enzymes (<5 × normal) with an AST:ALT >2:1. A severe elevation (e.g., AST 900, ALT 850) is typically seen in other hepatic conditions. An AST:ALT <2:1 (e.g., AST 50, ALT 120) or normal liver enzyme values (e.g., AST 20, ALT 33) would not be a typical pattern of alcohol-induced liver injury.

131. C) Serum albumin

Serum albumin is typically decreased in hepatocellular jaundice. Direct and indirect bilirubin are elevated in hepatocellular jaundice. Prothrombin time may be unchanged or increased if liver damage is severe.

132. A) Echocardiogram

Echocardiogram is the optimal diagnostic tool to confirm the presence and gradient of mitral valve regurgitation. EKG and chest CT are not valuable in identifying pulmonary valve stenosis. Cardiac catheterization can be used to identify coronary disease, but it is invasive and is not the best initial diagnostic tool of choice for mitral valve regurgitation.

133. A) Fluticasone (Flovent)

This patient's presentation is consistent with vasomotor rhinitis. The mainstay of treatment is an intranasal corticosteroid such as fluticasone (Flovent). Loratadine (Claritin) and fexofenadine (Allegra) are antihistamines that may be used for temporary control of symptoms but are not the best initial treatment. Antibiotics such as amoxicillin and clavulanate acid (Augmentin) treat various bacterial, not viral, infections.

134. A) Viral rhinitis

Viral rhinitis is typically characterized by rhinorrhea and erythematous nasal mucosa. Vasomotor rhinitis would typically present with pale or purplish mucosa. Because the patient is not presenting with additional symptoms or examination findings, such as fever, shortness of breath, or a productive cough, bacterial or viral pneumonia is an unlikely differential diagnosis.

135. C) Group A beta-hemolytic streptococcal infection

A differential diagnosis is developed by synthesizing subjective and objective data. Fever, sore throat, tender cervical nodes, and exudative tonsillopharyngitis are hallmark features of group A beta-hemolytic streptococcal infection. Squamous cell carcinoma typically presents as a lesion in the oral cavity. Oral candidiasis presents with curd-like exudate in the mouth without adenopathy or fever. Hairy leukoplakia appears as patches on the tongue and is not associated with the other symptoms.

136. A) Jugular venous examination

A jugular venous examination can assess for jugular vein distention. This can occur with emphysema and indicates chronic heart failure. A distended/bulging jugular vein signals that blood is backing up from the right side of the heart/superior vena cava into the jugular veins. Lincoln sign is used to diagnose Marfan syndrome and demonstrates excessive popliteal artery pulsation due to the hemodynamic effects of aortic regurgitation. An ankle-brachial index test is an exam that compares the blood pressure of the upper extremity to the lower extremity to assess for peripheral artery disease. When evaluating for a Cullen's sign, the AGACNP looks for a bluish discoloration of the periumbilical skin area that would be an indication of acute pancreatitis, which is not a relevant finding with a potential diagnosis of emphysema.

137. D) CT of abdomen and pelvis

CT of the abdomen and pelvis is often used to determine if cancer has invaded nearby lymph tissue. Digital rectal exams, 4Kscore PSA testing, and transrectal US are all recognized screening methods for prostate cancer itself but do not determine if cancer has spread to nearby organs or tissue.

138. D) Severe

A GCS score of 8 or less indicates a severe injury. A score of 9 to 12 indicates moderate injury, and a score of 13 to 15 indicates mild injury, with 15 being indicative of a patient who is alert, fully oriented, and following commands.

139. A) Insulin therapy should start simultaneously with fluid deficit correction.

It is critical that insulin therapy not be started without simultaneously correcting the fluid deficit; otherwise, an acute loss of vascular volume may occur. Fluid replacement beginning 2 or 4 hours later may result in worsening fluid volume deficit. Fluid replacement should always occur in conjunction with insulin administration regardless of whether clinical signs or symptoms of dehydration are present.

140. A) Visual analog scale

The visual analog scale depicts varying levels of pain intensity by using pictures of facial expressions. It is visual, allowing the patient to draw or mark an area that describes their current pain rating without the need for detailed instructions. Because the AGACNP and the patient do not share a common language, this may be the most concise method to gather a pain rating until an interpreter is available. The numeric rating scale requires some instruction on how it is used, waiting for the interpreter is not timely, and vital signs are not always reliable in assessing degree of pain; therefore, they are not the best methods for pain assessment in this patient.

141. B) Amoxicillin (Amoxil), rabeprazole sodium (Aciphex), and clarithromycin (Biaxin)

One standard first-line treatment for *H. pylori* is a triple therapy combination of a proton-pump inhibitor, amoxicillin (Amoxil), and clarithromycin (Biaxin). The combination of amoxicillin (Amoxil), rabeprazole sodium (Aciphex), and clarithromycin (Biaxin) meets those criteria. The combination of amoxicillin (Amoxil), ciprofloxacin (Cipro), and cimetidine (Tagamet); amoxicillin (Amoxil), metoclopramide (Reglan), and cimetidine (Tagamet); or amoxicillin (Amoxil), ciprofloxacin (Cipro), and sulfamethoxazole-trimethoprim (Bactrim) does not fit as a drug category combination for this standard first-line treatment.

142. B) Mafenide acetate 10% cream (Sulfamylon)

Mafenide acetate 10% cream (Sulfamylon) is highly soluble and penetrates eschar well to allow for debridement while keeping infection management in mind. Silver sulfadiazine 1% cream (Silvadene) and silver nitrate 0.5% in water have poor eschar penetration and therefore would not facilitate debridement, which is necessary to establish good wound bed preparation for wound healing. Triamcinolone 0.025% (Cinolar) is a topical steroid and does not facilitate debridement, which is required for the facilitation of healing in the presence of eschar.

143. B) Stage 3

Stage 3 is defined as an injury with full-thickness tissue loss, where subcutaneous fat may be visible, and undermining and tunneling may occur. Slough may also be present; however, slough fully obstructing the view of the wound bed would make the pressure injury unstageable. Bone, tendon, and muscle are not exposed as would be found in Stage 4. Stage 1 pressure injuries are intact areas with nonblanchable erythema.

144. A) Tissue-damaging heat production

Neutralizing chemical burns with another chemical is contraindicated because the procedure may generate heat and worsen the tissue injury. Initial treatment of chemical burns includes removing saturated clothing, brushing off any powdered chemical on the skin, and continuously irrigating the skin with water for 30 minutes. Chemical neutralization does not cause chemical adherence, which is created by the initial contact with the original caustic chemical. While some chemicals may crystallize on the surface of the skin, they do not do so within the dermis. Loss of motor function is not a result of neutralizing chemical burns with another chemical.

145. A) Akathisia

Many medications, including antipsychotic medications used to treat schizophrenia, can cause what is known as extrapyramidal side effects. Akathisia is a movement disorder characterized by a feeling of inner restlessness. Dystonia exhibits involuntary muscle contractions. Akinesia causes delayed or absent movement. Much more information would need to be gathered, including diagnostic testing, to diagnose this patient with Parkinson's disease.

146. A) Mechanical

Pain related to disk herniation is categorized as mechanical back pain. Causes of visceral back pain include abdominal aortic aneurysm, pancreatitis, nephrolithiasis, and pelvic inflammatory diseases. Neuropathic is not a classification of back pain. Sources of nonmechanical back pain include infections such as osteomyelitis, epidural abscess, paraspinal abscess, inflammatory arthritis, osteochondrosis, and back pain caused by cancer.

147. A) Irregular heart rate

In an intentional acute carbon monoxide overexposure in which the source of the poisoning and mechanism is confirmed, along with evaluating the patient's neurological functioning, the AGACNP should assess for signs and symptoms of heart arrhythmia and myocardial damage. Large exposure to carbon monoxide can cause arrhythmias and cardiac injury. Most likely, hyperglycemia will be found since it can naturally be induced by stress or produced by the initiated intravenous trauma therapy. Inhalation of chemicals and particles released in smoke from a fire, such as hydrogen chloride, phosgene, sulfur dioxide, toxic aldehyde chemicals, and ammonia, can cause smoke inhalation damage to the lungs. Since this patient's exposure was from carbon monoxide with no fire source, smoke inhalation would not be a finding. Rectal bleeding would not be a relevant manifestation in this patient.

148. B) Nerve conduction test

Nerve conduction testing is the gold standard for diagnosing carpal tunnel syndrome. Forced flexion of the wrist is the Phalen sign and has a positive predictive value of 76%. Ultrasound and two-view radiographs will not confirm compression of the medial nerve. An electromyogram measures the electrical activity of muscles when they are at rest and when they are being used. Nerve conduction studies measure how well and how fast the nerves can send electrical signals, which is how diagnosis is confirmed.

149. C) Smooth surface of the prostate

Normally, the prostate should have a smooth surface on palpation. Abnormal findings include tenderness or pain noted on palpation; an estimated size outside the parameters of 2 to 3 cm wide; or any irregularity, nodules, or masses noted on palpation.

150. D) It takes 2 to 4 weeks for the body to develop immunity.

The administration of most vaccinations induces a durable antibody response known as active immunity. It takes 2 to 4 weeks after vaccination for the body to develop immunity against the disease, and it has a duration of more than 3 months of effectiveness. Immunoglobin from pooled serum produces passive immunity.

151. A) Measurement of bone mineral density (BMD) at femoral neck only

The FRAX is a tool to assist in assessing a patient's 10-year risk for fracture and is useful in guiding treatment for patients at an increased fracture risk, especially those with osteopenia. Limitations include exclusion of vertebral spine BMD because the measurement is only of the femoral neck. Additionally, the FRAX tool does not include factors such as corticosteroid exposure or recent fractures at any location in the calculation.

152. C) Order a complete blood count

The amount of output collected suggests that the patient is actively bleeding. The AGACNP should assess the patient and their vital signs to determine status and then obtain blood for a complete blood count to assess hemoglobin and hematocrit levels. If the assessment suggests that the patient requires a transfusion, the AGACNP can order blood. The surgeon should be contacted if needed based on the findings.

153. C) 10 years

Barring any contraindication, adults who received their initial tetanus vaccine should receive a booster every 10 years. The influenza vaccine should be administered annually, and the pneumococcal vaccine should be received every 5 years for an appropriate immune response.

154. C) Appendectomy 10 days previously

Surgery performed within 14 days of stroke onset contraindicates the use of tPA per treatment guidelines. Patients who have suffered gastrointestinal or genitourinary bleeding within the past 21 days or a cerebral vascular accident within the past 3 months or who have a blood pressure greater than 185/110 mmHg are not candidates for tPA.

155. A) 3

The recommended treatment window for tPA is 3 hours from symptom onset. Six, 9, and 12 hours are all outside the therapeutic treatment window and are associated with increased risk of hemorrhagic transformation.

156. D) Cigarette smoking

Cigarette smoking is the most important modifiable risk factor associated with the development of COPD. Alcohol consumption has no clinical correlation to the development of COPD. Secondhand smoke exposure and environmental pollutant exposure are both associated with the development of COPD; however, they are less clinically significant in comparison with smoking.

157. A) "If I focus on diet and exercise, I may delay or prevent progression to diabetes."

Clinical research has shown that lifestyle modifications that focus on diet and exercise can slow or prevent the progression of DM. The statement "I am going to get diabetes no matter what" indicates that the patient is under the inaccurate impression that there is nothing they can do to alter their disease process. While starting a metformin (Glucophage) regimen can reduce the incidence of diabetes, it is less effective than lifestyle modification. A patient who continues their current dietary habits while implementing an exercise routine would only be addressing one of the lifestyle behaviors associated with development of DM.

158. C) Every 2 years

The U.S. Preventive Services Task Force recommends assessing lipid profiles every 5 years in adults age 40 to 75 years with no documented history of cardiovascular disease. Checking a patient's lipid profile every 6 months, yearly, or every 2 years would be outside of treatment guidelines for this patient.

159. D) 8.0%

The target HbA1C for older patients with limited life expectancy is 8% to 9%. The target HbA1C recommended for older adults with no underlying health conditions and an extended life expectancy is 7%. For older patients with extended life expectancy and few functional limitations, the recommended target is 7% to 7.5%. An HbA1C of 6.5% is not a recommended target for any patient population.

160. B) 2 to 6

Immunocompetent patients age 50 years or older should be given a second dose of the herpes zoster vaccine 2 to 6 months after initial immunization. Receiving the second dose after 12 months, 24 months, or 1 month does not align with current treatment guidelines.

161. B) 65 years

The U.S. Preventive Services Task Force recommends discontinuation of Pap smears in patients at age 65 years if they have had three consecutive negative cytology results. Ages 60, 70, and 75 years are all outside practice guidelines.

162. B) 26 years

The Centers for Disease Control and Prevention recommend that patients receive the HPV vaccine by the age of 26 years for maximum protection. Patients are eligible for vaccination up to the age of 45 years with a lesser protective effect.

163. A) Intramuscularly once

The Centers for Disease Control and Prevention recommend ceftriaxone (Recophin) 500 mg intramuscularly once for treatment of uncomplicated gonorrhea. Ceftriaxone (Recophin) 500 mg orally twice daily for 7 days, once daily for 7 days, and once daily for 14 days are not in accordance with treatment guidelines.

164. C) There is an increased risk of a cardiovascular thrombotic event.
In patients with and without CVD, the use of most NSAIDs is associated with an increased risk of adverse cardiovascular events, including death, myocardial infarction, heart failure, and stroke. The increased risk varies depending on the baseline cardiovascular risk of the patient, the NSAID chosen, and its dose. To minimize the risk for an adverse cardiovascular event in patients treated with an NSAID, it should be prescribed at the lowest effective dose for the shortest duration possible. Evidence does not show a correlation between use of NSAIDS and increase in blood sugar levels. Literature does support the use of NSAIDs for pain and inflammation reduction secondary to osteoarthritis.

165. B) Doxycycline (Doxycin) 100 mg orally twice daily for 7 days
The Centers for Disease Control and Prevention recommend treatment of chlamydia with doxycycline (Doxycin) 100 mg orally two times daily for 7 days. Alternative regimens include azithromycin (Zithromax) 1 g orally in a single dose or levofloxacin (Levaquin) 500 mg orally once daily for 7 days.

166. A) Varicella
Live vaccines, like the varicella vaccine, are contraindicated in patients who are HIV positive and symptomatic. Tetanus, hepatitis B, and pneumococcal vaccines are inactivated vaccines that are recommended for HIV patients.

167. B) Preparing for endotracheal intubation
Endotracheal intubation is the priority intervention because the patient is exhibiting signs of decreased responsiveness and impending respiratory failure. Scope of practice may vary based on the facility and/or the state; in some cases, intubation may need to be performed under direct supervision of a physician. Administration of flumazenil (Romazicon) would be second priority after establishing an airway. Charcoal is not indicated for overdose with alprazolam (Xanax) or other benzodiazepines. Laboratory studies are necessary but should be obtained after an airway has been secured and the patient has been stabilized.

168. A) Sulfamethoxazole/trimethoprim (Bactrim) 160/800 mg orally every 12 hours for 3 days
Sulfamethoxazole/trimethoprim (Bactrim) 160/800 mg orally every 12 hours for 3 days is the guideline-recommended first-line therapy for uncomplicated acute cystitis. Ciprofloxacin (Cipro) 250 mg orally every 12 hours for 3 days and levofloxacin (Levaquin) 250 mg orally every 24 hours for 3 days are considered second-line therapies. Cephalexin (Keflex) 500 mg orally every 6 to 12 hours for 7 days is a third-line therapy.

169. A) Macrocytic, normochromic

Folic acid deficiency is described as a macrocytic normochromic anemia. Microcytic hypochromic RBCs are seen in patients with iron-deficiency anemia. Hemolytic RBCs are seen in patients with sickle cell anemia. Normocytic normochromic RBCs are seen in patients with anemia of chronic disease.

170. A) Ceftriaxone (Rocephin) 500 mg intramuscularly once plus doxycycline (Doxycin) 100 mg orally twice a day for 10 days

The Centers for Disease Control and Prevention recommend treating male patients diagnosed with acute epididymitis, secondary to chlamydia, with ceftriazone (Rocephin) 500 mg intramuscularly once plus doxycycline (Doxycin) 100 mg orally twice daily for 10 days. Ceftriaxone (Rocephin) 250 mg intramuscularly once is not sufficient coverage for this infection. If enteritis is most likely caused by enteric organisms, doxycycline (Doxycin) would be replaced by levofloxacin (Levaquin) 500 mg orally once daily for 10 days. Levofloxacin (Levaquin) by itself is insufficient. Ofloxacin (Floxin) 300 mg orally every 12 hours for 10 days is not recommended for treatment of acute epididymitis secondary to chlamydia.

171. D) Epoetin alfa (Procrit)

Because this current oncology patient's hemoglobin is low, the AGACNP will want to ensure that the patient has been prescribed human erythropoietin (epoetin alfa). Epoetin alfa (Procrit) is used to prevent or treat anemia caused by chronic disease or by medication such as chemotherapy. Fondaparinux (Arixtra) is an anticoagulant used to treat and prevent blood clots. Gefitinib (Iressa) is a type of targeted cancer medication commonly used to treat certain types of breast and lung cancers. Ondansetron (Zofran) is a drug that prevents nausea and vomiting.

172. C) Low sensitivity, high specificity

The nitrite test has a low sensitivity (45% to 60%), which means that there is a high false-negative rate. This is because only certain strains of bacteria convert urine nitrate into nitrite. However, the specificity rate is high (85% to 98%), which means that the presence of nitrites in urine can be confidently interpreted as an infection.

173. A) Immunoglobulin A (IgA)

Recurrent sinus and pulmonary infections in a patient with a diagnosis of rheumatoid arthritis should raise suspicion for selective IgA deficiency, the most common type of primary immune deficiency. A CBC would not be helpful in this situation. ESR and CRP would likely be abnormal in rheumatoid arthritis patients, but these values are not diagnostic for immune deficiencies.

174. C) Gonorrhea

The patient is demonstrating signs and symptoms of gonorrhea. A vaginal yeast infection usually presents with complaints of intense itching. A urinary tract infection presents with complaints of pain or burning with urination, but usually not purulent vaginal discharge. Cervical cancer often presents with a watery and/or bloody discharge from the vagina.

175. B) Wash hands often

Frequent hand washing remains the best way to reduce the risk of hospital-acquired infections. There is no need to cook vegetables before eating. Wearing a face mask may be helpful in reducing the risk of airborne infections, but it is not as universally effective as handwashing. Prophylactic antibiotics are not necessarily indicated to prevent infection.

Practice Exam 2

6

1. A patient sustained a neurological head trauma and has been in the ICU for the past few days. The patient has been on supported on mechanical ventilation and continues to have altered mental status; now, urine output is exceeding 3 L/day. The patient is hypernatremic with a low urine osmolality of less than 300 mOsmol/kg. These findings are suggestive of which diagnosis?

   A. Syndrome of inappropriate antidiuretic hormone (SIADH)
   B. Solute diuresis
   C. Diabetes insipidus (DI)
   D. Primary polydipsia

2. Which of the following laboratory values is consistent with a diagnosis of syndrome of inappropriate antidiuretic hormone (SIADH)?

   A. Sodium level >135 mEq/L
   B. Serum osmolality <275 mOsmol/kg
   C. Urine osmolality <100 mOsmol/kg
   D. Urine sodium <20 mEq/L

3. A patient presents with a new onset of nocturia that has gradually gotten worse, keeping the patient up most of the night. The patient denies any prostate issues or new fever, dysuria, or urgency. The patient is hypernatremic with a urine osmolality of less than 300 mOsmol/kg. No elevation in urine osmolality is seen after administration of desmopressin; the urine osmolality remains less than 300 mOsmol/kg. This type of diabetes insipidus can be classified as which of the following?

   A. Complete nephrogenic
   B. Partial nephrogenic
   C. Complete central
   D. Partial central

4. A patient presents with polyuria. The patient reports, "I suddenly began urinating much more than usual a few days ago." The patient is hypernatremic with a low urine osmolality of less than 300 mOsmol/kg. Desmopressin is given to classify the type of diabetes insipidus. A rise in urine osmolality of more than 100% is seen over the next 2 hours. This type of diabetes insipidus can be classified as which of the following?

A. Complete nephrogenic
B. Partial nephrogenic
C. Complete central
D. Partial central

5. Which of the following is the cardinal diagnostic test for giant cell arteritis?

A. Doppler ultrasound (US) of the head and neck
B. Temporal artery biopsy
C. Occipital artery biopsy
D. CT angiography

6. A patient with a past medical history of schizophrenia presents with polyuria. The patient reports, "My mouth is always dry after taking my medications." Laboratory results reveal a low plasma sodium concentration with a low urine osmolality. These diagnostic findings are suggestive of which diagnosis?

A. Syndrome of inappropriate antidiuretic hormone (SIADH)
B. Solute diuresis
C. Diabetes insipidus
D. Primary polydipsia

7. When is the first ophthalmologic examination recommended in patients with type 2 diabetes according to the American Diabetes Association?

A. At the time of diagnosis
B. Within 5 years of diagnosis
C. Within 2 years of diagnosis
D. At routine eye exam

8. A 60-year-old patient presents with fever, new headache, and abrupt change in vision. The patient reports transient monocular visual loss. The patient also reports pain in their jaw. Based on this patient presentation, which diagnostic laboratory values can be expected?

A. Thrombocytopenia
B. Elevated albumin
C. Polycythemia
D. Elevated erythrocyte sedimentation rate and C-reactive protein

9. According to the American Academy of Ophthalmology, how often is screening for glaucoma recommended for a 50-year-old patient with a family history of vision loss from glaucoma?

A. Every 5 to 10 years
B. Every 2 to 4 years
C. Every 1 to 3 years
D. Every year

10. A patient presents with severe eye pain. The patient is reluctant to open the eye due to photophobia. The patient reports working on their house earlier that day and feeling something fall into their eye. After performing a visual acuity and fundus examination, which of the following diagnostic studies is indicated next?

A. Ultrasonography (US)
B. Fluorescein examination
C. CT scan
D. MRI

11. A patient presents with weakness, fatigue, and weight loss. Genetic testing is positive for the Philadelphia chromosome. Which of the following types of leukemia is most suggested by the presence of this chromosome?

A. Acute myeloid
B. Acute lymphocytic
C. Chronic lymphocytic
D. Chronic myeloid

12. A patient presents with a headache, severe eye pain, visual disturbances, and halos around lights. Physical assessment reveals conjunctival redness and cloudiness of the cornea. Emergent ophthalmologic examination is necessary. Which of the following diagnostic tests is indicated?

A. Dilated fundus examination
B. Measurement of intraocular pressure
C. Pachymetry
D. Fluorescein examination

13. A local apartment building caught on fire, leading to a mass influx of patients in the emergency department. An AGACNP working that day is trying to operate disaster triage of patients based on which ethical theory?

A. Justice
B. Utilitarianism
C. Autonomy
D. Nonmaleficence

14. A patient's caregiver tries to act in the best interest of the patient by making sure the patient's pain is controlled postoperatively. This is an example of which type of ethical principle?

A. Beneficence
B. Fidelity
C. Veracity
D. Justice

15. An example of patient medical abandonment is when the AGACNP:

A. Prepares for maternity leave but arranges for coverage for their patients
B. Prepares for withdrawal of ventilatory support from their patient
C. Refuses to see a patient after failure to pay for previous services
D. Provides notice to their patients before moving to a different state

16. The AGACNP working in hospice prescribes pain medications to a patient complaining of severe pain who is on comfort care. The use of narcotics to control this patient's discomfort is rationalized even if death may be hastened as a consequence of the pain control because of what principle?

A. Respect for autonomy
B. Physician-assisted suicide
C. American Nurses Association Code of Ethics
D. Double effect

17. A patient with necrotizing pancreatitis has been in the ICU for a long period of time and has not been progressing due to multiorgan failure. The AGACNP is considering the patient's prognosis and would like to plan a goals of care conversation with the family. The AGACNP knows a conflict may arise regarding whether or not to withdraw care if:

A. The AGACNP has not established a rapport with the family.
B. There is a lack of effective communication with the family.
C. The patient has a living will and durable power of attorney.
D. The AGACNP does not share the same values as the family.

18. The AGACNP is embarking on a research study and will be moving to a new location away from their clinical practice. Which of the following is necessary to avoid patient medical abandonment when terminating the patient–provider relationship?

A. Offer resources and recommendations about other AGACNPs who are accepting new patients and accept the patient's insurance
B. Provide an exact reason for the dismissal of the patient
C. Continue to provide treatment until the patient can secure care from another provider for up to 2 years
D. Notify the patient verbally during their next appointment; a formal letter is not necessary

19. How can the AGACNP maintain communication and establish rapport with a patient who is sedated and on mechanical ventilation in the ICU?

A. Ask the bedside nurse to communicate with the patient instead
B. Limit communication because this may cause the patient to wake up and become anxious
C. Use open-ended questions to better understand the patient's medical history
D. Verbally communicate to the patient before interventions and use appropriate touch during care

20. For critically ill patients admitted to the ICU, it is important for the AGACNP to meet the patient's support system (e.g., friends, caregivers) within the first few days after admission. The *most* important purpose of the initial meeting is to:

A. Answer questions regarding the patient's medical information
B. Identify the healthcare proxy
C. Begin to develop a trusting relationship
D. Limit family interaction unless it is initiated by the patient

21. The AGACNP will use therapeutic communication when discussing end-of-life decisions with family members by asking:

A. "What do you think we should do next to help your family member?"
B. "Have you ever talked to your family member about their wishes if they became critically ill?"
C. "Have you thought about what you would want if you were in the same situation as your family member?"
D. "What would your family member want in this situation?"

22. The AGACNP is planning a family meeting in order to inform the family of the patient's condition and prognosis, answer questions, and include them in the decision-making process. In most circumstances, who should be included within the family meeting?

A. Bedside nurse, chaplain, all family members, ICU attending
B. Respiratory therapist, social worker, ICU attending, all family members
C. Patient's healthcare power of attorney, ICU attending, bedside nurse
D. Palliative care team, limited family members, student nurse

23. The AGACNP uses the organizational error reporting system to report a "near-miss" patient incident. A unit of blood was ordered for a patient but was connected to the wrong patient's intravenous line. The error was detected before the transfusion was started. This is an example of which of the following Quality and Safety Education for Nurses initiatives?

A. Patient-centered care
B. Evidence-based practice
C. Quality improvement
D. Safety

24. Which of the following is the overall goal for the Quality and Safety Education for Nurses (QSEN) project?

A. To establish an ethical standard for the profession to guide nurses in ethical decision-making
B. To promote the formulation of clinical questions using PICO to evaluate the effectiveness of an intervention
C. To prepare future nurses with the knowledge, skills, and attitude necessary to continuously improve quality and safety in their healthcare systems
D. To assist with the licensing and credentialing processes for nurses

25. The AGACNP completes a four-step process for quality improvement. This involves an outline of objectives and desired outcomes, an implementation phase, assessment of data, and implementation of action. Which of the following continuous quality improvement (CQI) strategies describes this process?

A. Lean
B. Plan-Do-Study-Act (PDSA)
C. Six Sigma
D. Baldridge Criteria

26. An AGACNP leads a project to improve sleep quality in the ICU and prevent delirium. The AGACNP studied the impact of the initiation of a sleep hygiene bundle on sleep quality in the ICU and found an improvement in sleep duration and quality. This is an example of which of the following Quality and Safety Education for Nurses initiatives?

A. Quality improvement
B. Teamwork and collaboration
C. Evidence-based practice
D. Informatics

27. A patient with Parkinson disease is complaining about frequent falls, reporting that they feel unsteady while walking. Which of the following complementary therapies should the AGACNP recommend because it has been shown to improve motor issues and balance, and decrease the risk of falls in patients with Parkinson disease?

A. Massage therapy
B. Acupuncture
C. Hypnotherapy
D. Tai chi

28. An AGACNP develops a continuous quality improvement (CQI) project to improve handwashing and sanitizing practice to prevent infections. The AGACNP evaluates current practice in each department and then sets goals through the hospital for hand hygiene compliance. This is an example of which of the following?

A. Plan-Do-Study-Act (PDSA)
B. Patient-centered care
C. Internal benchmarking
D. Quality assurance

29. A patient with benign prostate hyperplasia (BPH) reports increased frequency, urgency, and difficulty starting urination. The patient reports taking an herbal supplement for the symptoms but cannot remember the name. Which of the following herbal supplements is commonly used in patients with BPH?

A. St. John's wort
B. Saw palmetto
C. Gingko biloba
D. Black cohosh

30. A patient with seasonal effective disorder (SAD) has been prescribed antidepressants but reports recurrent episodes of major depression. Which of the following complementary alternative therapies can be recommended for this patient?

A. Light therapy
B. Chiropractic manipulation
C. Music therapy
D. Healing touch

31. Which of the following herbal supplements can be used to treat nausea and motion sickness?

A. Echinacea
B. Evening primrose oil
C. Garlic
D. Ginger

32. A patient with depression reports compliance with their selective serotonin reuptake inhibitors (SSRIs) but reports new side effects of altered mental status, neuromuscular abnormalities, and autonomic hyperactivity. The AGACNP is concerned about serotonin syndrome from additional herbal supplement use causing a drug interaction. Which of the following herbal supplements can cause this type of interaction?

A. Saw palmetto
B. Ginger
C. St. John's wort
D. Ginseng

33. A young adult patient presents with an acute cystitis infection and describes dysuria at an 8 out of 10 on the pain scale. The AGACNP prescribes trimethoprim-sulfamethoxazole (Bactrim) to treat the infection. What else might the AGACNP include in the prescription?

A. Nitrofurantoin (Macrobid)
B. Ibuprofen (Motrin)
C. Acetaminophen with codeine
D. Phenazopyridine (Pyridium)

34. An older adult female patient presents with symptoms of frequency of urination and dysuria after a one-day history of lower left back pain that is radiating to the groin. Urinalysis reveals blood ++, protein+, pH 7. Which of the following is most likely the cause of the symptoms?

A. Appendicitis
B. Urinary tract infection (UTI)
C. Bladder cancer
D. Atrophic vaginitis

35. A patient presents with seasonal rhinitis and a dry cough. The patient has a history of congestive artery disease and hypertension and complains of excessive sneezing, rhinorrhea, and nasal congestion. Which of the following drugs would the AGACNP avoid prescribing?

A. Benzonatate
B. Guifenesin
C. Dextromethorphan
D. Phenylephrine

36. In which of the following genitourinary conditions would the AGACNP expect to find a positive Phren sign?

A. Testicular torsion
B. Acute epididymitis
C. Incarcerated hernia
D. Hydrocele

37. A patient with a history of myocardial infarction (MI) and hypertension presents with tinnitus. The physical examination shows no cause for the symptoms. Use of which of the following drugs could be the cause of the patient's tinnitus?

A. Beta-blocker
B. Aspirin
C. Calcium channel blocker
D. Statin

38. Nonsteroidal anti-inflammatory drugs are known to cause gastrointestinal (GI) bleeding. Which of the following drugs has a lowered risk of GI bleed?

A. Naproxen
B. Indomethacin
C. Celecoxib
D. Ketoralac

39. A patient presents with complaints of acute onset epigastric pain that radiates to the back. The pain is steady. The patient is experiencing nausea and vomiting and has a temperature of 101.4°F (38.5°C). The patient reports that lying supine makes the pain, worse but leaning forward helps to ease the pain. The AGACNP knows that the likely diagnosis is acute:

A. Diverticulitis
B. Pancreatitis
C. Appendicitis
D. Cholecystitis

40. A patient presents with a bleeding ulcer as a result of long-term use of nonsteroidal anti-inflammatory drugs (NSAIDs) to relieve pain. Which of the following drugs would be the best choice for treatment of bleeding ulcer?

A. Muscarinic antagonist
B. Bismuth
C. Famotidine
D. Misoprostol

41. A patient presents with watery diarrhea and signs of dehydration following a vacation outside of the United States. The patient exhibits confusion, tachypnea, and hypotension. Metabolic acidosis is suspected. Which of the following pH values is critical?

A. 7.5
B. 7.0
C. >7.60
D. 7.8

42. Which of the following laboratory results is consistent with a diagnosis of thalassemia anemia?

A. Macrocytic normochromic anemia, normal total iron-binding capacity
B. Microcytic hypochromic anemia, normal ferritin
C. Microcytic hyperchromic anemia, decreased alpha- and/or beta-globin chains
D. Microcytic hypochromic anemia, low serum ferritin

43. A patient presents with fatigue. A heart murmur is heard upon evaluation only at the cardiac apex. Which valve is most likely involved based on the location of the murmur?

A. Mitral
B. Tricuspid
C. Aortic
D. Pulmonic

44. In an adult patient with joint pain, which of the following diseases is systemic and not related to other diseases?

A. Gout
B. Osteoarthritis
C. Lupus
D. Spondylosis

45. A patient seen in the emergency department yesterday was treated with amoxicillin for streptococcal pharyngitis. The patient returns with reports of a flat, itchy, rash on the neck and chest area. What is the *priority* action?

A. Assess for respiratory compromise
B. Discontinue the medication
C. Provide a different prescription
D. Prescribe an antihistamine cream

46. A patient presents with a complaint of shortness of breath while walking short distances. The patient has no chronic conditions and does not take any medications. The AGACNP knows that which of the following symptoms is appropriate to inquire about during the cardiovascular review of systems?

A. Hematochezia
B. Abdominal pain
C. Orthopnea
D. Tinnitus

47. A patient who is right-handed complains of numbness in the thumb and 1, 2 digits of the right hand. The patient states that they frequently wake up in the night due to burning and numbness in the fingers and have to shake their hand to get the feeling back in the fingers. Which of the following tests would the AGACNP include in the physical exam?

A. McMurray
B. Phalen and Tinel
C. Apprehension
D. Drawer

48. A patient presents with trauma injury to the knee after a fall. The knee examination reveals significant forward translation of the tibia when the knee is in 15 degrees of flexion and external rotation at the hip. Which of the following maneuvers does this represent?

A. Lachman
B. Anterior drawer
C. Abduction stress
D. McMurray

49. Microcytosis is a term for red blood cells smaller than the normal range. Which of the following is a cause of microcytic anemia?

A. B_{12} deficiency
B. Folate deficiency
C. Iron-deficiency anemia
D. Megaloblastic anemia

50. During treatment of anaphylaxis, what site is used for the initial injection of epinephrine?

A. Deltoid muscle
B. Upper lateral thigh
C. Intravenous line
D. Abdomen

51. What document delineates the AGACNP's use of title and authorization for scope of practice, including prescriptive authority and disciplinary grounds?

A. State nurse practice acts
B. Best practice guidelines
C. Nursing dissertations
D. Credentialing agreements

52. Who mandates the AGACNP's scope of practice?

A. County chapter of the AGACNP council
B. State board of nursing
C. Federal government
D. Organization for which the AGACNP is employed

53. The AGACNP knows that credentials:

A. Are regulatory mechanisms to ensure accountability for competent practice
B. Establish the maximum level of acceptable performance
C. Diminish professional standards of practice
D. Are standards by which to measure quality of practice, service, or education

54. What determines the ability and extent of AGACNPs to prescribe medications, including controlled substances?

A. Drug Enforcement Agency (DEA)
B. State Board of Nursing via state nurse practice acts
C. Medicare guidelines
D. Hospital or clinic board of directors

55. An AGACNP refuses to accept responsibility for caring for an 8-year-old patient. Which of the following actions would help avoid a claim of patient abandonment?

A. Giving reasonable notice to the proper authority that the AGACNP lacks competence to carry out the assignment
B. Walking out without communicating with other providers or the director to minimize the number of people who are aware of the situation
C. Managing the care of the patient until a pediatric practitioner arrives
D. Asking the patient to leave the hospital and seek care elsewhere

56. Which of the following, granted by nongovernmental agencies, establish(es) that a person has met certain standards in a particular profession that signify mastery or specialized knowledge and skills?

A. Privileges
B. Credentials
C. Certification
D. Licensure

57. A hospital's risk management team is seeking to reduce risk in its organizations. Which of the following is *not* an important source of collected information that can help advance the efforts of a risk management team?

A. Incident reports
B. Satisfaction surveys
C. Material safety and data sheet
D. Complaints

58. A systematic effort to reduce an organization's risk begins with a formal, written risk management plan. Which of the following is *not* part of a written risk management plan?

A. Goals of the organization
B. Program's scope, components, and methods
C. Consequences for those who report sensitive information
D. Responsibility for implementation and enforcement

59. An AGACNP forgets to order a 12-lead EKG on a patient who has a complaint of chest pain. The patient subsequently dies of an acute myocardial infarction. What is this failure of the AGACNP called?

A. Negligence
B. Malpractice
C. Assault
D. Battery

60. During intubation, an AGACNP witnesses a paralytic agent being given prior to a sedating agent. Which of the following reports should be written?

A. Employee satisfaction survey
B. Incident report
C. Police report
D. Informed consent statement

61. An AGACNP is evaluating whether there is a correlation between time spent explaining discharge instructions and rate of readmissions. Which of the following values would indicate the absence of correlation?

A. –1
B. 0
C. 1
D. 100

62. Which of the following statements about the use of restraints is *not* accurate?

A. Restraints may be used to prevent a patient from harming themself or others.
B. The exact reason restraints have been ordered must be documented.
C. Safety checks of restraints must be routinely performed and documented.
D. The most severe form of restraint should be used initially and gradually scaled back to less severe restraint.

63. A patient becomes angry at their spouse and demands the spouse leave the room. After the spouse leaves, the AGACNP attempts to calm the patient, but the patient threatens to commit violent behavior toward the spouse as soon as they are discharged from the hospital. The AGACNP's most appropriate intervention is to:

A. Report the incident to the patient's spouse
B. Allow the patient to voice their anger
C. Notify the police department
D. Notify the charge nurse

64. A patient presents to the clinic after high-risk sexual behavior. The AGACNP orders screening for sexually transmitted infections, hepatitis, and HIV. The patient's HIV test result is positive. The AGACNP informs the patient and reports the result to:

A. Centers for Disease Control and Prevention
B. Other local hospitals
C. Local health department
D. The patient's sexual partner(s)

65. The AGACNP receives a call from police authorities regarding a patient on the medicine floor. They are asking for the patient's name and date of birth to aid in identifying a suspect in a homicide. What is the AGACNP's response?

A. Comply and provide requested information
B. Deny the request
C. Ask for the patient's written consent
D. Ask for a subpoena

66. The AGACNP is providing discharge instructions to a patient with renal calculi. The AGACNP knows that the education given to the patient must be:

A. Tailored to their educational level
B. Done quickly because their transportation is waiting
C. Generalized to fit many diseases processes
D. Written in the English language

67. What responsibility does the AGACNP have when suggesting herbal supplements to a patient who wishes to add them to their care regimen?

A. Understanding the potential for drug–herb and herb–herb interactions
B. Consulting with interprofessional team
C. Scheduling follow-up visits monthly to monitor patient outcomes
D. Referring to a doctor of osteopathy for initial consultation

68. The AGACNP is assessing an older adult who has been undergoing chemotherapy treatment for metastatic breast cancer. The patient reports feelings of agitation and anxiety related to the diagnosis but feels they are taking too many medications and do not want to add any more. The AGACNP suggests:

A. Therapeutic touch
B. Chakra balancing
C. Aromatherapy
D. Biofield energy medicine

69. The AGACNP is assessing a patient who reports signs and symptoms of both dementia and depression. Which action will the nurse take to ensure use of resources has been optimized while determining diagnosis?

A. Determining which tests will be least invasive
B. Weighing benefits of testing against the cost
C. Selecting testing that can be performed most quickly
D. Choosing testing based on insurance payment

70. When recommending integrative medicine to an older patient, which area will the AGACNP add as a focus of assessment?

A. Provider care and support
B. Health behaviors
C. Identification of least invasive, simplest therapies
D. Examination of mind–body treatment modalities

71. During an evaluation of the care plan, the AGACNP is discussing goals and outcomes that have not been met regarding diet and nutritional needs to maintain normal glucose levels. The patient is reluctant to make changes to their diet, stating that they like to eat ice cream every night before bed. To ensure that the standards of practice are met regarding evaluation, the AGACNP will first:

A. Make adjustments to the care plan based on their findings
B. Document the patient's response in standardized language and terminology
C. Communicate the effectiveness of the care plan to the patient and caregiver
D. Evaluate the effectiveness of the patient's support system

72. The AGACNP has completed an assessment of a patient with crushing injuries and severe burns on 55% of the body and has determined that the patient should be considered for transfer to a specialty hospital. In an effort to ensure that standards of practice regarding care management and planning are followed, the AGACNP will first:

A. Collaborate with interdisciplinary team to determine appropriate transition of care
B. Discuss the transition plan with the patient's family members and/or caregiver
C. Contact the specialty hospital to prepare for the transfer and transition of care
D. Complete the transfer paperwork and share it with the nursing staff

73. The AGACNP is assessing a patient for discharge home to recover from an automobile collision. Which tool does the AGACNP know provides the most encompassing information to direct care from a home health agency?

A. Katz Index
B. OASIS
C. Functional Index Measure
D. Minimum Data Sheet–ADL

74. When preparing a patient for discharge home following hip arthroplasty, the AGACNP has an obligation to:

A. Apply knowledge of organizational theories for provision of safe and effective care
B. Serve as resource for the design and development of a care program
C. Develop innovative solutions for addressing patient care
D. Collaborate with the interdisciplinary team on discharge teaching for home care

75. The Aviation Medical Assistance Act (AMAA) allows for the AGACNP to provide emergency care while in flight with what caveat?

A. Providers are not fully exempt from liability for damages
B. Providers must be familiar with on-flight medical equipment
C. All procedures and care should be reported to the Federal Aviation Administration
D. Providers are legally required to assist in health emergencies

76. The AGACNP is performing an assessment on a patient recently admitted to rehabilitation from a 28-day inpatient stay for crushing injuries. The patient is noted to have memory impairment with slight cognitive changes as well as changes in depth perception in the left eye. Which collaborative referral will the AGACNP initially make for this patient?

A. Physical therapy
B. Psychological evaluation
C. Occupational therapy
D. Ophthalmology evaluation

77. An older adult patient is being seen for the first time after being released from incarceration of 28 years. During the initial interview, the patient reports having "a lot of health problems" during incarceration, but the patient does not possess any medical records. Which action will the AGACNP take first to complete a full review of medical history?

A. Have the patient sign a release of medical records for institutional medical treatments
B. Contact the correctional medical provider for a copy of the Advanced Care Plan
C. Complete a full history and physical examination with advanced assessment
D. Evaluate for patient trauma during incarceration along with living conditions

78. An older adult patient being treated for hypertension, arthritis, hypercholesterolemia, and diabetes mellitus is planning a cruise that will take them to another country. How will the AGACNP *best* prepare this patient for their trip?

A. Develop a nutrition plan that can be provided to the cruise staff with a list of approved snacks and treats that the patient can indulge in.
B. Ensure that the patient has a stocked supply of insulin and needles along with a traveling biohazard container that can be discarded at the medical infirmary on the ship.
C. Collaborate with the patient on how to include daily exercise while on the ship to maintain consistent blood glucose levels.
D. Ensure that the patient has enough medication for their trip along with a list of all medications, dosages, pharmacy contact, and emergency contact information.

79. While preparing to discharge a patient who resides in two different homeless shelters, the AGACNP will assess the patient's functional status and ability to take medications using which tool?

A. Katz Index
B. OASIS
C. Brief Instrumental Functional Scale (BIFS)
D. Functional Index Measure (FIM)

80. The AGACNP is planning postoperative discharge for a patient who is self-reported homeless. The patient will need follow-up by a home health agency for wound care, activities of daily living, and ambulation. Which step will the AGACNP take to ensure that the patient has continuity of care?

A. Refer the patient to medical respite care
B. Request rapid rehousing during recovery
C. Contact a homeless shelter for a semi-permanent bed
D. Refer the patient to social services for case management

81. An older adult patient presents to the emergency department with nausea with severe abdominal pain, diaphoresis, and headache for the past 2 days. Upon further assessment, the patient reports feelings of anxiousness and inability to sleep through the night and rates overall pain status at 8/10. Patient vital signs are documented as blood pressure 122/68, pulse 72 and regular, respiratory rate 20 with clear lungs on auscultation, temperature 104.2°F (40.1°C). Based on these findings, what will the AGACNP do *first* for this patient?

A. Admit the patient for observation
B. Send the patient for CT scan of the head
C. Refer the patient to rehabilitation
D. Order dronabinol (Syndros) and gabapentin (Neurontin) for the patient

82. An older adult patient recently diagnosed with neuropathy reports taking tetrahydrocannabinol (THC) 8 mg a day. What will the AGACNP do to ensure safe administration of this new therapeutic approach?

A. Review current medications for interactions
B. Have the patient decrease the dosage to 5 mg
C. Educate the patient on the side effects of THC
D. Explain to the patient that THC provides only temporary relief and prescribed medications should be continued

83. Which tool has been identified as a framework for practitioner guidance when intervening in elder mistreatment?

A. Geriatric Injury Documentation Tool (Geri-IDT)
B. Abuse Intervention Model (AIM)
C. Elder Mistreatment Multidisciplinary Teams (EM-MDT)
D. Functional Independence Measure (FIM)

84. During a routine examination of an older adult patient, the AGACNP notices bruising around the patient's wrist. When questioned, the patient states that their young-adult grandson has just started living with them and grabbed them by the wrist in an effort to keep them from falling. Upon further evaluation, the AGACNP learns that the grandson came to the patient from a drug rehabilitation program. What increased risk should the AGACNP further evaluate?

A. Altered cognition
B. Risk for falls
C. Elder mistreatment
D. Social isolation

85. An older adult who is hard of hearing is accompanied by their adult child while in the emergency department for abdominal pain. The patient is ruled in for having an acute abdomen. The surgeon explains to the adult child in private that the patient will be brought to the operating room; however, due to the patient's other comorbidities, including severe chronic obstructive pulmonary disease and multivessel coronary artery disease, the patient's perioperative mortality is high. The patient hears none of this but signs consent for surgery. The patient right violated by the surgeon is the right to:

A. Medical treatment in an emergency

B. Informed consent

C. Refuse care

D. Continuity of care

86. An older adult patient with decisional capability is informed while in the hospital that the next day the patient will receive a heart catheterization due to elevations in the patient's troponins. The procedure and risks have been fully explained. The patient states, "I'm not doing that." The patient is practicing the right to:

A. Refuse care

B. Emergency treatment

C. Confidentiality

D. Informed consent

87. The AGACNP is examining a patient and notes a sacral pressure injury with full-thickness skin loss. What stage does the AGACNP assign to this injury?

A. 1

B. 2

C. 3

D. 4

88. A patient has the right to confidentiality with some exceptions. Which of the following would require patient confidentiality protection?

A. Suicide threat

B. Homicide threat

C. HIV/AIDS

D. Hepatitis A

89. The AGACNP evaluates an older adult patient who presents with acute and fluctuating cognitive impairment. The AGACNP documents this condition as:

A. Delirium
B. Dementia
C. Amnesia
D. Medication-related side effects

90. What assessment tool can be used to evaluate gait and balance?

A. Romberg
B. Timed Up and Go
C. Nuclear stress test
D. MRI of spine

91. The AGACNP is educating an older adult patient and their family on risk factors for developing pressure injuries. What does the AGACNP indicate as the primary risk factor?

A. Immobility
B. Incontinence
C. Malnutrition
D. Friction

92. The AGACNP is seeing a patient who reports multiple falls occurring first thing in the morning upon standing up from bed. What does the AGACNP suspect as the most likely cause of the falls?

A. Vision impairment
B. Environmental hazards
C. Lower extremity weakness
D. Postural hypotension

93. Which medication is associated with tinnitus if administered too quickly and is not recommended to be administered faster than 40 mg/min?

A. Intravenous (IV) cefazoline (Ancef)
B. IV morphine
C. IV furosemide (Lasix)
D. 0.9% normal saline IV solution

94. A patient presents to the emergency department with severe dyspnea, wheezing, and hives following an insect sting. Which pharmacologic agent is indicated first?

A. Epinephrine
B. Lorazepam
C. Albuterol
D. 0.9% normal saline IV solution

95. A patient presents with complaints of fatigue and weakness. Upon flexion of the neck, the patient complains of an electric shock-like sensation that goes down the spine. The visual exam is concerning for optic neuritis. These physical exam findings are suggestive of which of the following diagnoses?

A. Multiple sclerosis
B. Myasthenia gravis
C. Guillain-Barré syndrome
D. Trigeminal neuralgia

96. A patient presents with a severe headache and nausea. Physical assessment is significant for a fever, nuchal rigidity, and spontaneous flexion of the hips during passive flexion of the neck. A head CT is obtained, and then a lumbar pressure is performed. Considering these findings, what does the AGACNP anticipate when reviewing the cerebrospinal fluid (CSF) results?

A. Increased glucose concentration
B. Elevated protein concentration
C. Decreased opening pressure
D. Minimal white blood cells

97. Which of the following assessment findings is seen with Cushing triad?

A. Arrythmias, apnea, bradycardia
B. Tachycardia, hypotension, widened pulse pressure
C. Hyperglycemia, hyperreflexia, tachycardia
D. Irregular respirations, widened pulse pressure, bradycardia

98. The AGACNP assesses a patient who is ambulating with short steps and a shuffling, unstable gait with minimal arm swing. The patient has a stooped posture, moves slowly, and appears unsteady on their feet. The AGACNP notices hand tremors at rest, and the patient's face appears "mask-like." These physical exam findings are concerning for which type of diagnosis?

A. Alzheimer disease
B. Guillain-Barré syndrome
C. Multiple sclerosis
D. Parkinson disease

99. A patient presents with complaints of low back pain radiating down both legs and difficulty voiding. During the neurological assessment, the AGACNP also notes bilateral lower extremity motor weakness with diminished sensation. There is no motor dysfunction in the upper extremities. Considering this clinical presentation, the AGACNP anticipates which type of spinal cord disorder?

A. Brown-Sequard syndrome
B. Cauda equina syndrome
C. Central cord syndrome
D. Spondylolisthesis of C2

100. A rugby player presents to the emergency department with diminished motor function to the extremities after being knocked down during a game. A neurological assessment reveals minimal movement of the lower extremities that is slightly increased compared with the upper extremities. These physical exam findings are suggestive of which type of spinal cord injury?

A. Anterior cord syndrome
B. Brown-Sequard syndrome
C. Central cord syndrome
D. Complete cord syndrome

101. A patient with a spinal cord injury who is quadriplegic presents with restlessness and anxiety. Upon physical exam, the AGACNP notices diaphoresis, hypotension (blood pressure of 80/45 mmHg), and bradycardia (heart rate of 52 beats/min). Hemodynamic parameters are significant for cardiac output of 2 L/min, cardiac index of 1 L/min, and systemic vascular resistance (SVR) of 500 dyn·s/cm^5. The AGACNP is concerned for which type of shock?

A. Hypovolemic
B. Cardiogenic
C. Obstructive
D. Neurogenic

102. A patient presents following a skiing accident. During the physical assessment, the AGACNP notices decreased sensation below the nipple line. These findings are suggestive of a spinal injury at or above which of the following levels?

A. Cervical 8
B. Lumbar 5
C. Thoracic 4
D. Sacral 1

103. Which of the following evaluates for lumbar radiculopathy?

A. Straight leg raise
B. Spurling test
C. Extension-rotation test
D. Empty can test

104. Which of the following tests evaluates cerebellar function?

A. Pronator drift
B. Stereognosis
C. Finger-to-nose test
D. Graphesthesia

105. A patient presents with bilateral lower extremity weakness. The AGACNP's physical examination is significant for a grade 1 motor strength to the patient's bilateral lower extremities, along with a grade 1+ to the Achilles and patellar tendons. The patient reports a viral illness about 2 weeks ago. Based on these physical exam findings, what should the AGACNP order next?

A. Methylprednisolone
B. Physical therapy
C. Pulmonary function test
D. Oseltamivir

106. A patient presents complaining of unilateral burning and stabbing facial pain. During the assessment, the AGACNP notices that the pain is localized to the cheek and chin area and worsens while the patient is talking and swallowing. The AGACNP is concerned for which of the following?

A. Multiple sclerosis
B. Trigeminal neuralgia
C. Myasthenia gravis
D. Parkinson disease

107. A patient presents with an acute sudden onset of altered mental status. The patient states that they got up to urinate during the night and developed sudden weakness of their face and arm. During the assessment, the AGACNP notes a facial droop, ataxia, nystagmus, and right-sided weakness. Cardiac auscultation reveals a fast-paced irregular rhythm with a murmur. Based on these physical exam findings, the AGACNP is concerned for which of the following stroke types?

A. Intracerebral hemorrhage
B. Ischemic (thrombotic)
C. Subarachnoid hemorrhage
D. Ischemic (embolic)

108. A patient presents with an abrupt onset of a sudden, severe headache while mowing the lawn. No focal neurologic deficits are appreciated on the neurologic assessment. Past medical history is significant for hypertension and alcohol abuse. Based on these physical exam findings, the AGACNP is *most* concerned for which of the following stroke types?

A. Intracerebral hemorrhage

B. Ischemic (thrombotic)

C. Subarachnoid hemorrhage

D. Ischemic (embolic)

109. A patient presents with acute right-sided weakness, aphasia, and a facial droop. Which of the following diagnostic tests is the priority to obtain *first* to guide further treatment decisions?

A. MRI of the brain without contrast

B. CT of the head without contrast

C. MRI of the brain with contrast

D. CT angiography

110. A patient presents with an acute change in neurologic status. The assessment is significant for homonymous hemianopia, transient aphasia, and hemiparesis. Within 24 hours, no focal deficits are noted on further assessments. These physical exam findings are suggestive of which of the following?

A. Transient ischemic attack

B. Intracerebral hemorrhage

C. Subdural hematoma

D. Subarachnoid hemorrhage

111. A patient presents with symptoms of a focal seizure. The patient has not lost consciousness, but during the assessment the AGACNP notices that the patient is having speech difficulties. Based on these findings, the AGACNP is concerned for a seizure beginning in which area of the brain?

A. Occipital cortex

B. Motor cortex

C. Parietal cortex

D. Frontal lobe

112. A rapid response team is called to the patient's room due to concern for a seizure. Upon arrival, the AGACNP assessment is significant for impaired consciousness and sudden muscle stiffening in the upper and lower extremities. These findings are suggestive of which type of generalized seizure?

A. Absence

B. Myoclonic

C. Tonic

D. Atonic

113. The AGACNP is called to bedside of a patient who recently experienced a focal motor seizure. The family is concerned that the patient may be experiencing another seizure because the patient is still confused. Physical assessment findings are significant for weakness of the right arm and an altered level of consciousness. These findings likely represent which of the following?

A. Postictal period

B. Aura

C. Generalized status epilepticus

D. Myoclonic seizure

114. The AGACNP assesses a patient with findings suggestive of a generalized seizure. The motor movements are significant for rhythmic jerking muscle contractions in the patient's bilateral arms, neck, and face. These findings are concerning for which type of seizure?

A. Myoclonic

B. Clonic

C. Tonic

D. Atonic

115. A patient with a previous history of a spinal cord injury at T5 presents to the emergency department complaining of a headache and anxiety. The physical assessment is significant for diaphoresis, flushing above the nipple line, hypertension (blood pressure 190/115 mmHg), and bradycardia (heart rate 45 beats/min). Based on these physical exam findings, what should the AGACNP order next?

A. Bladder scan and intermittent catheterization
B. Strict bedrest in supine position until vital signs improve
C. 10 mg of labetalol (Trandate) intravenously
D. Warm blanket therapy for temperature management

116. A patient presents after a direct injury to the head. During the physical assessment, the AGACNP notices clear fluid draining from the patient's nose and periorbital ecchymosis. These findings are concerning for which type of injury?

A. Epidural hematoma
B. Subdural hematoma
C. Basilar skull fracture
D. Cerebral contusion

117. Which of the following is the *most* common causative organism for an acute complicated urinary tract infection?

A. *Escherichia coli* (*E. coli*)
B. *Klebsiella*
C. Methicillin-sensitive *Staphylococcus aureus* (MSSA)
D. Methicillin-resistant *S. aureus* (MRSA)

118. The AGACNP is called to the bedside to assess an older adult patient who was admitted for a urinary tract infection. Per the RN, the patient developed a sudden onset of confusion. Mental status has been fluctuating over the past few hours. The patient has not had previous episodes of confusion or memory impairment. Upon assessment, the patient is alert and oriented only to self and has urinary incontinence. These findings are suggestive of which of the following?

A. Dementia
B. Alzheimer disease
C. Lewy body dementia
D. Acute delirium

119. Which of the following is the *preferred* test to distinguish prerenal disease from acute tubular necrosis (ATN) as the cause of acute kidney injury?

A. Fractional excretion of sodium (FENa)
B. Urinalysis
C. Blood urea nitrogen/serum creatinine ratio
D. Serum creatinine trend

120. Which of the following is a cause of prerenal disease in acute kidney injury?

A. Nephrotoxic agents
B. Dehydration
C. Renal calculi
D. Benign prostatic hypertrophy

121. Which of the following laboratory tests is warranted in all patients being evaluated for benign prostatic hypertrophy (BPH)?

A. Urine culture
B. Urinalysis
C. Serum creatinine
D. Prostate-specific antigen (PSA)

122. Which of the following is the *most* common type of stone formation in patients with nephrolithiasis?

A. Uric acid
B. Struvite
C. Calcium
D. Cystine

123. Which of the following is not commonly seen in chronic kidney disease (CKD) alone?

A. Edema
B. Hypertension
C. Oliguria
D. Weakness/fatiguability

124. Which of the following is the current recommendation for screening of prostate cancer?

A. All men ages 55 to 69 years should engage in shared decision-making regarding screening.

B. All men 50 years or older should be screened with a prostate-specific antigen (PSA) test and a digital rectal examination.

C. All men ages 55 to 69 years old should undergo a digital rectal examination.

D. All men older than 70 years should be screened due to the increased risk of advanced disease.

125. Which of the following is one of the components used to stage chronic kidney disease (CKD) in order to guide management and identify risk for progression and complications?

A. Albuminuria

B. Serum creatinine

C. Blood urea nitrogen

D. Urine output

126. Which of the following presentations warrants a nephrology evaluation in an adult patient with newly identified chronic kidney disease (CKD)?

A. Estimated glomerular filtration rate (eGFR) <40 mL/min/1.73 m^2

B. Family history of systemic autoimmune disease

C. Diabetes mellitus

D. Pregnancy

127. A patient hospitalized in the ICU presents with an acute change in altered mental status. The patient is found to have an elevated white blood cell count and lactate level. Urinalysis is positive for pyuria and bacteriuria. Urine culture and susceptibility testing are pending. The patient is febrile, hypotensive, and tachycardic. Which of the following antimicrobial agents is indicated?

A. Ceftriaxone 1 g intravenous (IV) once daily

B. Ciprofloxacin 500 mg orally twice daily

C. Meropenem 1 g IV every 8 hours plus vancomycin 15 mg/kg IV every 12 hours

D. Amoxicillin-clavulanate 875 mg orally twice daily

128. A patient with a past medical history of hypertension and diabetes is postoperative day 2 following a total hip replacement. The patient has been recovering well on the orthopedic floor but today has a fever and is complaining of dysuria and urinary frequency and urgency. Urinalysis is significant for pyuria and bacteriuria. The patient's vital signs are otherwise stable, and they deny other signs of systemic illness. The patient denies a history of any recent broad-spectrum antimicrobial use, travel, and health care exposures. Which of the following antimicrobial agents is indicated?

A. Vancomycin 15 mg/kg intravenous (IV) every 12 hours
B. Ceftriaxone 1 g IV once daily
C. Nitrofurantoin 100 mg orally twice daily
D. Trimethoprim-sulfamethoxazole one double-strength tablet orally twice daily

129. The pneumococcal vaccination is recommended for which of the following patients?

A. 55-year-old adult with chronic obstructive pulmonary disease (COPD)
B. 60-year-old adult with hypertension
C. 58-year-old adult with a family history of multiple myeloma
D. 62-year-old adult who has a history of cigarette smoking but quit 10 years ago

130. Which of the following is an absolute contraindication to the placement of a urethral catheter?

A. Urethral stricture
B. Recent urinary tract surgery
C. Presence of an artificial sphincter
D. Presence of blood at the meatus

131. Which of the following patients is at an increased risk for meningococcal disease?

A. Adult from the United States who is vacationing in Ireland
B. American high school student who is a transgender female
C. Person with HIV infection in the United States with a low CD4 count
D. College student living in a private apartment in a small U.S. city

132. It recommended for most adults to start receiving routine vaccination for herpes zoster at how many years of age?

A. 40
B. 50
C. 60
D. 20

133. *Healthy People 2030* is a national health-promotion and disease-prevention initiative. Which of the following is one of the overarching goals?

A. Reduce the cost of medications
B. Increase the number of patients with medical insurance
C. Decrease amount of emergency department visits and wait times
D. Achieve health equity and eliminate disparities

134. Which of the following is a means of acquiring passive immunity?

A. Being exposed to a disease, which causes infection
B. Receiving a vaccination
C. Feeding formula to an infant
D. Treating a disease with intravenous immune globulin

135. An adult patient presents following a motorcycle crash. The hospital treatment course is significant for a splenectomy and open reduction and internal fixation (ORIF) of right femur fracture. Which of the following vaccines are indicated upon discharge?

A. 20-valent pneumococcal conjugate vaccine (PCV20)
B. Herpes zoster vaccination
C. PCV20 followed by 23-valent pneumococcal polysaccharide vaccine (PPSV23) >4 weeks later
D. Human papillomavirus (HPV) vaccination

136. A 60-year-old patient had a colonoscopy this year, the results of which were normal. The patient has no personal or family history of colon cancer. When asked when the patient needs to follow up with additional screening, the AGACNP recommends:

A. Annual fecal immunochemistry testing (FIT)
B. Flexible sigmoidoscopy every 2 years
C. CT colonography every 3 years
D. Colonoscopy screening every 5 years

137. A patient presents with a fever and lower abdominal pain with pelvic discomfort. Acute cervical motion and adnexal tenderness are noted on bimanual pelvic examination. Which of the following tests should be performed on this patient?

A. Pregnancy test
B. C-reactive protein
C. Urine culture
D. Papanicolaou stain

138. A patient asks the AGACNP when they should have their first Pap test. At which time should cervical screening be initiated?

A. At the start of sexual activity
B. At age 21 years
C. At the start of menstruation
D. At age 18 years

139. A male patient presents with reports of an unusual craving for ice. Laboratory results are significant for hemoglobin 10 g/dL, hematocrit 30%, mean corpuscular volume (MCV) 74 fL, and mean corpuscular hemoglobin concentration (MCHC) 30%. These findings are suggestive of which type of anemia?

A. Thalassemia
B. Folic acid deficiency
C. Iron-deficiency anemia
D. Pernicious anemia

140. A male patient presents after a syncopal fall at home. Laboratory results are significant for hemoglobin 10 g/dL, hematocrit 30%, mean corpuscular volume (MCV) 72 fL, and mean corpuscular hemoglobin concentration (MCHC) 28%. Based on these lab values, this anemia is classified as:

A. Microcytic, hyperchromic
B. Microcytic, hypochromic
C. Macrocytic, normochromic
D. Macrocytic, hypochromic

141. A patient presents with fatigue, symmetric paresthesias, numbness, and gait problems. Past medical history is significant for diabetes mellitus for which the patient has been prescribed metformin for the past 5 years. Laboratory studies are significant for macrocytic anemia with mild pancytopenia. Serum level B_{12} is 150 pg/mL, and folate is 5 ng/mL. These findings are suggestive of which type of anemia?

A. Vitamin B_{12} deficiency
B. Thalassemia
C. Iron-deficiency anemia
D. Pernicious anemia

142. A patient with a past medical history significant for alcohol use disorder presents after being found on the ground. The patient has fatigue, dyspnea, and jaundice. The patient denies paresthesia, numbness, or gait problems. Laboratory studies are significant for a macrocytic anemia with mild pancytopenia. Serum level B_{12} is 315 pg/mL, and folate is 1.5 ng/mL. These findings are suggestive of which type of anemia?

A. Thalassemia
B. Iron-deficiency anemia
C. Vitamin B_{12} deficiency
D. Folic acid deficiency

143. A patient presents with a fasting blood glucose of 150 mg/dL but denies polyuria, polydipsia, weight loss, and blurry vision. Hemoglobin A1C is 5.5%. The patient is concerned that they have diabetes. Based on this information, which of the following is indicated next?

A. No further tests are required; diagnosis is confirmed based on fasting blood glucose
B. Fasting blood glucose should be repeated on a subsequent day for confirmation
C. Because the hemoglobin A1C is 5.5%, no additional tests are required
D. The hemoglobin A1C should be rechecked on a subsequent day for confirmation

144. Which of the following is included within the American Diabetes Association criteria for the diagnosis of diabetes mellitus?

A. Hemoglobin A1C >6.5%
B. Fasting plasma glucose >140 mg/dL
C. Two-hour plasma glucose >250 mg/dL during an oral glucose tolerance test
D. Random plasma glucose > 80 mg/dL in patient with symptoms of hyperglycemia

145. Which of the following diagnostic values are consistent with a diagnosis of metabolic syndrome according to the National Cholesterol Education Program Adult Treatment Panel III (ATP III) criteria?

A. Fasting blood glucose 150 mg/dL, high-density lipoprotein (HDL) cholesterol 35 mg/dL in a male patient, triglyceride level 120 mg/dL
B. Triglyceride level 160 mg/dL, waist circumference 80 cm (31.5 in) in a female patient, blood pressure 150/95 mmHg
C. Blood pressure 140/90 mmHg, HDL cholesterol 50 mg/dL in a female patient, fasting blood glucose 95 mg/Dl
D. Waist circumference 110 cm (43 in) in a male patient, fasting blood glucose 126 mg/dL, blood pressure 155/90 mmHg

146. Which of the following laboratory results is consistent with a diagnosis of prediabetes according to the American Diabetes Association criteria?

A. Hemoglobin A1C 5.5%
B. Fasting plasma glucose 128 mg/dL
C. Hemoglobin A1C 5.9%
D. Blood glucose of 135 mg/dL 2 hours post 75-g oral glucose tolerance test

147. A patient presents with polydipsia, polyuria, and weight loss with hyperglycemia (random plasma glucose >200 mg/dL) and ketonemia. Which of the following can be used to distinguish type 1 from type 2 diabetes mellitus?

A. Body mass index (BMI)
B. Pancreatic autoantibodies
C. Glycosylated hemoglobin (A1C)
D. Fasting plasma glucose

148. A patient presents complaining of thirst, polyuria, weight loss, and blurry vision. The random plasma blood glucose is 226 mg/dL. Which of the following is indicated next?

A. No further tests are required; diagnosis is confirmed based on random blood glucose and presenting symptoms
B. Plasma blood glucose should be repeated on a subsequent day for confirmation of diagnosis
C. Hemoglobin A1C should be checked to confirm diagnosis
D. An oral glucose tolerance test should be performed to confirm diagnosis

149. A male patient presents with a waist circumference of 100 cm (about 39 in), neck circumference of 38 cm (15 in), blood pressure of 150/90 mmHg, fasting blood glucose of 140 mg/dL, and triglyceride level of 160 mg/dL. The patient has a past medical history of type 2 diabetes, obstructive sleep apnea, chronic kidney disease, and hypertension. The patient meets criteria for metabolic syndrome based on what diagnostic parameters?

A. Neck circumference, blood pressure, fasting blood glucose
B. History of type 2 diabetes, blood pressure, triglyceride level
C. Fasting blood glucose, waist circumference, history of obstructive sleep apnea
D. Blood pressure, fasting blood glucose, triglyceride level

150. A patient with type 1 diabetes reports waking up with elevated blood glucose levels. The patient denies evening or night-time snacking and reports following their insulin regimen of basal and bolus insulin. Which of the following can assist with diagnosis and treatment for this patient's fasting hyperglycemia?

A. Obtain a blood glucose level before the patient eats dinner
B. Perform an oral glucose tolerance test in the morning
C. Check the blood glucose level at 3 a.m.
D. Assess the glycosylated hemoglobin (A1C) level

151. A patient presents with polyuria, polydipsia, lethargy, and fatigue that started a few days ago. Upon physical assessment, focal neurologic symptoms are noted; the patient is found to have hemiparesis and is difficult to arouse. Vital signs are significant for heart rate of 120 beats/min, blood pressure of 95/54 mmHg, respiratory rate of 18 breaths/min, and oxygen saturation of 98% on 2 L nasal cannula. Which of the following tests can assist in diagnosis based on this patient's presentation?

A. Serum beta-hydroxybutyrate
B. Plasma osmolality
C. Arterial blood gas
D. Serum bicarbonate

152. A patient presents with polyuria, polydipsia, weakness, abdominal pain, and fatigue that began this morning. Upon physical assessment, the patient is hyperventilating; a fruity breath odor, decreased skin turgor, dry oral mucosa, and tachycardia are noted. No focal deficits are present. Which of the following tests can assist in diagnosis based on this patient's presentation?

A. Anion gap
B. Lipid level
C. Plasma osmolality
D. Serum creatinine

153. A patient presents with clinical symptoms of hyperglycemia and Kussmaul respirations. The patient's laboratory results are significant for blood glucose level 300 mg/dL, sodium 135 mEq/L, chloride 105 mEq/L, potassium 5.2 mmol/L, phosphate 3 mg/dL, and serum bicarbonate 10 mEq/L During the diagnostic workup for diabetic ketoacidosis (DKA), the anion gap can be calculated as:

A. 5
B. 15
C. 18
D. 20

154. Which of the following laboratory results is often seen in patients presenting with diabetic ketoacidosis (DKA)?

A. Hypernatremia
B. Decreased blood urea nitrogen and serum creatinine concentration
C. Hyperkalemia
D. Hypophosphatemia

155. A patient presents with an elevated blood glucose and reports polyuria, polydipsia, weakness, fatigue, and altered mental status. The patient appears hypovolemic on physical exam with dry oral mucosa, decreased skin turgor, tachycardia, and hypotension. How might elevated blood glucose differ in the presence of diabetic ketoacidosis (DKA) versus hyperosmolar hyperglycemic state (HHS)?

A. There would be no difference; blood glucose is equally elevated in patients with DKA and patients with HHS
B. Blood glucose may exceed 1,000 mg/dL in HHS, but it is generally less than 800 mg/dL in patients with DKA
C. Blood glucose may exceed 800 mg/dL in DKA, but it is generally within the range of 350 to 500 mg/dL in HHS
D. Elevation in blood glucose does not vary based on the patient presentation and normal blood glucose range

156. A patient presents with polyuria, polydipsia, fatigue, lethargy, and hemianopsia. The patient's laboratory results are significant for blood glucose level 990 mg/dL, sodium 135 mEq/L, chloride 100 mEq/L, potassium 5.3 mmol/L, phosphate 3 mg/dL, and serum bicarbonate 22 mEq/L During the diagnostic workup of hyperosmolar hyperglycemic state (HHS), the effective plasma osmolality can be calculated as:

A. 325
B. 300
C. 320
D. 295

157. Primary hypothyroidism is based on which of the following diagnostic results?

A. Low serum thyroid-stimulating hormone (TSH) concentration and low serum free thyroxine (T4) concentration
B. High serum TSH concentration and high serum free T4 concentration
C. Low serum TSH concentration and high serum free T4 concentration
D. High serum TSH concentration and low serum free T4 concentration

158. The diagnostic finding suggestive of the "dawn phenomenon" is blood glucose of:

A. 200 mg/dL at 1900
B. 90 mg/dL at 0700
C. 250 mg/dL at 0700
D. 110 mg/dL at 1900

159. On a routine physical exam, a patient is found to have a thyroid nodule. A full history and physical exam is performed, along with a neck ultrasonography. Laboratory results reveal a thyroid-stimulating hormone (TSH) of 0.2 mU/L. Which of the following diagnostic tests is the next best step in evaluation?

A. Fine needle aspiration of thyroid
B. Thyroid scintigraphy
C. Measurement of serum calcitonin concentration
D. CT scan of the neck

160. A patient presents with symptoms of anxiety, palpitations, fatigue, and insomnia. On physical examination, extremities are warm and moist, periorbital edema is noted, and the patient is tachycardic. There is diffuse thyroid gland enlargement upon palpitation. Which of the following diagnostic laboratory values can be expected in this patient?

A. High thyroxine (T4) and/or triiodothyronine (T3) concentrations, low thyroid-stimulating hormone (TSH) concentration
B. Low T4 and/or T3 concentration, low TSH concentration
C. High T4 and/or T3 concentration, high serum TSH concentration
D. Low T4 concentration, high TSH concentration

161. A patient presents with reports of fatigue, cold intolerance, weight gain, and constipation. Physical examination is notable for bradycardia; coarse, dry skin; and slowed deep tendon reflexes. Which of the following diagnostic laboratory values can be expected in this patient?

A. Low serum thyroid-stimulating hormone (TSH) concentration and a high serum free thyroxine (T4) concentration
B. Low serum TSH concentration and a low serum free T4 concentration
C. High serum TSH concentration and a high serum free T4 concentration
D. High serum TSH concentration and a low serum free T4 concentration

162. On a routine physical exam, a patient is found to have a thyroid nodule. A full history and physical exam is performed, along with a neck ultrasonography, which reveals a solid hypoechoic nodule of 2 cm with irregular margins. Laboratory results reveal a thyroid-stimulating hormone (TSH) of 6.2 mU/L. Which of the following diagnostic tests is the *next best step* in evaluation?

A. Thyroid scintigraphy
B. Measurement of serum calcitonin concentration
C. Fine needle aspiration of thyroid (FNA)
D. CT scan of the neck

163. A patient presents with reports of increasing central obesity, hypertension, facial swelling, striae, menstrual irregularities, and a decreased libido. Which of the following is an appropriate initial test for diagnostic workup?

A. Early-morning salivary cortisol
B. Overnight 1 mg dexamethasone suppression test
C. 48-hour urinary free cortisol excretion
D. Late-night serum cortisol

164. A patient presents with anxiety, diaphoresis, fine tremors, weight loss despite an increased appetite, and exophthalmos. An electrocardiogram reveals a new onset of atrial fibrillation. Which of the following is the *best* initial diagnostic test for this patient presentation?

A. Thyroid-stimulating hormone (TSH)
B. Free thyroxine (T4)
C. Free triiodothyronine (T3)
D. Blood glucose level

165. Which of the following electrolyte abnormalities may be reflected in a patient with Addison disease?

A. Hypokalemia
B. Hyperglycemia
C. Hyponatremia
D. Hypocalcemia

166. Which of the following laboratory results may be reflected in a patient with Cushing syndrome?

A. Hypoglycemia
B. Hyperkalemia
C. Leukocytosis
D. Hypercalcemia

167. Which of the following would differentiate primary from secondary adrenal insufficiency?

A. ACTH
B. Serum cortisol
C. Corticotropin-releasing hormone test
D. Insulin-induced hypoglycemia test

168. A patient admitted to the ICU develops tachycardia, hypotension, cool extremities, weak peripheral pulses, and altered mental status. Laboratory findings are consistent with hyponatremia and hypoglycemia. Hyperpigmentation is noted in the buccal mucosa. Which of the following diagnostic tests is suggestive of adrenal insufficiency?

A. Salivary cortisol concentration at 8 a.m. of more than 5.8 ng/mL
B. Serum cortisol measurement at 4 p.m. of 7 mcg/dL
C. Serum cortisol measurement at 10 p.m. of 4.5 mcg/dL
D. Serum cortisol concentration at 6 a.m. of less than 3 mcg/dL

169. A patient presents with weakness, anorexia, myalgias, and arthralgias. Hyperpigmentation is not present. Laboratory values include serum sodium level of 130 mEq/L, potassium of 4.0 mmol/L, and blood glucose of 90 mg/dL. Diagnostic workup reveals a low cortisol and low ACTH level. A corticotropin-releasing hormone (CRH) test reveals an exaggerated and prolonged ACTH response. These diagnostic findings are suggestive of which type of adrenal insufficiency?

A. Primary
B. Secondary
C. Tertiary
D. Adrenal crisis

170. A patient presents with fatigue, weakness, and muscle and joint pain. Laboratory values are significant for serum sodium of 131 mEq/L, and the patient's blood sugar is 67 mg/dL. A basal plasma ACTH, cortisol 60 minute, and ACTH 250 mcg stimulation test are performed. The patient has a low cortisol and low ACTH level. Which of the following diagnostic tests can be used to differentiate the type of adrenal insufficiency this patient is likely experiencing?

A. High-dose 250 mcg ACTH stimulation test
B. Corticotropin-releasing hormone test
C. Urinary cortisol measurement
D. Insulin-induced hypoglycemia test

171. A patient presents with decreased mental status, hypothermia, hypotension, and bradycardia. The patient is minimally responsive. Family reports that the patient takes a medication every day for their thyroid. Along with emergency resuscitation and support, which laboratory test would aid in diagnosis of this patient?

A. Urinary cortisol measurement
B. Serum cortisol measurement
C. Insulin-induced hypoglycemia test
D. Corticotropin-releasing hormone test

172. A patient presents with fatigue, weight loss, nausea, skin hyperpigmentation, and postural hypotension. Laboratory values are significant for serum sodium level of 131 mEq/L, potassium of 5.2 mmol/L, and hemoglobin value of 9.0 g/dL. Diagnostic workup reveals a low cortisol and a very high plasma ACTH level. These diagnostic findings are suggestive of which type of adrenal insufficiency?

A. Primary
B. Secondary
C. Tertiary
D. Adrenal crisis

173. A patient presents with an episodic headache, sweating, tachycardia, and sustained hypertension. An incidentally discovered solid, hypervascular adrenal mass with cystic and hemorrhagic changes was noted on the patient's last CT scan. Which of the following is the *first-line test* for this patient's presentation?

A. 24-hour urine fractionated metanephrines
B. Genetic testing for multiple endocrine neoplasia type 2
C. 24-hour urine fractionated catecholamines
D. Plasma fractionated metanephrines

174. A patient presents with a decreased mental status, hypothermia, hypotension, and bradycardia. The patient is minimally responsive, but the AGACNP notes the presence of a thyroidectomy scar during the physical assessment. Which of the following diagnostic laboratory values can be expected based on this patient presentation?

A. High serum thyroxine (T4) concentration
B. High blood glucose level
C. High serum thyroid-stimulating hormone (TSH) concentration
D. High serum cortisol level

175. A patient presents with an episodic headache, sweating, tachycardia, and sustained hypertension. Biochemical tests have confirmed the diagnosis of a pheochromocytoma. Which of the following additional diagnostic tests would be indicated next?

A. CT of the abdomen and pelvis
B. Kidney, ureter, and bladder x-ray
C. Total body nuclear imaging
D. Image-guided needle biopsy

Practice Exam 2 Answers

1. C) Diabetes insipidus (DI)

In general, polyuria is defined as a urine output greater than 3 L/day in adults. A patient has DI when they are hypernatremic with a urine osmolality of less than 300 mOsmol/kg. Solute diuresis occurs in patients who are hypernatremic with a urine osmolality greater than 600 mOsmol/kg. SIADH causes impaired water excretion due to the inability to suppress the secretion of antidiuretic hormone. SIADH should be suspected in a patient who presents with hyponatremia, hypo-osmolality, urine osmolality above 100 mOsmol/kg, and urine sodium concentration usually above 40 mEq/L. Primary polydipsia is caused by a primary increase in water intake, most often seen in middle-aged female patients and in those with psychiatric illnesses. Certain medications can lead to the sensation of dry mouth. Because the patient has been intubated on mechanical ventilation, this diagnosis is less likely.

2. B) Serum osmolality <275 mOsmol/kg

SIADH causes impaired water excretion due to the inability to suppress the secretion of antidiuretic hormone. SIADH should be suspected in a patient who presents with hyponatremia (sodium level below 135 mEq/L), hypo-osmolality (normal range 275 to 290 mOsmol/kg), urine osmolality above 100 mOsmol/kg, and urine sodium concentration usually above 40 mEq/L.

3. A) Complete nephrogenic

The response to exogenous desmopressin and the patient history can help classify the type of diabetes insipidus. Central diabetes insipidus is a result of deficient secretion of antidiuretic hormone (ADH), which may be idiopathic or caused by trauma, pituitary surgery, or hypoxic or ischemic encephalopathy. Nephrogenic diabetes insipidus is due to a defect in the renal tubules resulting in renal insensitivity to ADH. Nocturia in the absence of other causes (e.g., prostatic enlargement, urinary tract infection) is often the first indicator of diabetes insipidus. Central diabetes insipidus usually has an abrupt onset in comparison to the more gradual onset seen in acquired nephrogenic diabetes insipidus or primary polydipsia. Regarding the desmopressin test, for complete nephrogenic diabetes insipidus, no elevation in urine osmolality will be seen, and the urine osmolality is <300 mOsmol/kg. For partial nephrogenic diabetes insipidus, a small (up to 45%) elevation in urine osmolality will be seen, but it remains <300 mOsmol/kg. A rise in urine osmolality of more than 100% can be seen in patients with complete central diabetes insipidus, and an increase in urine osmolality of 15% to 50% to a level >300 mOsmol/kg can be seen in patients with partial central diabetes insipidus.

4. C) Complete central

The response to exogenous desmopressin and patient history can help classify the type of diabetes insipidus. Central diabetes insipidus is a result of deficient secretion of antidiuretic hormone (ADH), which may be idiopathic or caused by trauma, pituitary surgery, or hypoxic or ischemic encephalopathy. Nephrogenic diabetes insipidus is due to a defect in the renal tubules resulting in renal insensitivity to ADH. Central diabetes insipidus usually has an abrupt onset in comparison to the more gradual onset seen in acquired nephrogenic diabetes insipidus or primary polydipsia. In regard to the desmopressin test, for complete nephrogenic diabetes insipidus, no elevation in urine osmolality will be seen and the urine osmolality is <300 mOsmol/kg. For partial nephrogenic diabetes insipidus, a small (up to 45%) elevation in urine osmolality will be seen, but it remains <300 mOsmol/kg. A rise in urine osmolality of more than 100% can be seen in patients with complete central diabetes insipidus, whereas an increase in urine osmolality of 15% to 50% to a level >300 mOsmol/kg can be seen in patients with partial central diabetes insipidus.

5. B) Temporal artery biopsy

Giant cell arteritis is diagnosed based on histopathologic proof or evidence from imaging exams. Clinical presentation can only raise the suspicion of diagnosis. The cardinal diagnostic procedure is the temporal artery biopsy; nonnecrotizing panarteritis is the typical histopathologic finding. Doppler US of the head, neck, and upper extremities can be a useful initial diagnostic procedure. While it often serves as a substitute for a temporal artery biopsy, it requires a skilled technique. Further, the biopsy remains an essential diagnostic measure for the evaluation of suspected giant cell arteritis. Imaging with CT or CT with angiography, MRI or magnetic resonance angiography, and positron emission tomography can be useful for identification of large vessel giant cell arteritis in patients who have had a negative temporal artery biopsy or for postdiagnostic imaging evaluation in patients with cranial arteritis. Temporal arteries are biopsied as they are most accessible for diagnosis; it is rare to biopsy other arteries (e.g., occipital, facial) unless there are specific signs of inflammatory involvement.

6. D) Primary polydipsia

A low plasma sodium concentration in a patient who has polyuria strongly suggests water overload secondary to primary polydipsia. Primary polydipsia, also known as psychogenic polydipsia, is caused by a primary increase in water intake, most often seen in middle-aged female patients and in those with psychiatric illnesses because certain medications (e.g., phenothiazine) can lead to the sensation of dry mouth. The patient has persistent thirst, nonadherence to fluid restriction, and development of hyponatremia. SIADH also presents with hyponatremia, but with an increased urine osmolality. A patient has diabetes insipidus when they are hypernatremic with a low urine osmolality of less than 300 mOsmol/kg. Solute diuresis occurs in patients who are hypernatremic with a urine osmolality greater than 600 mOsmol/kg.

7. A) At the time of diagnosis

For patients with type 2 diabetes, an initial comprehensive eye examination by an ophthalmologist or optometrist is recommended at the time of diagnosis with dilated fundus examination or retinal photography. Since type 2 diabetes has an insidious onset, some patients may already have retinopathy at the time of diagnosis of hyperglycemia. For patients with type 1 diabetes, an initial comprehensive examination is recommended within 5 years of diagnosis. It is less likely for patients with type 1 diabetes (younger than 30 years) to develop retinopathy. If retinopathy is present, routine follow-up should be at least yearly; if absent, routine follow-up is recommended at least every 2 years.

8. D) Elevated erythrocyte sedimentation rate and C-reactive protein

The diagnosis of giant cell arteritis should be suspected in a patient older than 50 years who has at least one or more of the following symptoms in the setting of an elevated erythrocyte sedimentation rate and C-reactive protein: new headache or change in characteristics of headache, abrupt onset of visual changes, jaw claudication, unexplained fever, and signs of vascular abnormalities (e.g., limb claudication, asymmetric blood pressures). While laboratory data can aid in the evaluation of giant cell arteritis, they are not specific for definitive diagnosis. Even so, in most patients with giant cell arteritis, erythrocyte sedimentation rate and C-reactive protein are nearly always elevated. Patients are likely to experience a systemic inflammation and often present with a normochromic normocytic anemia (rather than polycythemia), thrombocytosis (rather than thrombocytopenia), a reduced (not elevated) albumin, increased fibrinogen, and abnormal liver function tests.

9. C) Every 1 to 3 years

It is suggested that individuals undergo periodic comprehensive eye evaluations by an ophthalmologist to evaluate for glaucoma starting at age 40 years. For adult patients without risk factors for eye disease, a comprehensive eye exam should be performed every 5 to 10 years in patients younger than 40 years, every 2 to 4 years in patients 40 to 54 years, every 1 to 3 years in patients 55 to 64 years, and every 1 to 2 years in patients older than 65 years. For patients with risk factors for glaucoma (e.g., known family history of glaucoma), a comprehensive eye examination should be performed every 1 to 2 years in patients younger than 40 or older than 55 years, and every 1 to 3 years in patients age 40 to 54 years old.

10. B) Fluorescein examination

The patient presents with signs and symptoms consistent with a corneal abrasion (severe eye pain, reluctance to open the eye due to photophobia and/or foreign body sensation). The patient's history of something falling or flying into the eye is another clue to identify the etiology of the abrasion. Fluorescein examination is used to confirm the diagnosis of a corneal abrasion after completion of visual acuity, penlight, and fundus assessment. Fluorescein staining and examination with Wood's light or a slit-lamp can identify surface eye injuries, such as corneal abrasions. More detailed imaging such as a CT scan of the orbits is the preferred imaging study for patients with serious traumatic eye injuries. Specifically, an orbital CT scan is indicated for patients with an open globe, intraocular, or intraorbital foreign body; traumatic optic neuropathy; orbital fracture; or orbital compartment syndrome. While bedside US of the globe and orbit may provide rapid detection of serious eye injuries, a working diagnosis of a corneal abrasion can be made based on this patient's history, physical findings, and lack of signs of a more serious disorder. An MRI is not the preferred initial imaging modality due to the length of time it takes, and it may be contraindicated in patients who have a metal foreign body.

11. D) Chronic myeloid

Chronic myeloid leukemia (CML) is a myeloproliferative neoplasm that causes dysregulation production and uncontrolled proliferation of mature and maturing granulocytes. The fusion of two genes, *BCR* (on chromosome 22) and *ABL1* (on chromosome 9) results from a reciprocal translocation between chromosomes, causing the abnormal Philadelphia chromosome. While there are other Philadelphia chromosome-positive malignancies, all patients with CML have evidence of the Philadelphia chromosome, the *BCR:ABL1* fusion gene, or its product, the *BCR:ABL1* fusion mRNA. Therefore, the presence of this abnormal chromosome strongly suggests CML.

12. B) Measurement of intraocular pressure

This patient is presenting with signs and symptoms of acute primary-angle closure glaucoma. The clinical presentation often includes decreased vision, halos around lights, headache, severe eye pain, nausea, and vomiting. Clinical signs that suggest a rapid increase in intraocular pressure include conjunctival redness, corneal edema or cloudiness, a shallow anterior chamber, and a mid-dilated pupil (4 to 6 mm) that reacts poorly to light. Diagnosis begins with emergent examination of both eyes by an ophthalmologist, including the following tests: visual acuity, evaluation of the pupils, measurement of intraocular pressure, slit-lamp examination of the anterior segments, visual field testing, gonioscopy, and undilated fundus examination. Pupillary dilation can exacerbate angle-closure glaucoma and should be deferred when diagnosis is suspected. Fluorescein examination is used to confirm the diagnosis of a corneal abrasion after completion of visual acuity, penlight, and fundus assessment. Because the patient is presenting with clinical signs and symptoms concerning for angle-closure glaucoma, this diagnosis is less likely, and therefore this test is not indicated. Pachymetry is the measurement of corneal thickness that is indicated in patients with suspected or diagnosed open-angle glaucoma to further evaluate their risk of development and progression.

13. B) Utilitarianism

Utilitarianism considers that the right act is the one that produces the greatest good for the greatest number of people. While disaster triage can cause moral distress, an understanding of utilitarianism can help AGACNPs make decisions in such a mass casualty situation. Justice is the duty to be fair. Autonomy is the duty to respect an individual's thoughts and actions. Nonmaleficence is the duty to do no harm.

14. A) Beneficence

Beneficence mandates all clinicians and caregivers to act in the best interest of their patients. Making sure the patient's pain is under control postoperatively is an example of promoting a patient's well-being. The principle of veracity is the duty to be truthful. Fidelity is the duty to remain faithful and keep commitment to the patient. Justice is the duty to be fair.

15. C) Refuses to see a patient after failure to pay for previous services

Patient abandonment involves withdrawing from an established clinician–patient relationship without giving reasonable notice or providing a competent replacement. Refusing to see a patient after failure to pay for previously received medical services is an example of intentional abandonment. Inadvertent abandonment may occur if there is miscommunication regarding call coverage or negligence that occurs through scheduling errors. The patient can be inadvertently abandoned if the AGACNP is unavailable for long periods of time without notifying the patient or arranging for emergency coverage. A termination letter must be sent to the patient with reasonable notice and with arrangements and recommendations to other providers who may accept the patient and their insurance. Withdrawal of mechanical ventilation is not abandonment because the AGACNP continues the therapeutic relationship with the patient after extubation or transfers the care to another provider if discharging the patient from the ICU. The AGACNP continues to provide medical treatments for palliative management following the withdrawal of ventilation.

16. D) Double effect

The principle of double effect differentiates effects that are intended from those that are foreseeable though unintended. It explains how the bad consequences of an action can be considered ethically justified if the original intention was to do good. For this patient, the principle of double effect is upheld as long as the intention is to control the patient's discomfort even if death may occur as a consequence of the pain control (due to the side effects of respiratory depression, hypotension, etc.). The unintended side effect does not make the use of pain medicine unethical. Respect for autonomy involves regarding an individual's thoughts and actions. It upholds that the patient has a right to participate in medical decision-making. Physician-assisted suicide is legal only in certain states and involves facilitating a patient's death by providing the necessary means and/or information to enable the patient to perform the life-ending act. The principle of double effect does not provide moral justification for physician-assisted suicide. The American Nurses Association has established the Code of Ethics for Nurses, which sets the ethical standard for the profession and provides a guide for nurses to use in ethical analysis and decision-making. This code provides helpful discussions and ethical morals to guide decision-making, but the doctrine of double effect is the specific ethical principle applied in this case.

17. B) There is lack of effective communication with the family

Conflicts may occur when there is disagreement on whether to continue or withdraw ventilatory support. The three main reasons conflicts occur are lack of effective communication, lack of emotional support, and value conflicts. Many patients, caregivers, and families lack the skills to communicate and understand complex medical information, which can cause anxiety and confusion. The AGACNP must remember that the information should be presented in such a way that patients and families understand and are able to ask questions within a reasonable timeframe. Inadequate emotional support may also contribute to conflict due to stress, guilt, and uncertainty about decisions. Value conflicts can arise if the AGACNP is not respectful of the patient's values; the AGACNP does not have to have the same values in order to understand the patient's values. A patient's living will and durable power of attorney for healthcare can prevent conflict because it relays the patient's wishes and preferences for end of life. An established rapport can be helpful during a difficult conversation; however, it is not a requirement to avoid conflict, as long as the AGACNP uses therapeutic communication techniques.

18. A) Offer resources and recommendations about other AGACNPs who are accepting new patients and accept the patient's insurance

When terminating the patient–provider relationship, it is recommended to send a termination letter to the patient by certified mail with a return receipt requested. It is advised to provide the patient with an explanation for termination, but an exact reason is not required and is up to the provider's discretion. It is recommended to continue to provide treatment and medication refills for a reasonable period of time, such as 30 to 90 days, until the patient can secure care from another provider. Providing resources and recommendations to the patient about other physicians who may accept the patient and their insurance is necessary. Transferring records to the new provider upon patient authorization is necessary to avoid lapses in care.

19. D) Verbally communicate to the patient before interventions and use appropriate touch during care

Even when sedated, patients are still likely able to hear and can respond to those speaking to them. It is important to perform a neurological assessment on patients who are sedated to assess any changes in mental status. The AGACNP should use a gentle voice to arouse the patient, communicate with them, assess their ability to follow simple commands, and evaluate their responsiveness. Asking the bedside nurse to communicate on the behalf of the AGACNP is not appropriate and would not facilitate the AGACNP's establishing a rapport with the patient. Avoidance of communication is also not appropriate because the patient should be assessed and updated as appropriate. Open-ended questions may be difficult for the patient to answer with an endotracheal tube. Using "yes or no" questions may be more helpful to elicit information from the patient until they are better able to communicate.

20. C) Begin to develop a trusting relationship

The purpose of the initial meeting with families is to begin to develop a trusting relationship, provide emotional support, explain the medical situation, and elicit the patient's values and preferences. While answering questions and identifying the healthcare proxy can be helpful for future decision-making and may often be accomplished during the meeting, it is often not the goal of the first meeting. In certain situations, patients may ask the AGACNP not to provide information to family members. Depending on the case, that may be appropriate; however, for most critically ill patients in the ICU, decision-making by a family member or healthcare proxy is often needed due to the patient's critical illness. Avoidance of communication and interaction can cause confusion and frustration for the family.

21. B) "Have you ever talked to your family member about their wishes if they became critically ill?"

End-of-life discussions can be difficult, and the specific language used is particularly critical. The AGACNP should guide family members to what they believe the patient would think if they could speak. Therefore, rather than asking vaguely "What do you think we should next to help your family member?" the AGACNP may ask, "What do you think your family member would say if they were able to right now?" Specific questions such as "Have you ever talked to your family member about their wishes if they became critically ill?" are helpful because they probe the family members to be better able to predict what the patient would say in this situation. It is natural to ask the patient's family what the patient "would want" in regard to their end-of-life values. However, this language can lead to unrealistic suggestions and focus too much on treatment options rather than goals. It is recommended to ask what the patient would "say" or "think" about the situation, which often then leads to a discussion of goals and values. Asking the family member their own thoughts and values regarding end-of-life care strays away from the patient's perspective, and the focus should be on the patient. The AGACNP may offer, "It's okay if what you would say in this situation varies from your what your family member would say. However, I respect your ability to focus on the patient's perspective."

22. A) Bedside nurse, chaplain, all family members, ICU attending

The meeting should be open to all family members (at least all those who are involved in the patient's care) as this allows them to hear the same information to decrease misunderstandings and allow all varying views to be heard. If applicable, the patient's healthcare power of attorney should be present, but all family members who have visited or called should be offered the opportunity to attend. While all relevant healthcare providers are encouraged to attend, this often does not apply to the respiratory therapist and student nurse, whose attendance is often not necessary or appropriate unless certain circumstances permit their presence. The primary care clinician (often the AGACNP) and the ICU attending (and sometimes the ICU fellow) should be present. The bedside nurse caring for the patient should be included because nurses frequently establish a close relationship with the family. A social worker, a chaplain, and palliative care consultation teams may be valuable additions to the meeting to assist with the decision-making process.

23. D) Safety

The safety initiative minimizes the risk of harm to patients and providers by way of system effectiveness and individual performance. A culture of safety is created with open communication strategies and organizational error reporting systems. It is important for the AGACNP to communicate observations or concerns related to hazards and errors to patients and use organizational error reporting systems for near-miss and error reporting. Patient-centered care focuses on the patient and on providing compassionate and coordinated care based on respect for the patient's preferences, values, and needs. Evidence-based practice involves the use of best current evidence with clinical expertise and patient and family preferences to deliver optimal patient care. Quality improvement monitors the outcomes of care and uses improvement methods to design and test changes to continuously improve the quality and safety of health care systems.

24. C) To prepare future nurses with the knowledge, skills, and attitude necessary to continuously improve quality and safety in their healthcare systems

QSEN is an initiative aimed at providing future nurses with the knowledge, skills, and attitudes necessary to ensure continuous improvement in quality and safety of their respective healthcare systems. QSEN identifies, funds, and promotes education across six key competences: patient-centered care, teamwork and collaboration, evidence-based practice, quality improvement, safety, and informatics. The American Nurses Association has established the Code of Ethics for Nurses, which sets the ethical standard for the profession and provides a guide for nurses to use in ethical analysis and decision-making. While evidence-based practice is one of the key competencies of QSEN, formulation of clinical questions using PICO is not the overall goal of the project. Assisting with licensure and credentialing is not the overall goal of QSEN.

25. B) Plan-Do-Study-Act (PDSA)

CQI involves the improvement of processes, safety, and patient care. Strategies for CQI involve Lean, Six Sigma, PDSA, and Baldridge Criteria. PDSA is also known as the Deming cycle. This four-step process for quality improvement involves the planning stage to identify objectives and desired outcomes; the "do" phase for implementation of the plan; the study phase where results are gathered and studied to determine the effect; and the "act" stage to implement the new-found data into practice. Lean is a process of improving value to customers and employees with a focus on the reduction of waste. Six Sigma, referring to six standard deviations from the mean, is focused on reducing error rates. Baldridge Criteria focus on improving the entire organization with implementation of a culture based on CQI.

26. A) Quality improvement

Quality improvement monitors the outcomes of care and uses improvement methods to design and test changes to continuously improve the quality and safety of healthcare systems. The AGACNP is participating in a quality improvement project to seek information about outcomes of care and use quality measures to evaluate the effect of change and improve care. Teamwork and collaboration involve functioning effectively within nursing and interprofessional teams, using open communication, maintaining mutual respect, and promoting shared decision-making to improve patient care. Evidence-based practice involves the use of best current evidence with clinical expertise and patient/family preferences to deliver optimal patient care. Informatics uses information and technology to communicate, manage knowledge, mitigate error, and support decision-making.

27. D) Tai chi

Complementary and alternative medicine refers to treatments that are used along with, or in place of, conventional medicine. Originating in China, Tai chi is a form of mind-body exercise that involves martial arts, meditation, and dance-like movements. The use of tai chi has been found to decrease the risk of falls and improve motor balance. It has the potential to slow down the progression of symptoms of Parkinson disease and delay the introduction of levodopa. Additionally, a meta-analysis has found that tai chi reduces anxiety. While massage therapy, acupuncture, and hypnotherapy are also mind and body practices that may help to relieve stress, tai chi has been shown to specifically assist with balance issues in patients with Parkinson disease.

28. C) Internal benchmarking

Benchmarking works to develop specific goals for CQI projects by comparing performance or core measures in similar settings. The four core principles of benchmarking are maintaining quality, improving customer satisfaction, improving patient safety, and continuous improvement. Internal benchmarking, specifically, compares departments or divisions within the same hospital or clinic. This helps examine a particular set of measures across those locations. PDSA is a four-step process for quality improvement, which involves a planning stage to identify objectives and desired outcomes, a do phase for implementation of the plan; a study phase where results are gathered and studied to determine the effect; and an act stage to implement the newly found data into practice. Patient-centered care is one of the Quality and Safety Education for Nurses initiatives. Patient-centered care focuses on the patient and on providing compassionate and coordinated care based on respect for the patient's preferences, values, and needs. Quality assurance is a process for evaluating the care of patients using established standards of care to ensure quality.

29. B) Saw palmetto

Historically, extracts of the fruit from saw palmetto (*Serenoa repens*), the American dwarf palm tree, have been commonly used to treat BPH. However, further education by the AGACNP is needed because saw palmetto is not recommended for treating patients with BPH symptoms. Large high-quality trials have not shown saw palmetto to be effective for the treatment of BPH. St. John's wort has been used for the management of depression; however, there is inconsistent evidence for its efficacy, so it is not recommended for treating patients with depression. Ginkgo biloba has been studied for the treatment and prevention of memory issues, cognitive impairment, and dementia. Black cohosh is an herbal therapy used for the management of hot flashes.

30. A) Light therapy

SAD involves episodes of major depression, mania, or hypomania that regularly occur during particular seasons. Winter depression is the most prevalent form of SAD; it causes unipolar depression that begins in the fall or winter. First-line therapy for patients with winter depression involves an antidepressant drug therapy in addition to artificial light (bright light therapy, dawn simulation, or both). While healing touch, chiropractic manipulation, and music may alleviate symptoms associated with depression, several randomized trials have found that bright light therapy is especially efficacious for patients with SAD. Additional adjunctive interventions for patients with SAD include sleep hygiene, daily walks outside, aerobic exercise, enhanced indoor lighting with regular lamps, and dawn simulation.

31. D) Ginger

Ginger has been shown to have some antiemetic efficacy in various situations that may elicit nausea and vomiting (e.g., postoperative, chemotherapy, motion sickness, pregnancy). Patients with nausea are suggested to consume ginger-containing foods (e.g., ginger lollipops, ginger tea, foods or drinks containing ginger root or syrup). Echinacea can be used for the treatment and prevention of nonspecific upper respiratory infection. Evening primrose oil can be used in menopause to treat hot flashes, as well as for the treatment of atopic dermatitis as an alternative medicine remedy. Garlic can be used to improve indigestion and may even be associated with a reduced risk of colonic adenomas. While garlic is often used for lipid management, it is not advised due to safety concerns and lack of high-quality evidence.

32. C) St. John's wort

The use of St. John's wort in combination with antidepressants should be avoided to reduce the potential for serotonin syndrome. Symptoms of serotonin excess include agitation, hyperthermia, diaphoresis, tachycardia, and neuromuscular disturbances. Use of St. John's wort with SSRIs can cause a drug interaction and may contribute to serotonin syndrome. Ginger can be used for its antiemetic efficacy, and ginseng can be used as an adaptogen to increase overall physical and mental well-being. However, ginkgo, ginseng, and garlic can alter coagulation and increase the risk of bleeding. Ginseng can also alter glucose control. Saw palmetto may be used for benign prostatic hypertrophy but can cause mild side effects of headache, nausea, and dizziness.

33. D) Phenazopyridine (Pyridium)

Phenazopyridine (Pyridium) may be prescribed in conjunction with an antibiotic for painful urinary tract infections. It has a local anesthetic action on the urinary mucosa. Ibuprofen (Motrin) and acetaminophen with codeine are analgesics and do not exert an effect on urinary mucosa. Nitrofurantoin (Macrobid) is an antibiotic and would not be added to the current trimethoprim-sulfamethoxazole (Bactrim) regimen.

34. B) Urinary tract infection (UTI)

The patient is showing symptoms characteristic of lower UTI. Appendicitis would involve pain on the right side. Bladder cancer typically involves hematuria without pain, and atrophic vaginitis can cause dysuria but not lower back pain.

35. D) Phenylephrine

Phenylephrine is contraindicated in patients with congestive artery disease and hypertension. It is a sympathomimetic agent that can cause adverse cardiovascular effects. Benzonatate, guifenesin, and dextromethorphan are all safe to use in a patient with a cardiac history.

36. B) Acute epididymitis

A positive Prehn sign, or relief of pain upon elevation of the scrotum, is associated with acute or chronic epididymitis. Elevation of the scrotum would not lead to relief of pain in testicular torsion, incarcerated hernia, or hydrocele.

37. B) Aspirin

Patients with a history of MI may take daily aspirin to help prevent future myocardial infarction and other health issues. Early symptoms of acute aspirin toxicity include tinnitus, and aspirin is the only drug known to cause tinnitus. Although a patient with a history of MI and hypertension may also take a beta-blocker, calcium channel blocker, or statin, these medications do not have the side effect of tinnitus.

38. C) Celecoxib

Use of COX-2 inhibitors such as celecoxib presents a lower risk of GI bleeding than use of COX-1 inhibitors. Naproxen, indomethacin, and ketoralac are all COX-1 inhibitors.

39. B) Pancreatitis

Most patients with acute pancreatitis have acute onset of persistent, severe epigastric and left upper quadrant abdominal pain. The pain persists for several hours to days and may be partially relieved by sitting up or bending forward. Pain from acute diverticulitis, appendicitis, and cholecystitis is not relieved by sitting up or bending forward.

40. D) Misoprostol

Misoprostol, a prostaglandin analog, is used specifically to treat NSAID-induced ulcers. Muscarinic antagonists are bronchodilators, bismuth may be used to treat nausea and diarrhea, and famotidine is used to treat heartburn.

41. B) 7.0

Metabolic acidosis is a clinical disturbance defined by a pH less than 7.35.

42. B) Microcytic hypochromic anemia, normal ferritin

In all of the thalassemia syndromes (except with asymptomatic carriers), microcytic hypochromic anemia is present. Alpha- and beta-thalassemia are hemoglobinopathies caused by a reduction of alpha-globin chains or beta-globin chains, leading to an imbalance in the alpha-to-beta ratio. Iron-deficiency anemia is also characterized by a microcytic hypochromic anemia. However, ferritin is low and total iron-binding capacity is high in iron-deficiency anemia, whereas these levels are often normal in thalassemia.

43. A) Mitral
Mitral valve sounds are usually heard best at and around the cardiac apex.

44. C) Lupus
Lupus is a systemic disease; one symptom of lupus may be joint pain. Gout, osteoarthritis, and spondylosis are not considered systemic diseases.

45. B) Discontinue the medication
The patient's rash suggests an allergy to amoxicillin. The priority action would be to discontinue the medication to prevent worsening of the symptoms. A new prescription would then be provided, and a topical antihistamine cream may also be administered for the rash. The patient would also be assessed for respiratory involvement, but that action would not be the priority action.

46. C) Orthopnea
Orthopnea is the occurrence of dyspnea while the patient is lying down. It improves when the patient sits up. Orthopnea is part of the cardiovascular review of systems that may indicate congestive heart failure. Inquiry about hematochezia, abdominal pain, and tinnitus would not be part of the cardiovascular review.

47. B) Phalen and Tinel
The patient is presenting with classic signs of carpal tunnel syndrome. The Phalen and Tinel tests are used in the examination to diagnose carpal tunnel syndrome. The McMurray and drawer tests are used to assess the knee, and the apprehension test is used for the shoulder.

48. A) Lachman
The Lachman test is performed to evaluate the anterior cruciate ligament. The knee is placed in 15 degrees of flexion and external rotation of the hip. The anterior drawer test involves pulling the tibia forward, the abduction stress test consists of placing the knee in thirty degrees of flexion and adducting the ankle, and the McMurray test involves bringing the knee to full flexion and laterally rotating the tibia.

49. C) Iron-deficiency anemia
There are three common causes of microcytosis or microcytic anemia: iron-deficiency anemia, anemia of chronic disease/anemia of inflammation, and thalassemia.

50. B) Upper lateral thigh

Epinephrine should be injected only in the middle of the outer side of the thigh. It can be injected through clothing if necessary in an emergency.

51. A) State nurse practice acts

The state nurse practice acts authorize boards of nursing in each state to establish statutory authority for licensure of RNs. States also vary in specific practice requirements, such as certifications. Best practice guidelines, nursing dissertations, and credentialing agreements do not dictate the scope of practice for AGACNPs.

52. B) State board of nursing

The state board of nursing mandates the AGACNP scope of practice based on legal allowances in each state, according to and delineated by individual State Nurse Practice Acts.

53. A) Are regulatory mechanisms to ensure accountability for competent practice

Credentialing is necessary to ensure that safe healthcare is provided by qualified individuals. Credentials encompass required education, licensure, and certification to practice as an AGACNP. They establish the minimum, not maximum, levels of acceptable performance. Credentials enhance (not diminish) professional standards of practice. Authoritative statements by which to measure quality of practice, service, or education are known as Standards of Advanced Practice.

54. B) State Board of Nursing via state nurse practice acts

The level of prescriptive authority that nurses in advanced practice have is dependent on the state practice acts set forth by the State Board of Nursing. The DEA has ruled that nurses in advanced practice may obtain registration numbers, but it does not determine the ability or extent of their prescribing authority. Medicare guidelines and a hospital or clinic board of directors do not determine what AGACNPs may or may not prescribe.

55. A) Giving reasonable notice to the proper authority that the AGACNP lacks competence to carry out the assignment

By giving reasonable notice that they cannot care for the patient, the AGACNP gives the patient (and the family) time to find other, more qualified caregivers for that patient. Determination of patient abandonment may depend on many factors, including: (1) whether the practitioner accepted the patient assignment, (2) whether the practitioner provided reasonable notice before terminating the practitioner–patient relationship, and (3) whether reasonable arrangements could have been made to continue patient care when the adequate notification was given. An AGACNP should not agree to manage care of a pediatric patient in the interim if the AGACNP is not certified to treat that age group; nor should they walk out or ask the patient to leave.

56. C) Certification

A certification establishes that a person has achieved mastery in a particular profession. It is often required for licensure in most states and reimbursement by most insurers. Credentials and privileges are both part of the process by which an AGACNP is granted permission to practice in an inpatient setting. Licensure is granted by a governmental body.

57. C) Material safety and data sheet

A material safety and data sheet is a document that lists information relating to occupational safety and health for the use of various substances and products. While it is important (and mandatory) to have, it is not a component that can help advance the success of a risk management team. Incident reports are the most common method of documentation for risk management. Satisfaction surveys are an important way to identify problems before they develop into actual incidents of claims. Complaints are another key source of potential risk management information.

58. C) Consequences for those who report sensitive information

A risk management plan articulates guarantees of confidentiality and immunity from retaliation for those who report sensitive information; it does not seek to impose consequences on them. A written risk management plan will include the goals of the organization; the program's scope, components, and methods; and who is responsible for implementation and enforcement of the plan.

59. A) Negligence

Negligence is the failure of an individual to do what a reasonable person would do, resulting in injury to the patient. It is a form of carelessness. Malpractice implies professional misconduct with an unreasonable lack of skill or infidelity or illegal/immoral conduct that results in patient harm. Assault is an intentional act by one person that creates an apprehension in another of an imminent harmful or offensive contact. Battery is an illegal, willful, angry, violent, or negligent striking of a person, their clothes, or anything with which they are in contact.

60. B) Incident report

An incident report should be written after such an event in the hopes of addressing all of the issues that led up to the problem or incident. Incident report policies should be designed by the risk management team and include persons authorized to complete a report, persons responsible for reviewing a report, immediate actions needed to minimize the effects of the report's event, and security and storage of completed incident report forms. Employee satisfaction surveys are helpful for identifying problems before they develop into actual incidents. A police report would not be filled out because no actual harm came to the patient as the result of the medicines being given out of order by mistake. Informed consent is a statement that indicates that a patient has received adequate instruction or information regarding aspects of care to make a prudent, personal choice.

61. B) 0

In evaluating correlation, the measure of the interdependence between two random variables ranges in value from −1 to +1. A measure of 0 indicates the absence of correlation; there is no correlation between the time spent explaining discharge instructions and the rate of readmissions. The measure of −1 indicates a perfect negative correlation; more time spent explaining discharge instructions would result in fewer readmissions. The measure of +1 indicates a perfect positive correlation; more time spent explaining discharge instructions would result in more readmissions.

62. D) The most severe form of restraint should be used initially and gradually scaled back to less severe restraint.

The least severe form of restraint should always be used first, not the most severe form. Restraints may be used to prevent a patient from harming themself or others, but the specific reasons for ordering the restraints must be documented, and safety checks of the restraints must be performed and documented as well.

63. C) Notify the police department

This patient is clearly threatening violence against their spouse, so the AGACNP must notify the police. Reporting the incident to the spouse or the charge nurse does not ensure that the appropriate authorities are notified. Allowing the patient to voice their anger without proper notification will not mitigate the situation or help prevent violent behavior from the patient.

64. C) Local health department

Providers are required to report positive HIV test results to their local health department. Reporting to the Centers for Disease Control and Prevention, other local hospitals, and the patient's sexual partner(s) is not required.

65. A) Comply and provide requested information

Police authorities may request protested health information, such as name and date of birth, for the purpose of identifying or locating a potential suspect or fugitive. Denying the request would be inappropriate because the police are allowed to obtain this information; the patient's written consent or a subpoena is not needed.

66. A) Tailored to their educational level

When the AGACNP is providing any kind of patient education, it must be customized to fit the patient's educational level. Reviewing instructions quickly may lead to missed information or miscommunication. Generalized instructions are not as helpful as goal-oriented, specific instructions. Educational materials must be written in the patient's native language, which may not be the English language.

67. A) Understanding the potential for drug–herb and herb–herb interactions

It is important for the AGACNP to understand all aspects of interactions between prescribed medications and herbal and supplemental therapies, including both upregulation and downregulation of cytochrome P450 isoenzymes. While consulting with the interprofessional team and scheduling followup visits are important, they would not be a responsibility of the AGACNP when it comes to recommending complementary and alternative therapy. Referring to a doctor of osteopathy is not necessary because the AGACNP can provide this form of treatment.

68. C) Aromatherapy

Aromatherapy has been determined to be beneficial in calming patients experiencing anxiety related to palliative care therapies due its anxiolytic effect. Although therapeutic touch, chakra balancing, and biofield energy medicine are all complementary alternatives, they involve some touching or activity that may increase anxiety levels in some patients.

69. B) Weighing benefits of testing against the cost

Use of resources involves finding the most appropriate and effective way to treat the patient with a reasonable amount of cost. Therefore, weighing the benefits of the tests needed against the cost would be the most appropriate action. While choosing tests that are less invasive is important in some patients, this is not the most optimal method of implementing use of resources, nor is selecting testing that would be performed most quickly or based on insurance payments.

70. B) Health behaviors

Integrative medicine incorporates not only disease and symptoms, but also overall health and health behaviors such as exercise, social supports, nutrition, and spiritual beliefs. Exploring provider care and support is important but is not specific to the integrative medicine assessment. Identification of the least invasive, simplest therapies and mind-body treatment modalities is part of determining treatment options, not assessment.

71. D) Evaluate the effectiveness of the patient's support system

The first step the AGACNP will take is to assess the patient's support system to ensure that the patient is set up for success in making both cognitive and behavioral changes. Once this is done, the AGACNP will make adjustments and communicate the importance and effectiveness of the care plan. Documentation will not be done until the AGACNP has completely evaluated all systems, outcomes, and support.

72. A) Collaborate with interdisciplinary team to determine appropriate transition of care

The care planning and management standards of practice should be followed, and the AGACNP should first collaborate with the interdisciplinary team to determine which next steps for transferring the patient are appropriate for safe transition and continuity of care. Once this has been established, the AGACNP will discuss the plan with the patient's family members and/or caregiver. Providing that the family is in agreement, the AGACNP would then make preparations with the nursing staff and the specialty hospital for a smooth transition.

73. B) OASIS

The OASIS functional assessment tool provides information on both activities of daily living (ADLs) and instrumental activities of daily living (IADLs) and is useful in determining functioning for patients receiving assistance from home care agencies. The Katz Index, Minimum Data Sheet–ADL, and Functional Index Measure are all valuable tools for patients in long-term care facilities and cover assessment of many areas of care, including elimination and pressure sores.

74. D) Collaborate with the interdisciplinary team on discharge teaching for home care

When planning for discharge, it is the AGACNP's obligation based on scope of practice to collaborate with the interdisciplinary team to ensure that the patient has had all discharge teaching for at-home care. Applying knowledge or organizational theories, serving as a resource for care programs, and developing innovative solutions all fall under areas of practice that do not apply directly to patient care.

75. A) Providers are not exempt from liability

The AMAA was put in place to provide clarity on providers' response to needs for on-flight assistance in medical emergencies and to provide protection to the caregiver as long as the care was delivered "in good faith" without "gross negligence." However, the caregiver may be liable for damages if "gross negligence or willful misconduct" is determined. While is it wise for the provider to understand and recognize the medical equipment on the aircraft, this is not a caveat of the AMAA. Likewise, documentation is important in all care, but it is not a requirement under the AMAA to report to the Federal Aviation Administration. Providers are not legally obligated to volunteer to help in emergencies, though there may be an ethical obligation.

76. C) Occupational therapy

Occupational therapists are part of the interdisciplinary team that works with patients who have cognitive, sensory, and perception impairments. Physical therapy would be instrumental for patients with mobility issues. Psychological evaluation would be indicated for potential mental illness, and ophthalmology evaluation would be needed if depth-perception does not improve with occupational therapy.

77. B) Contact the correctional medical provider for a copy of the Advanced Care Plan

The first step will be to contact the chief correctional medical officer to gain information about the patient's medical care during incarceration, including the Advanced Care Plan that should have been provided to the patient upon release. There is no need at this time to have the patient sign a release of records as this would have already been done before leaving the facility. Completing a full history is not the first step, nor is evaluating the patient for trauma.

78. D) Ensure that the patient has enough medication for their trip along with a list of all medications, dosages, pharmacy contact, and emergency contact information.

The patient should be prepared with an ample supply of medication, a full list of all medications and doses along with the pharmacy contact information, and an emergency contact list to keep with them at all times in the event of an emergency. While discussing nutrition and exercise with the patient is important, developing a plan for the cruise staff is not needed, and exercise regimens are not the most important preparation. Also, ensuring that the patient has an ample supply of insulin administration equipment is important, but it is not the only preparation needed and thus is not the best preparation.

79. C) Brief Instrumental Functional Scale (BIFS)

For patients who are homeless, BIFS is most appropriate to determine their ability to engage in completing applications for benefits, budgeting money, finding an attorney, and taking medications as prescribed. The Katz Index and OASIS are tools used for assessing more fundamental activities of daily living. The FIM is a comprehensive tool intended to measure level of disability and the associated level of assistance required.

80. A) Refer the patient to medical respite care

The AGACNP should refer and prepare the patient for medical respite care, which is a form of temporary posthospitalization care with supportive services when patients who are homeless cannot return to shelters or their living environment. Rapid housing is temporary assistance for those who are experiencing barriers to housing that will be alleviated with some assistance. Contacting the homeless shelter would not be an appropriate action because shelters are not set up to care for a recovery patient. Social services would be contacted if medical respite care is unavailable. They would not be contacted for regular case management, but only for intensive case management that is all encompassing for those with specific medical needs.

81. D) Order dronabinol (Syndros) and gabapentin (Neurontin) for the patient

The patient is exhibiting signs of cannabis withdrawal syndrome or withdrawal from another substance, so the AGACNP will first order dronabinol (Syndros) for nausea and abdominal pain and gabapentin (Neurontin) to reduce risk of seizure activity from withdrawal and increased body temperature. The patient may need to be admitted for observation and CT scan of the head, but this would occur after patient has been stabilized and their immediate needs have been addressed. Referring the patient to rehabilitation for substance use disorder may be an action taken later in the process.

82. A) Review current medications for interactions

The AGACNP will review all medications currently being taken by the patient to ensure that there are no potential interactions, such as with sedation medication. THC can have a stronger effect on older adults, so interactions must be reviewed. Decreasing dosing is not necessarily indicated, and the side effects would have been explained previously by the prescriber. Decreasing dosing also does not ensure safe administration. Explaining that THC provides only temporary relief is not the appropriate action, and prescribed medications may need to be adjusted or even stopped, rather than continued, if there is potential for adverse reactions.

83. B) Abuse Intervention Model (AIM)

The AIM has been proposed as the most effective tool to guide practitioners in understanding and intervening based on three risk factor domains: characteristics of vulnerable adults, characteristics of the trusted other or perpetrator, and living care environments. The Geri-IDT is used for documenting findings, and EM-MDTs provide a varied approach to assessing for elder mistreatment. The FIM is intended to determine the level of assistance required by a patient with disability.

84. C) Elder mistreatment

The patient is at risk for elder mistreatment based on the evidence presented regarding changes in living conditions and a grandson with a history of substance use. Monitoring for altered cognition and risk for falls is important but has not been demonstrated to be necessary. It has not been demonstrated that the patient is at risk for social isolation.

85. B) Informed consent

Informed consent implies that a patient has received adequate instructions or information about all aspects of care to make a prudent, personal choice regarding treatment. This includes the provider discussing all of the benefits and risks with the patient so they can make a truly informed decision. By explaining these benefits and risks to the family member but not to the patient and then allowing the patient to sign the consent form, the surgeon has violated this right. The right to medical care in an emergency implies that life-saving measures must be taken to the point of stabilization, regardless of the patient's ability to pay for treatment. The patient's right to refuse care is not presently the issue, although if the patient knew all of the risks of surgery, perhaps they would elect not to proceed. Continuity of care refers to a patient's ability to choose future relationships with healthcare providers.

86. A) Refuse care

Patients must be advised at the time of their admission to a federally funded institution such as a hospital, or nursing home that they have a right to refuse care. Care that may be refused includes any, some, or all care, as long as the patient has competence. The right to medical care in an emergency implies that life-saving measures must be taken to the point of stabilization, regardless of the patient's ability to pay for treatment. Here, a procedure is being offered, and the patient is choosing to refuse it. The right to confidentiality stems from the provider–patient relationship, in which the patient trusts that the provider will not allow others to know the particulars of the patient's illness or situation. Informed consent is a state indicating that a patient has received adequate instruction or information regarding aspects of care to make a prudent, personal choice regarding such treatment. This patient has already received this information.

87. C) 3

A pressure injury with full-thickness skin loss is considered a stage 3 pressure injury. Stage 1 is characterized by nonblanchable erythema of intact skin, stage 2 by partial-thickness skin loss and exposed dermis, and stage 4 by full-thickness skin and tissue loss.

88. D) Hepatitis A

Exceptions to confidentiality include imminent danger to the patient or others (as in suicide or homicide threat) and certain infectious diseases. Reportable sexually transmitted infections include HIV/AIDS, human papillomavirus, genital herpes, chlamydia, gonorrhea, and syphilis.

89. A) Delirium

Delirium is a condition in which an individual exhibits acute and fluctuating cognitive impairment. Dementia is a gradual, progressive course of cognitive impairment. Amnesia refers to memory loss. Delirium may occur from medication side effects, but the patient has not reported medication use.

90. B) Timed Up and Go

The Timed Up and Go test is a quick assessment tool that can be used to identify gait and balance issues in older adults. The Romberg test evaluates neurologic impairment in balance. The nuclear stress test identifies cardiac abnormalities. MRI of the spine can identify physiologic abnormalities in the vertebra and spinal column.

91. A) Immobility

Immobility is the primary risk factor for developing pressure injuries. Incontinence, malnutrition, and friction are other risk factors that can also contribute to developing pressure injuries, but they are not the primary risk factor.

92. D) Postural hypotension

Falls that occur upon standing up, particularly after one is supine for a long period of time, are likely due to postural hypotension. While it is possible that vision impairment, environmental hazards, and lower extremity weakness are contributing factors, the most likely cause of falls in this patient is postural hypotension.

93. C) IV furosemide (Lasix)

Rapid infusion of loop diuretics such as furosemide (Lasix) is associated with tinnitus, which may be permanent. Typically, a bolus is administered no faster than 40 mg/min. IV cefazoline (Ancef) can lead to nausea, vomiting, and possible diarrhea as side effects. IV morphine can lead to respiratory depression if administered too quickly. Normal saline may be administered quickly without concern for tinnitus, although care must still be taken to avoid volume overload.

94. A) Epinephrine

First-line pharmacologic treatment in anaphylaxis is epinephrine. Treating the underlying etiology in an attempt to improve oxygenation and restoration of tissue perfusion is the basic goal of therapy. Anxiolytics such as lorazepam assist with anxiety but will not treat the underlying etiology. Albuterol will act to dilate the bronchioles but does not prevent or relieve upper airway edema, hypotension, or shock. Normal saline solution has no effect on anaphylactic response.

95. A) Multiple sclerosis

Although there are no physical exam findings specific to multiple sclerosis, there are a few that are highly characteristic of the disease, including optic neuritis, Lhermitte sign (a sudden, shock-like sensation that passes down the spine and may radiate to arms and legs), internuclear ophthalmoplegia, fatigue, and heat sensitivity (Uhthoff phenomenon). Myasthenia gravis also causes skeletal muscle weakness, in addition to isolated ocular symptoms of ptosis and/diplopia; patients may also present with bulbar symptoms (dysarthria, dysphagia, and fatigable chewing) as well as proximal limb weakness alone. The clinical features of Guillain-Barré syndrome include progressive and symmetric muscle weakness with absent or depressed deep tendon reflexes. Trigeminal neuralgia involves sudden, usually unilateral, severe, brief, stabbing, recurrent episodes of pain in the distribution of one or more branches of the fifth cranial (trigeminal) nerve.

96. B) Elevated protein concentration

This patient is presenting with the cardinal features (fever, nuchal rigidity, altered mental status) concerning for bacterial meningitis. In addition, the Brudzinski sign to examine for meningeal irritation is positive. A head CT should be obtained prior to a lumbar puncture in adults to exclude a mass lesion or increased intracranial pressure. The typical CSF findings in a patient with bacterial meningitis include a white blood cell count of 1,000 to 5,000 mcL (range of <100 to >10,000) with neutrophils usually greater than 80%, protein of 100 to 500 mg/dL (1,000 to 5,000 mg/L), and glucose of <40 mg/dL (2.22 mm/L; with a CSF-to-serum glucose ratio of $\leq$0.4). The opening pressure is generally elevated in patients with bacterial meningitis.

97. D) Irregular respirations, widened pulse pressure, bradycardia

Cushing triad is seen in patients with critically elevated intracranial pressure (ICP), especially in the later phase of increased ICP when the patient is close to brain death. Cushing triad involves severe hypertension, most notably with an increased systolic pressure resulting in a widened pulse pressure, bradycardia, and respiratory irregularity due to medullary dysfunction. This phenomenon occurs during herniation and is considered a late sign of increased ICP. Since these patients are critically ill, hyperglycemia, arrythmias, and changes in reflexes may be present; however, these conditions are not part of Cushing triad.

98. D) Parkinson disease

The common features of Parkinson disease are tremor (typically described as pill-rolling), bradykinesia (generalized slowness of movement), rigidity (increased resistance to passive movement), and postural instability (an impairment of centrally mediated postural reflexes that causes a feeling of imbalance). Other features include hypomimia (masked facial expression) and a shuffling, short-stepped gait. The clinical features of Guillain-Barré syndrome include progressive and symmetric muscle weakness with absent or depressed deep tendon reflexes. While there are no clinical exam findings unique to multiple sclerosis, there are a few that are highly characteristic of the disease, including optic neuritis, Lhermitte sign (a sudden, shock-like sensation that passes down the spine and may radiate to arms and legs), internuclear ophthalmoplegia, fatigue, and heat sensitivity (Uhthoff phenomenon). Alzheimer disease is characterized by cognitive decline, neuropsychiatric and behavioral symptoms, and neurologic deficits.

99. B) Cauda equina syndrome

Cauda equina syndrome is caused by damage to the lumbosacral nerve roots within the spinal canal at the level of L1 to L5. The term cauda equina is Latin for "horse's tails," which describes the collection of nerve roots that are distal to conus medullaris. Symptoms include low back pain accompanied by pain radiating into one or both legs; motor weakness of the lower extremities; bladder and rectal sphincter paralysis; and sensory loss of the affected nerve roots. The patient likely does not have Brown-Sequard syndrome as there is no ipsilateral loss of motor function. This is also not likely to be central cord syndrome, which is characterized by a loss of motor function in the upper extremities that is greater than that of the lower extremities. Spondylolisthesis of C2 involves the fracture of the pedicle of the axis, usually from a hyperextension injury. Regardless of the marked anterior displacement of C2 on C3, if the victim survives the initial injury, a spinal cord injury may be minimal or absent. Therefore, patients with spondylolisthesis of C2 often present with neck pain but no neurological deficits.

100. C) Central cord syndrome

Central cord syndrome can occur in athletes as a result of a hyperextension injury causing increased pressure on the central cord. It is characterized by loss of motor function in the upper extremities that is greater than that of the lower extremities because the most central portions of the spinal tracts contain fibers from the upper extremities. Symptoms also include bladder dysfunction and variable sensory loss below the level of injury. Anterior cord syndrome involves injury to the spinothalamic tract and is characterized by immediate onset of complete motor paralysis and loss of pain, perception of light touch, and temperature sensation. The patient retains fine touch, vibration, pressure, and proprioception sensation distal to the injury. Brown-Sequard syndrome is a rare spinal injury characterized by ipsilateral loss of motor function, vibration, and proprioception below the level of the lesion and contralateral loss of pain and temperature sensation. Complete cord syndrome involves transection of the spinal cord resulting in complete loss of motor, sensory, and autonomic function below the level of the lesion or trauma.

101. D) Neurogenic

Neurogenic shock, a type of distributive shock, is common in patients with severe traumatic brain injury and spinal cord injury. It is caused by an interruption of autonomic pathways, causing decreased vascular resistance and altered vagal tone. The interruption of descending sympathetic fibers in the thoracic and cervical cord produces vasodilation below the level of injury and, subsequently, hypotension. Bradycardia can result due to interruption in sympathetic outflow to the heart while parasympathetic outflow remains intact via the vagus nerve. In most cases of severe distributive shock (e.g., sepsis, neurogenic shock), both cardiac output and SVR are often reduced. Cardiac output is the product of heart rate and stroke volume; it is the amount of fluid in liters per minute that the heart pumps into systemic circulation. Normal values range from about 4 to 8 L/min; therefore, a cardiac output of 2 L/min is considered low. Cardiac output is generally measured using the cardiac index, which takes into account a patient's body surface area; normal values range from 2.5 to 4 L/min. SVR is the resistance provided by the systemic circulation against which the left ventricle must pump blood. It is determined by vessel length, blood viscosity, and vessel diameter. Normal values range from about 900 to 1400 dyn·s/cm^5; therefore, a value of 500 dyn·s/cm^5 is low. In general, hypovolemic, cardiogenic, and obstructive shock are characterized by a low cardiac output and a compensatory increase in the SVR in an attempt to maintain perfusion to vital organs. Hypovolemic shock is often a result of hemorrhagic (internal/external bleeding) or nonhemorrhagic losses (e.g., severe dehydration). Cardiogenic shock often results from a cardiomyopathic cause (e.g., myocardial infarction) or is due to an arrythmia (e.g., sustained ventricular tachycardia) or mechanical abnormality (e.g., acute valvular rupture). Obstructive shock is often the result of a pulmonary vasculature issue (e.g., pulmonary embolism), or it may be due to a mechanical cause of decreased preload (e.g., tension pneumothorax, pericardial tamponade).

102. C) Thoracic 4

A sensory assessment is performed using dermatome levels in patients with spinal cord injuries. The pathways for various sensory modalities can be used to localize spinal lesions because they cross at different levels in the nervous system. Sensation at the level of the nipple line is indicative of a spinal lesion at thoracic 4. The cervical 6 nerve root transmits sensation from the thumb to the index finger, which travels via cervical root 7 to the middle finger and to the fourth and fifth fingers via the cervical 8 root. Of note, an injury at C4 or above likely requires mechanical ventilation. The lumbar 5 dermatome provides sensation to the large toe and the lateral lower leg while the sacral 1 includes the small toe and sole.

103. A) Straight leg raise

The straight leg raise helps to identify lumbar radiculopathy. With the patient supine, the clinician raises the patient's extended leg on the symptomatic side with the foot dorsiflexed, being mindful that the patient is not actively helping to lift the leg. The result of straight leg raising causes an increase in dural tension in the low lumbar and high sacral levels. The Spurling test and the extension-rotation test are special tests of the cervical spine. The Spurling test looks to identify if a nerve root is being compressed because of intervertebral disc pathology. The extension-rotation test is best used to rule out facet joint etiology. The empty can test identifies supra-spinatus weakness because of a tear, impingement, or nerve injury.

104. C) Finger-to-nose test

The finger-to-nose test allows the clinician to test the accuracy of movements to assess for cerebellar function. Other coordination tests include rapid alternating movements, finger tapping, and heel-to-shin testing. Pronator drift is also a motor examination, but it assesses an upper motor neuron pattern of weakness that causes the arm to pronate and drift downward when the patient is asked to hold it extended with palms up. Stereognosis and graphesthesia are sensory examinations. Stereognosis assesses for the ability to identify a familiar object by touch (such as a key or a coin in the patient's hand). Graphesthesia tests the ability of the patient to identify the shape or number drawn in their palm with the blunt end of an applicator.

105. C) Pulmonary function test

These examination findings are suggestive for Guillain-Barré syndrome. Typical clinical features include progressive and symmetric muscle weakness with absent or depressed deep tendon reflexes. Often, patients may have sensory symptoms and dysautonomia. Supportive care is indicated for all patients, and monitoring for deterioration of neurologic, respiratory, cardiovascular, and autonomic status is essential. Neuromuscular weakness can cause respiratory failure, so specific clinical features and thresholds on pulmonary function tests allow for the detection of those who may need intubation due to high risk of respiratory failure. Glucocorticoids are not recommended for patients with Guillain-Barré syndrome as there is no evidence indicating any benefit. Immunotherapy therapy with either intravenous immune globulin or plasma exchange may be indicated. While physical therapy is important for rehabilitation and long-term management, it is not the priority right now. Guillain-Barré syndrome is often provoked by a preceding infection, but antiviral therapy is not indicated for treatment.

106. B) Trigeminal neuralgia

Trigeminal neuralgia is characterized by recurrent paroxysmal sharp pain radiating into one or more branches of the trigeminal nerve (ophthalmic, maxillary, and mandibular). It is caused by small artery compression of the trigeminal nerve, causing demyelination of the trigeminal nerve root. This produces the features of unilateral facial pain in the chin or cheek. The common features of Parkinson disease are tremor (typically described as pill-rolling), bradykinesia (generalized slowness of movement), rigidity (increased resistance to passive movement), and postural instability (an impairment of centrally mediated postural reflexes that cause a feeling of imbalance). Other features include hypomimia (masked facial expression) and a shuffling, short-stepped gait. While there are no clinical exam findings unique to multiple sclerosis, there are a few that are highly characteristic of the disease, including optic neuritis, Lhermitte sign (a sudden, shock-like sensation that passes down the spine and may radiate to arms and legs), internuclear ophthalmoplegia, fatigue, and heat sensitivity (Uhthoff phenomenon). Myasthenia gravis also causes skeletal muscle weakness, in addition to isolated ocular symptoms of ptosis and/diplopia; patients may also present with bulbar symptoms (dysarthria, dysphagia, and fatigable chewing) as well as proximal limb weakness alone.

107. D) Ischemic (embolic)

Embolic strokes often arise from a source in the heart, aorta, or large vessels. Symptoms have a sudden onset but may improve quickly. Cardiac findings, especially atrial fibrillation, murmurs, and cardiac enlargement, suggest a cardiac-origin embolism. Embolic strokes can be precipitated by getting up at night to urinate or by sudden coughing or sneezing. A thrombotic stroke is less likely because thrombotic strokes often present with fluctuating symptoms, varying between normal and abnormal, progressing in a stepwise fashion with some periods of improvement. A subarachnoid hemorrhage is less likely because the patient does not report a headache (which is an invariable symptom). An intracerebral hemorrhage is less likely because in contrast to brain embolism and subarachnoid hemorrhage, the neurologic symptoms of an intracerebral hemorrhage do not begin abruptly and are not maximal at onset.

108. C) Subarachnoid hemorrhage

A subarachnoid hemorrhage stroke is characterized by an abrupt onset of a sudden, severe headache. Headache is an invariable symptom and, often, the sudden increase in pressure causes a cessation in activity. However, there are usually no significant focal neurologic sign changes. Risk factors are significant for smoking, hypertension, moderate to heavy alcohol use, genetic susceptibility, and substance use. While a headache can also be noted in an intracerebral hemorrhage, it is more common in a subarachnoid hemorrhage. If present, the onset is typically more gradual, with a progression of minutes to hours in most patients. Hemorrhagic strokes are often precipitated by physical activity, while thrombotic strokes are not. The onset of an ischemic (thrombotic) stroke may vary, with stuttering progression and periods of improvement. While a sudden onset is also seen with embolic strokes, this patient does not have any other focal deficits typically seen with ischemic strokes: abrupt onset of hemiparesis, visual field deficits, facial droop, ataxia, nystagmus, aphasia, motor weakness, or decreased level of consciousness. Additionally, embolic strokes are often associated with a history of heart disease (e.g., atrial fibrillation, valvular disease, recent myocardial infarction).

109. B) CT of the head without contrast

Noncontrast head CT is the preferred imaging study for early and initial acute stroke evaluation due to its availability, rapid scan times, and sensitivity for intracranial hemorrhage or mass lesion. An initial noncontrast CT scan can confirm the ability to proceed with administration of tPA, if indicated. Further workup, including CT angiography or MRI, may be subsequently performed, but a noncontrast head CT is the priority due to its speed of acquisition and increased access. MRI reliably detects intracranial hemorrhage and is superior for the detection of acute ischemic stroke, but it is not as readily available and is more limited by patient contraindications or intolerance. A CT angiography is often performed during further evaluation to detect intracranial large vessel stenosis and occlusions.

110. A) Transient ischemic attack

A transient ischemic attack is a sudden onset of a focal neurologic symptom or sign lasting less than 24 hours. This is caused by a transient decrease in blood supply to the brain, spinal cord, or retina. A subarachnoid hemorrhage is less likely because the patient does not report a headache (which is an invariable symptom). An intracerebral hemorrhage is less likely because in contrast to brain embolism and subarachnoid hemorrhage, the neurologic symptoms for an intracerebral hemorrhage do not begin abruptly and are not maximal at onset. A subdural hematoma may present with similar clinical manifestations of weakness, numbness, and visual impairment, but the timeline of symptoms resolving within 24 hours is specific to a transient ischemic attack.

111. D) Frontal lobe

In general, seizures can be classified as to whether the onset of electrical activity involves a focal region of the brain or both sides of the brain simultaneously (generalized). The location of the seizure in the brain and the amount of cortex involved can produce varying clinical manifestations of seizures. A seizure that begins in the frontal lobe—responsible for emotional regulation, speech production, and problem-solving—may cause sudden speech difficulties. A seizure that begins in the occipital cortex, responsible for visual reception and interpretation, may cause flashing lights. A seizure that begins in the motor cortex will produce rhythmic jerking movements of the face, arm, or leg on the opposite side of the body to the involved cortex. A seizure that begins in the parietal cortex, responsible for body orientation and sensory discrimination, may cause distortion of spatial perception.

112. C) Tonic

Subtypes of generalized seizures include tonic-clonic seizures (also known as grand mal seizures and the most common type); absence seizures; and clonic, myoclonic, tonic, and atonic seizures (also called drop seizures). Tonic seizures are characterized by sudden muscle stiffening and are often associated with impaired consciousness. Absence seizures usually occur during childhood and are characterized by sudden staring with impaired consciousness. Myoclonic seizures consist of sudden, brief muscle contractions that may occur singly or in clusters; however, impaired consciousness is not common. Atonic seizures produce the opposite effect of tonic seizures and cause sudden loss of control of the muscles, most often the legs, causing patients to collapse to the ground.

113. A) Postictal period

After a seizure, the postictal period is the transition from the ictal state back to the patient's baseline level. It is not uncommon for patients to remain confused and have suppressed alertness. Focal neurologic deficits may be present, such as weakness of a hand, arm, or leg that appears following a focal motor seizure involving the one side of the body. The postictal state may last only seconds or as long as hours depending on the part of the brain affected, the length of the seizure, the medications received, and the patient's age. An aura is often described as the warning symptom that the patient experiences at the beginning of a seizure. While auras are focal seizures that can cause symptoms, they do not interfere with consciousness. Generalized status epilepticus is less likely because the clinical manifestations are confined to focal movement of one arm, rather than generalized bilateral tonic-clonic movements. A myoclonic seizure is a type of generalized seizure, characterized by sudden, brief muscle contractions that may occur singly or in clusters; impaired consciousness is not common.

114. B) Clonic

Clonic seizures cause rhythmic jerking muscle contractions that usually involve the arms, neck, and face. Tonic seizures are characterized by sudden muscle stiffening and are often associated with impaired consciousness. Myoclonic seizures consist of sudden, brief muscle contractions that may occur singly or in clusters; impaired consciousness is not common. Atonic seizures cause the sudden loss of control of the muscles, most often the legs, which causes patients to collapse to the ground.

115. A) Bladder scan and intermittent catheterization

Patients with a spinal cord injury above T6 may experience chronic medical complications, such as autonomic dysreflexia. This involves the loss of coordinated autonomic responses to demands on heart rate and vascular tone. Symptoms include headache, diaphoresis, increased blood pressure, flushing, piloerection, blurred vision, nasal obstruction, anxiety, and nausea. Some patients may experience bradycardia while others experience tachycardia. Once this complication is suspected, management includes finding and correcting the source of the noxious inciting stimuli. Bladder distention and fecal impaction are common causes; therefore, a bladder scan and intermittent catheterization should be performed. If present, the urinary catheter should be assessed for obstruction. The patient should be turned so that a rectal examination can be performed. The patient should not be kept supine; instead, the patient should be sat upright to orthostatically lower the blood pressure. Depending on the severity and the response to these interventions, rapid onset and short duration antihypertensive agents may be indicated to reduce the patient's blood pressure, such as nitrates, nifedipine, and intravenous (IV) hydralazine. However, IV labetalol (Trandate) should be avoided when the patient is bradycardic. While patients with spinal cord injury often lose thermoregulatory function and can develop poikliothermia (an inability to internally regulate body temperature), it is of a higher priority to remove all noxious stimuli at this time. Any restrictive and tight-fitting clothing or blankets should be removed until symptoms improve.

116. C) Basilar skull fracture

Basilar skull fractures involve at least one of the five bones that compose the base of the skull: the cribriform plate of the ethmoid bone, orbital plate of the frontal bone, petrous and squamous portion of the temporal bone, and sphenoid and occipital bones. Clinical signs can often be used for diagnosis and may include retroauricular or mastoid ecchymosis (Battle sign), periorbital ecchymosis ("raccoon eyes"), cerebrospinal fluid leakage from nose (rhinorrhea) and ears (otorrhea), and hemotympanum (blood behind the tympanic membrane). While similar neurological deteriorations may occur with epidural hematoma, subdural hematoma, and cerebral contusion, rhinorrhea and periorbital ecchymosis are specific clinical signs for a basilar skull fracture.

117. A) *Escherichia coli* (*E. coli*)

The most frequent causative organism for an acute complicated urinary tract infection is *E. coli*. While other uropathogens include Enterobacterales (e.g., *Klebsiella* and *Proteus* species), *Pseudomonas*, *Enterococci*, and *Staphylocci* (both MSSA and MRSA), the most frequent cause is *E. coli*. It is important to note that the prevalence of a particular pathogen over another depends on the host.

118. D) Acute delirium

Delirium is an acute, sudden, and transient onset of clouded sensorium with a disturbance in consciousness and altered cognition. The condition typically develops over a short period of time and tends to fluctuate over the course of the day. Often, the disturbance is precipitated by a medical condition or by polypharmacy, infection, dehydration, immobility, malnutrition, substance intoxication, or a medication side effect. In contrast, dementia is a persistent, progressive, and gradual form of memory loss with significant cognitive impairment in at least one of the cognitive domains (learning and memory, language, executive function, complex attention, perceptual-motor function, social cognition). Dementia with Lewy bodies is characterized by core clinical features such as cognitive fluctuations, visual hallucinations, rapid eye movement sleep disorder, and parkinsonism. Alzheimer disease also has cognitive deficits, but symptoms progress insidiously.

119. A) Fractional excretion of sodium (FENa)

The three major diagnostic approaches to distinguish prerenal disease from ATN are urinalysis, FENa, and the response to fluid repletion in patients who have evidence of volume depletion (the gold standard to diagnose prerenal disease). The urinalysis is often normal or nearly normal in patients with prerenal disease; while hyaline casts may be seen, this is not a specific finding. The classic urinalysis of ATN indicates muddy brown granular, epithelial cell casts, and free epithelial cells. However, neither the absence nor the presence of these urinary findings excludes or establishes the diagnosis of ATN; therefore, the value of urinalysis in distinguishing between prerenal and ATN may vary among patients. FENa is the preferred test because it includes the urine-sodium concentration, measures only sodium handling (the fraction of the filtered sodium load that is excreted), and is not affected by changes in urinary output. For patients with prerenal disease, the FENa is often less than 1%, and for patients with ATN, the FENa is typically above 2%. While the blood urea nitrogen/serum creatinine ratio is often greater in prerenal disease (20:1) compared with ATN (which is often normal at 10 to 15:1), this ratio cannot reliably differentiate prerenal disease from ATN. Lastly, the rise of the serum creatinine concentration tends to increase progressively in patients with ATN. A slower rise with periodic fluctuations is more suggestive of prerenal disease, but this trend cannot reliably distinguish one from the other.

120. B) Dehydration

Prerenal disease is often a consequence of true volume depletion in the setting of hypovolemia caused by dehydration, hemorrhage, or renal (diuretics) or gastrointestinal (vomiting, diarrhea) fluid loss. Nephrotoxins are a common cause of acute tubular necrosis, a form of intrarenal acute kidney injury. Postrenal acute kidney injury (often referred to as obstructive nephropathy) is frequently a result of prostatic disease (hyperplasia or cancer), renal calculi, clots, neurogenic bladder, and medications that cause urinary retention.

121. B) Urinalysis

A urinalysis should be obtained in all patients being evaluated for BPH to identify pyuria, glucosuria, proteinuria, ketonuria, or bacteria. If present, these may indicate alternative diagnoses and therefore the need for further evaluation. In addition, a post-void residual volume should be obtained in all patients presenting with BPH symptoms to evaluate for retention. Urine culture, serum creatinine, and PSA tests are not needed for diagnosis and are not routinely performed. However, these additional laboratory tests may be helpful to obtain in certain patients. A urine culture is not needed unless there is other evidence to suggest a urinary tract infection. If renal impairment is suspected, a serum creatinine can be obtained. While PSA may be elevated with BPH and can assist in the assessment of prostate volume when considering the use of a 5-alpha reductase inhibitor, it is not needed for diagnosis. Additionally, a histologic confirmation is not needed for diagnosis, and prostate biopsy is indicated only if there is a concern for prostate cancer.

122. C) Calcium

Calcium stones occur in approximately 80% of patients with nephrolithiasis; most are composed of calcium oxalate and less often of calcium phosphate. While uric acid, struvite (magnesium ammonium phosphate), and cystine stones can occur, calcium stones are the most common.

123. C) Oliguria

Patients with CKD often present with signs and symptoms as a result of diminished kidney function (such as edema or hypertension) or prolonged kidney failure (such as weakness, fatigability, anorexia, vomiting, pruritis, and even encephalopathy and seizures in advanced stages). However, an abnormally reduced urine output (seen with oliguria or anuria) is not a common presentation with CKD alone. Often, this indicates some component of acute kidney injury superimposed on the chronic disease.

124. A) All men ages 55 to 69 years old should engage in shared decision-making regarding screening.

In 2018, the U.S. Preventive Services Task Force (USPSTF) made the following recommendations: Men who are 55 to 69 years old should engage in shared decision-making about whether they choose to be screened. A deciding factor involves individual patient preferences and health history; the potential benefits must be balanced against the potential harms, including the risks of false-positive tests, prostate biopsy, anxiety, over-diagnosis, and treatment complications. Screening involves a PSA blood test. A digital rectal examination is not recommended as a screening test due to its low sensitivity and specificity for detecting prostate cancer. The USPSTF does not recommend PSA-based screening for prostate cancer in men 70 years and older.

125. A) Albuminuria

Staging CKD allows for risk stratification for progression and complications and guides treatments and the intensity of monitoring and patient education. CKD is staged according to cause of disease, glomerular filtration rate, and albuminuria. Serum creatinine, blood urea nitrogen, and urine output are not used to stage disease progression of CKD.

126. D) Pregnancy

A nephrology evaluation is often based on the patient's specific health history, physical examination, laboratory results, and imaging, as well as other diagnostic tests and family history. Specifically, indications for consultation include eGFR <30 mL/min/1.73 m^2, persistent urine albumin to creatinine ratio ≥300 mg/g (34 mg/mmol), persistent urine to protein creatinine ratio ≥500 mg/g (56.5 mg/mmol), abnormal urine microscopy, personal history of systemic autoimmune disease, large cystic kidneys, history of multiple myeloma or monoclonal gammopathy, evidence of relatively rapid loss of kidney function (reduction in eGFR >5 mL/min/1.73 m^2 per year or decline >25%), single kidney with eGFR <60 mL/min/1.73 m^2, inability to identify a presumed cause of CKD (especially in younger patients), difficult-to-manage laboratory abnormalities or complications of various medications, resistant hypertension, recurrent or extensive nephrolithiasis, pregnancy, and confirmed or presumed hereditary kidney disease (such as polycystic kidney disease, Alport syndrome, or autosomal dominant interstitial kidney disease).

127. C) Meropenem 1 g IV every 8 hours plus vancomycin 15 mg/kg IV every 12 hours

A broad-spectrum antimicrobial regimen for acute complicated urinary tract infection is indicated for patients who are critically ill (e.g., with severe sepsis or requiring an ICU admission) or who have a suspected urinary tract obstruction. An antipseudomonal carbapenem (imipenem or meropenem) is used to cover extended-spectrum beta-lactamase–producing organisms and *Pseudomonas aeruginosa*, as well as vancomycin to cover methicillin-resistant *Staphylococcus aureus*. Ceftriaxone and ciprofloxacin are often indicated for other hospitalized patients who are not critically ill. Amoxicillin-clavulanate may be indicated in the outpatient setting but is not generally used in hospitalized patients for acute complicated urinary tract infection. For outpatients, if there is no risk for multidrug-resistant organisms but there is concern for an adverse effect with fluroquinolones, one dose of a long-acting parenteral agent (e.g., ceftriaxone, ertapenem, gentamicin, tobramycin) can be given followed by amoxicillin-clavulanate.

128. B) Ceftriaxone 1 g IV once daily

For hospitalized patients who are not critically ill nor at risk for an infection with a multidrug-resistant gram-negative organism, ceftriaxone 1 g IV once daily is recommended. Multidrug-resistant gram-negative urinary tract infections should be suspected in any patient with a history of the following within the past 3 months: a previous multidrug-resistant gram-negative urinary isolate or a fluoroquinolone-resistant *Pseudomonas aeruginosa* isolate; inpatient stay at a healthcare facility; use of a fluoroquinolone, trimethoprim-sulfamethoxazole, or broad-spectrum beta-lactam; and/or travel to areas with high rates of multidrug-resistant organisms. Hospitalized patients with critical illness warranting intensive care for sepsis or urinary tract obstruction should receive an antipseudomonal carbapenem (imipenem or meropenem) in addition to vancomycin. Nitrofurantoin is generally avoided in the setting of acute complicated urinary tract infections as it does not achieve adequate levels outside the bladder. Trimethoprim-sulfamethoxazole may be indicated in the outpatient setting but is not generally used in hospitalized patients for acute complicated urinary tract infection. For outpatients, if there is no risk for multidrug-resistant organisms but there is concern for an adverse effect with fluroquinolones, one dose of a long-acting parenteral agent (e.g., ceftriaxone, ertapenem, gentamicin, tobramycin) can be given followed by trimethoprim-sulfamethoxazole.

129. A) 55-year-old adult with chronic obstructive pulmonary disease (COPD)

The pneumococcal vaccination is recommended for all adults older than 65 years old, as well as adults ages 19 to 64 years who are at risk for infection, such as those with predisposing medical conditions like alcohol use disorder; chronic heart disease (including congestive heart failure and cardiomyopathies, excluding hypertension); chronic lung disease (e.g., COPD, emphysema, asthma); chronic liver disease; diabetes mellitus; sickle cell anemia, or current cigarette smoking. Also included are those at increased risk of meningitis and those with a personal history of an immunocompromising condition (e.g., HIV infection, Hodgkin disease, leukemia, lymphoma, multiple myeloma, solid organ transplant, chronic kidney disease).

130. D) Presence of blood at the meatus

The presence of a urethral injury is the only absolute contraindication to the placement of a urethral catheter. This is evidenced by the presence of blood at the meatus or gross hematuria associated with trauma. Evaluation and urologic consultation should be performed first. Urethral stricture, recent urinary tract surgery, and the presence of an artificial sphincter are relative contraindications to urethral catheterization. Often a urologist is consulted to assist with insertion and/or management.

131. C) Person with HIV infection in the United States with a low CD4 count

Risk factors for meningococcal disease include a previous viral infection, household crowding, and smoking. Certain groups are at an increased risk, such as those with persistent complement component deficiencies, those who use complement inhibitors, those with asplenia (including sickle cell disease), those living with HIV infection, biologists exposed to *Neisseria meningitidis*, travelers to countries where the disease is hyperendemic or epidemic (specifically sub-Saharan Africa), college students living in residence halls and miliary recruits (likely due to the overcrowded living conditions), and men who have sex with men.

132. B) 50

Routine vaccination for herpes zoster is recommended for adults starting at age 50 years or older. A two-dose series of recombinant zoster vaccine (RZV) (Shingrix) 2 to 6 months apart is recommended regardless of previous herpes zoster or history of zoster vaccine live. RZV (Shingrix) is also recommended for adults ages 19 years and older who are immunodeficient.

133. D) Achieve health equity and eliminate disparities

The objective of *Healthy People 2030* is to guide national health-promotion and disease-prevention efforts to improve the health of the nation. The U.S. Department of Health and Human Services has released a new initiative every decade since 1980 with new objectives to monitor progress and motivate action. A goal of *Healthy People 2030* is to accomplish health equity, eliminate disparities, and improve the health of all people.

134. D) Treating a disease with intravenous immune globulin

Passive immunity occurs via antibody-containing products such as immune globulin, which can be given for treatment of certain diseases. Passive immunity also occurs when antibodies to a disease are given, such as when a newborn acquires passive immunity through the placenta and breast milk. Active immunity occurs after exposure to a disease that triggers the immune system to produce antibodies. It can be acquired through natural immunity (exposure to the disease itself) or vaccine-induced immunity (via the introduction of a killed or weakened form of the disease during vaccination).

135. A) 20-valent pneumococcal conjugate vaccine (PCV20)
All patients with impaired splenic function should receive vaccinations against *Streptococcus pneumoniae, Haemophilus influenzae* type b, and *Neisseria meningitidis;* COVID-19; and seasonal influenza virus, in addition to all age-appropriate vaccinations. PCV20 alone can be given without supplementation. If a lesser valent pneumococcal conjugate vaccine (e.g., 15-valent PCV, 13-valent PCV) is given, it should be followed by PPSV23 >8 weeks later. In the United States, the HPV vaccine is not approved after age 45 years. Herpes zoster vaccination is indicated for adults age 50 years or older but is not specifically indicated for those with impaired splenic function.

136. A) Annual fecal immunochemistry testing (FIT)
According to the U.S. Preventive Services Task Force, it is recommended that adults age 45 to 75 years be screened for colorectal cancer. The recommended intervals for colorectal cancer screening tests for asymptomatic adults who are at average risk of colorectal cancer (i.e., no prior diagnosis of colorectal cancer, adenomatous polyps, or inflammatory bowel disease; no personal diagnosis or family history of known genetic disorders that increase risk colorectal cancer) are as follows: high-sensitivity guaiac-based fecal occult blood test or FIT every year, stool DNA-FIT every 1 to 3 years, CT colonography every 5 years, flexible sigmoidoscopy every 5 years, flexible sigmoidoscopy every 10 years + FIT every year, and/or colonoscopy screening every 10 years.

137. A) Pregnancy test
These findings are presumptive of a clinical diagnosis of pelvic inflammatory disease (PID). For all patients suspected of having PID, the following tests should be obtained: pregnancy test (to rule out ectopic pregnancy and complications of intrauterine pregnancy); microscopy of vaginal discharge (to assess for increased white blood cells); nucleic acid amplification tests for *Neisseria gonorrhoeae, Chlamydia trachomatis,* and *Mycoplasma genitalium;* HIV screening, and serologic testing for syphilis (to rule out sexually transmitted infections that share similar risk factors with PID). While erythrocyte sedimentation rate and C-reactive protein can often be obtained to assess severity, these tests have poor sensitivity and specificity for the diagnosis of pelvic inflammatory disease. A urinalysis, not urine culture, should be done in patients with urinary symptoms. Hepatitis B virus testing may be indicated depending on the patient's risk history. A Papanicolaou stain is used for cervical cancer screening and is not indicated at this time.

138. B) At age 21 years
Cervical cancer screening should begin at age 21 years with cervical cytology every 3 years. It is not recommended to screen for cervical cancer in patients younger than 21 years, regardless of the age of initiation of sexual activity or menstruation cycle.

139. C) Iron-deficiency anemia

Iron-deficiency anemia is significant for low hemoglobin and hematocrit, low red blood cell count, low absolute reticulocyte count, low MCV, and low MCHC. The patient's hemoglobin and hematocrit values are below the normal range for male patients (hemoglobin 13.6 to 16.9 g/dL and hematocrit 40% to 50%). The MCV is 74, which is below the normal range of 80 to 100 fL, indicating a microcytic anemia. The MCHC is also below the normal range of 32% to 36%; so a level of 30% indicates that this anemia is hypochromic. Pagophagia (pica for ice) is considered a specific finding for iron deficiency. Thalassemia is also characterized by a microcytic hypochromic anemia, but pica is not generally seen. Folic acid deficiency is characterized by macrocytic and normochromic anemia, while macrocytosis is often seen with pernicious anemia, along with decreased serum B_{12} levels.

140. B) Microcytic, hypochromic

This patient is experiencing a microcytic, hypochromic anemia seen in iron-deficiency anemia and thalassemia. The patient's hemoglobin and hematocrit values are low, indicating anemia (normal range for hemoglobin in male patients is 13.6 to 16.9 g/dL, and normal hematocrit in male patients is 40% to 50%). The normal range for MCV, the average volume size of the red blood cell, is 80 to 100 fL. A level of 72 fL indicates a decreased MCV or microcytosis. Macrocytic anemia would be seen if the value was higher than 100 fL. The normal range for MCHC, the average hemoglobin concentration per red blood cell, is 32% to 36%; therefore, a level of 28% indicates a decreased MCHC, indicating that this anemia is hypochromic. Hyperchromic would be indicated by a value higher than 36%.

141. A) Vitamin B_{12} deficiency

Vitamin B_{12} and folic acid deficiency should be suspected in a patient presenting with macrocytic anemia with mild pancytopenia, hyper-segmented neutrophils, and an underlying condition or diet associated with deficiency. A normal value for vitamin B_{12} is >300 pg/mL, whereas, a normal folate level is >4 ng/mL. A vitamin B_{12} level below 200 pg/mL is consistent with deficiency. An adverse effect of long-term use of metformin (and other biguanides) is reduced absorption of vitamin B_{12} secondary to altered calcium hemostasis. In as early as 3 to 4 months after starting treatment with metformin, low serum vitamin B_{12} levels can be seen; however, symptomatic deficiency is likely to present after 5 to 10 years of therapy. For patients receiving metformin, it is recommended to undergo annual monitoring for vitamin B_{12} deficiency.

142. D) Folic acid deficiency

Vitamin B_{12} and folic acid deficiency should be suspected in a patient presenting with macrocytic anemia with mild pancytopenia, hyper-segmented neutrophils, and an underlying condition or diet associated with deficiency. A normal value for vitamin B_{12} is >300 pg/mL, whereas a normal folate level is >4 ng/mL. A folate level <2 ng/mL is considered deficient. Folate acid deficiency is often a consequence of nutritional deficiency as seen frequently in patients with alcoholism; substance use; poor dietary intake (often seen in individuals with excessive alcohol use with corresponding reductions in dietary intake of folate-rich foods such as fresh vegetables and grains); malabsorption (e.g., celiac disease, inflammatory bowel disease); use of certain medications (e.g., methotrexate, sulfasalazine); and increased requirement states (e.g., pregnancy). A microcytic (not macrocytic) hypochromic anemia is seen in iron-deficiency anemia and thalassemia.

143. B) Fasting blood glucose should be repeated on a subsequent day for confirmation

Diabetes can be diagnosed based on American Diabetes Association criteria. These includes hemoglobin A1C >6.5%; fasting plasma glucose >126 mg/dL; 2-hour plasma glucose >200 mg/dL during an oral glucose tolerance test; and random plasma glucose >200 mg/dL in a patient with classic symptoms of hyperglycemia. In the absence of hyperglycemia symptoms, the diagnosis of diabetes must be confirmed on a subsequent day by repeat measurement, repeating the same test for confirmation. If two different tests are available and are concordant for the diagnosis of diabetes, additional testing is not needed. However, if two different tests are discordant, the test that is diagnostic for diabetes (in the case, fasting blood glucose) should be repeated to confirm the diagnosis.

144. A) Hemoglobin A1C >6.5%

Hemoglobin A1C >6.5% is within the criteria for the diagnosis of diabetes mellitus. The test should be performed in a laboratory using a method that is National Glycohemoglobin Standardization Program certified and standardized to the Diabetes Control and Complications Trial Assay. Fasting plasma glucose >126 mg/dL, in which fasting is defined as no caloric intake for at least 8 hours, is diagnostic for diabetes. A 2-hour plasma glucose >200 mg/dL during an oral glucose tolerance test, as identified by the World Health Organization, using a 75 g glucose load is within the criteria. In a patient with classic symptoms of hyperglycemia (polydipsia, polyuria, weight loss, blurry vision) or hyperglycemic crisis, a random plasma glucose >200 mg/dL is considered a part of the diagnostic criteria.

145. D) Waist circumference 110 cm (43 in) in a male patient, fasting blood glucose 126 mg/dL, blood pressure 155/90 mmHg

Diagnostic criteria for metabolic syndrome includes more than three of the following abnormalities: fasting blood glucose >100 mg/dL; HDL cholesterol <40 mg/dL in men and <50 mg/dL in women or drug treatment for low HDL cholesterol; triglycerides >150 mg/dL or drug treatment for elevated triglycerides; waist circumference >102 cm in men or >88 cm in women; and hypertension as defined by blood pressure >130/85 mmHg or drug treatment for hypertension.

146. C) Hemoglobin A1C 5.9%

A hemoglobin A1C of 5.7 to 6.5% is prediabetes; a level >6.5% is diagnostic for diabetes. The diagnosis of prediabetes is based on impaired fasting glucose, impaired glucose tolerance, and hemoglobin A1C. A fasting blood glucose of 100 to 125 mg/dL is considered prediabetes. A fasting plasma glucose >126 mg/dL is diagnostic for diabetes. Two-hour plasma glucose value during a 75-g oral glucose tolerance test between 140 and 199 mg/dL is considered prediabetes.

147. B) Pancreatic autoantibodies

A diagnosis of diabetes has been made based on the clinical symptoms and hyperglycemia. Often, patients with type 1 diabetes have one or more pancreatic autoantibodies, indicating autoimmune destruction of pancreatic beta cells (type 1A diabetes). While rare, type 1B diabetes can occur in patients with no detectable autoantibodies. The following pancreatic autoantibodies can be measured: glutamic acid decarboxylase 65, IA2 (the 40K fragment of tyrosine phosphatase), insulin, and ZnT8 (zinc transporter). Additionally, there is a strong association with the presence of human leukocyte antigens (i.e., HLA-DR3 or HLA-DR4) in patients with type 1 diabetes. BMI cannot distinguish type 1 from type 2 diabetes; about 20% of 25% of patients with type 1 diabetes may be overweight at diagnosis but can experience recent history of weight loss as well. Glycosylated hemoglobin and fasting plasma glucose would be helpful in the diagnosis of diabetes but do not differentiate between type 1 and type 2.

148. A) No further tests are required; diagnosis is confirmed based on random blood glucose and presenting symptoms

Diabetes can be diagnosed based on the American Diabetes Association criteria. These include hemoglobin A1C >6.5%; fasting plasma glucose >126 mg/dL; a 2-hour plasma glucose >200 mg/dL during an oral glucose tolerance test; and a random plasma glucose >200 mg/dL in a patient with classic symptoms of hyperglycemia. The diagnosis of diabetes mellitus is often made when a patient presents with the classic symptoms of hyperglycemia (thirst, polyuria, weight loss, blurry vision) in conjunction with a random blood glucose value of 200 mg/dL or higher. No additional tests are required in patients with symptomatic hyperglycemia. In the absence of hyperglycemia symptoms, the diagnosis of diabetes must be confirmed on a subsequent day by repeat measurement, performing the same test for confirmation. If two different tests are available and are concordant for the diagnosis of diabetes, additional testing is not needed. However, if two different tests are discordant, the test that is diagnostic of diabetes should be repeated to confirm the diagnosis.

149. D) Blood pressure, fasting blood glucose, triglyceride level

Diagnostic criteria for metabolic syndrome includes more than three of the following abnormalities: fasting blood glucose >100 mg/dL or drug treatment for elevated glucose; high-density lipoprotein (HDL) cholesterol <40 mg/dL in men and <50 mg/dL in women or drug treatment for low HDL cholesterol; triglycerides >150 mg/dL or drug treatment for elevated triglycerides; waist circumference >102 cm (about 40 in) in men or >88 cm (about 35 in) in women; and hypertension as defined by blood pressure >130/85 mmHg or drug treatment for hypertension. Metabolic syndrome is not defined by neck circumference, history of type 2 diabetes, or obstructive sleep apnea.

150. C) Check the blood glucose level at 3 a.m.

The patient is likely experiencing the "dawn phenomenon," often a cause of the diurnal secretion patterns of hormones. An increased release of growth hormone at midnight to 2 a.m. can combat the actions of insulin in the early morning hours, increasing blood glucose in the morning. Treatment often includes increasing basal insulin dosing after assessing blood glucose levels beginning at least 3 to 4 hours after the last meal or snack and insulin bolus, as well as 3 a.m. testing. The patient should already be checking blood glucose before dinner to assess bolus dosing of insulin. Performing an oral glucose tolerance test in the morning and obtaining glycosylated hemoglobin (A1C) would not be helpful in diagnosis to guide treatment.

151. B) Plasma osmolality

The patient exhibits clinical symptoms of marked hyperglycemia and signs concerning for hyperosmolar hyperglycemic state (HHS). Symptoms in patients with HHS develop more insidiously, with polyuria and polydipsia occurring for a few days before patients present to the hospital. Neurologic symptoms often develop as the degree of hyperglycemia worsens. These include lethargy, focal signs (such as hemiparesis or hemianopsia), obtundation, and/or seizures. Physical assessment often reveals signs of volume depletion, including decreased skin turgor, dry axillae and oral mucosa, low jugular venous pressure, tachycardia, and, if severe, hypotension. Diabetic ketoacidosis (DKA) and HHS primarily differ according to the presence of ketoacidosis and the degree of hyperglycemia. In HHS, the serum glucose concentration may exceed 1,000 mg/dL, and the plasma osmolality may reach 380 mOsmol/kg. Plasma osmolality is always elevated (typically > 320 mOsmol/kg) in patients with HHS but not in patients with DKA. Often, serum bicarbonate is normal (>20 mEq/L) or only mildly reduced in HHS (in comparison with patients with DKA, in which it is often markedly reduced). An arterial blood gas is often indicated only if the serum bicarbonate is substantially reduced or hypoxia is present. Most patients with HHS have an admission pH of >7.30. Three ketone bodies are produced in DKA (not HHS): one ketoacid (acetoacetic acid), one hydroxyacid (beta-hydroxybutyrate), and one natural ketone (acetone).

152. A) Anion gap

The patient is presenting with clinical symptoms of marked hyperglycemia. Often in patients with diabetic ketoacidosis (DKA), symptoms evolve rapidly, over a 24-hour period. While neurologic symptoms are more common in hyperosmolar hyperglycemic state (HHS), hyperventilation and abdominal pain are primarily seen only in patients with DKA. Physical assessment will often reveal signs of volume depletion (common in both DKA and HHS), including decreased skin turgor, dry axillae and oral mucosa, low jugular venous pressure, tachycardia, and, if severe, hypotension. Patients with DKA often present with a fruity breath odor and Kussmaul respirations, deep respirations reflecting the compensatory hyperventilation. The combination of hyperglycemia, anion gap metabolic acidosis, and ketonemia are diagnostic for DKA. Patients in DKA often present with a serum anion gap greater than 20 mEq/L; the elevated anion gap metabolic acidosis is a result of the accumulation of beta-hydroxybutyric and acetoacetic acids. Serum anion gap can be calculated by serum sodium subtracted from the sum of serum chloride and bicarbonate. Patients in DKA or HHS may both present with hyperlipidemia and lactescent serum, so obtaining a lipid level panel would not specifically help with diagnosis of DKA. Plasma osmolality is always elevated (typically >320 mOsmol/kg) in patients with HHS but not in patients with DKA. Most patients with uncontrolled hyperglycemia have acute elevations in blood urea nitrogen and serum creatinine and reduction in glomerular filtration rate, often as a result of hypovolemia. This level is not diagnostic for DKA.

153. D) 20

The calculation for serum anion gap is serum sodium – (serum chloride + bicarbonate); therefore, the anion gap is 135 – (105 + 10) = 20. Patients with moderate DKA often present with serum bicarbonate 10 to <15 mEq/L and anion gap > 12 mEq/L. However, the serum anion gap is often greater than 20 mEq/L (normal range 3 to 10 mEq/L) in patients with DKA; this elevated anion gap metabolic acidosis is caused by the accumulation of beta-hydroxybutyric and acetoacetic acids.

154. C) Hyperkalemia

In most patients with diabetic ketoacidosis (DKA), potassium levels are elevated on admission secondary to the shift of potassium from the intracellular fluid to the extracellular fluid caused by hyperosmolality and insulin deficiency. Careful monitoring of potassium is important during treatment because insulin therapy will shift potassium back into cells, lowering potassium concentration. Most patients with DKA present with mild hyponatremia; the increase in plasma osmolality created by hyperglycemia pulls water out of the cells, reducing the plasma sodium concentration. Most patients with uncontrolled hyperglycemia have acute elevations in blood urea nitrogen and serum creatinine and reduction in glomerular filtration rate, often as a result of hypovolemia. At presentation, serum phosphate is usually normal to high due to insulin deficiency and metabolic acidosis, which causes a shift of phosphate out of the cells, and because of extracellular fluid volume contraction.

155. B) Blood glucose may exceed 1,000 mg/dL in HHS, but it is generally less than 800 mg/dL in patients with DKA

Both DKA and HHS are characterized by uncontrolled hyperglycemia. In patients with HHS, there is little or no ketoacid accumulation, the serum glucose concentration is usually >600 and may often exceed 1,000 mg/dL, the plasma osmolality may reach 380 mOsmol/kg, and neurologic abnormalities may be seen. In contrast, patients with DKA present with anion gap metabolic acidosis, ketonemia, and hyperglycemia. However, the serum glucose concentration is usually less than 800 mg/dL and commonly between 350 to 500 mg/dL. Elevation in blood glucose may vary based on patient presentation. There are cases in which the serum glucose concentration may exceed 900 mg/dL in patients who are comatose with DKA (although this is not as common). Additionally, some patients in DKA may be euglycemic, particularly those with poor oral intake, treatment with insulin prior to hospital arrival, pregnancy, or treatment with sodium-glucose co-transporter 2 (SGLT2) inhibitors.

156. A) 325

In patients with HHS, the plasma osmolality is always elevated. The effective plasma osmolality is the portion of total osmolality that is generated by sodium salts and glucose. For patients with HHS, effective osmolality is often >320 mOsmol/kg (normal range 275 to 295 mOsmol/kg). Effective osmolality can be estimated by the following equation: [2 × Na (mEq/L)] + [glucose (mg/dL) ÷ 18]; therefore [2 × 135] + [990 ÷ 18] = 270 + 55 = 325 mOsmol/kg. Effective plasma osmolality does not include "ineffective" osmoles, such as urea, which is rapidly permeable across most cell membranes, and its accumulation does not induce major water shifts between the intracellular spaces and the extracellular water space.

157. D) High serum TSH concentration and low serum free T4 concentration

Primary hypothyroidism is characterized by a high serum TSH concentration and a low serum free T4 concentration. Subclinical hypothyroidism is seen in patients with a high serum TSH concentration and a normal serum free T4 concentration. Hyperthyroidism is characterized by a low TSH concentration and high free T4 and T4 concentration.

158. C) 250 mg/dL at 0700

Fasting hyperglycemia is characteristic of the "dawn phenomenon," which is often caused by the diurnal secretion patterns of hormones. An increased release of the growth hormone at midnight to 2 a.m. can combat the actions of insulin in the early morning hours, increasing blood glucose in the morning. Treatment often includes increasing basal insulin dosing after assessing blood glucose levels beginning at least 3 to 4 hours after the last meal or snack and insulin bolus. The patient should also be questioned regarding any evening snacking and bedtime insulin bolusing for food and/or correction of hyperglycemia because insufficient coverage can also cause fasting hyperglycemia.

159. B) Thyroid scintigraphy

Thyroid nodules are often noted by the patient, during routine physical examinations, or when incidentally noted during imaging. For all patients with a thyroid nodule, initial evaluation includes a history and physical examination, measurement of serum TSH, and ultrasound to confirm the presence of nodularity and additional nodules and to assess the features. If the serum TSH concentration is low (<0.4 mU/L), there is an increased possibility that the nodule is hyperfunctioning, and thyroid scintigraphy should be performed next to determine the functional status of the nodule. If the TSH concentration is normal or high, and the nodule meets sonographic criteria for sampling, the next step in evaluation is an ultrasound-guided fine needle aspiration biopsy. The routine measurement of serum calcitonin in patients with nodular thyroid disease is not recommended. While a CT scan may indicate a thyroid nodule during routine imaging, it is not indicated at this time for further evaluation.

160. A) High T4 and/or T3 concentrations, low TSH concentration

Hyperthyroidism causes symptoms of anxiety, emotional lability, weakness, tremor, palpitations, heat intolerance, increased perspiration, and weight loss despite a normal or increased appetite. The skin is usually warm and moist, and hair may be thin and fine. Tachycardia is common, along with systolic hypertension. Tremors, muscle weakness, and hyperreflexia may be noted. In patients with Graves' disease (an autoimmune disease consisting of hyperthyroidism), exophthalmos, periorbital and conjunctival edema, and a thyroid goiter may be present. All patients with low serum TSH and high free T4 and/or T3 concentrations have primary hyperthyroidism. Most patients with hyperthyroidism caused by Graves' disease or nodular goiter have greater increases in serum T3 than in serum T4. This is a result of a disproportionate increase in thyroidal T3 secretion and increased extrathyroidal conversion of T4 to T3. Patients with hypothyroidism often present with fatigue, cold intolerance, weight gain, constipation, dry skin, myalgia, menstrual irregularities, a goiter, bradycardia, diastolic hypertension, and a delayed relaxation phase of the deep tendon reflexes, among other symptoms. Primary hypothyroidism is characterized by a high serum TSH concentration and a low serum free T4 concentration. Subclinical hypothyroidism is seen in patients with a high serum TSH concentration and a normal serum free T4 concentration.

161. D) High serum TSH concentration and a low serum free T4 concentration

The clinical manifestations presented are characteristic of thyroid hormone deficiency. Patients often present with fatigue, cold intolerance, weight gain, constipation, dry skin, myalgia, menstrual irregularities, a goiter, bradycardia, diastolic hypertension, and a delayed relaxation phase of the deep tendon reflexes among others. Primary hypothyroidism is characterized by a high serum thyroid-stimulating hormone (TSH) concentration and a low serum free T4 concentration. Subclinical hypothyroidism is seen in patients with a high serum TSH concentration and a normal serum free T4 concentration. Hyperthyroidism causes symptoms of anxiety, emotional lability, weakness, tremor, palpitations, heat intolerance, increased perspiration, and weight loss despite a normal or increased appetite. Hyperthyroidism is characterized by a low TSH concentration and high free T4 and T4 concentration.

162. C) Fine needle aspiration of thyroid (FNA)

Thyroid nodules are often noted by the patient, during routine physical examinations, or when incidentally noted during imaging. For all patients with a thyroid nodule, initial evaluation includes a history and physical examination, measurement of serum TSH, and ultrasound to confirm the presence of nodularity and additional nodules and to assess the features. If the TSH concentration is normal or high, and the nodule meets sonographic criteria for sampling, the next step in evaluation is an ultrasound-guided FNA biopsy. An FNA biopsy is the most accurate method for evaluating thyroid nodules and selecting patients for thyroid surgery. A nodule meets sonographic criteria for sampling if it is solid and hypoechoic and >1.5 cm (as determined by the largest dimension). A biopsy should be performed in solid and hypoechoic modules if they are >1 to 1.5 cm with at least one of the following features: irregular margins, microcalcifications, taller-than-wide shape, macrocalcifications, or peripheral calcifications. A thyroid scintigraphy is indicated if the serum TSH concentration is low (<0.4 mU/L), in order to determine the functional status of the nodule. The routine measurement of serum calcitonin in patients with nodular thyroid disease is not recommended. Although a CT scan may indicate a thyroid nodule during routine imaging, it is not indicated during further evaluation of the nodule.

163. B) Overnight 1 mg dexamethasone suppression test

A high index of suspicion for hypercortisolism can be made based on the multiple progressive features suggestive of Cushing syndrome. These include the most common signs and symptoms: striae, decreased libido, obesity/weight gain, menstrual changes, facial plethora/round face, hirsutism, hypertension, ecchymoses, lethargy, dorsal fat pad, and abnormal glucose tolerance. Initial testing includes two or three of the following: late-night salivary cortisol (two measurements), 24-hour urinary free cortisol excretion (two measurements), or overnight 1 mg dexamethasone suppression test. The low-dose dexamethasone test is a standard test used to differentiate patients with Cushing syndrome of any cause from patients who do not have Cushing syndrome. The late-night serum cortisol test relies on the fact that the normal evening nadir in serum cortisol is preserved in patients with obesity and depression but not in patients with Cushing syndrome. Because this test is less convenient than the late-night salivary cortisol test, it is not routinely used in practice.

164. A) Thyroid-stimulating hormone (TSH)

This patient is presenting with symptoms suggestive of hyperthyroidism, which is diagnosed based on thyroid function tests. In particular, isolated symptoms of unexplained weight loss, new-onset atrial fibrillation, myopathy, menstrual disorders, and gynecomastia should lead to an evaluation of hyperthyroidism in all patients. The best initial test is serum TSH in a patient in whom there is a clinical suspicion of hyperthyroidism. It is very unlikely that a patient would have primary hyperthyroidism if the TSH level is normal. Once a low TSH level is obtained, many institutions and laboratories have automatic protocols to assess serum free T4 and T3 afterwards. While a blood glucose level may be necessary since the patient is presenting with diaphoresis (which is concerning for hypoglycemia), consideration of all of the symptoms presented as a whole are more suggestive of hyperthyroidism rather than a blood glucose irregularity.

165. C) Hyponatremia

In the majority of patients (about 70% to 80%) with adrenal insufficiency (Addison disease), hyponatremia is found. This electrolyte abnormality is reflective of both sodium loss and volume depletion caused by mineralocorticoid deficiency and increased vasopressin secretion caused by cortisol deficiency. Hyperkalemia, rather than hypokalemia, often occurs due to hypoaldosteronism (since one of the major functions of aldosterone is to promote the urinary excretion of dietary potassium). Mild hyperchloremic acidosis often occurs in conjunction with hyperkalemia. However, not all patients develop hyperkalemia; patients may often have normal potassium levels due to aldosterone-independent regulation of potassium secretion by the distal nephron. Hypoglycemia, rather than hyperglycemia, occurs in adults with secondary adrenal insufficiency secondary to ACTH deficiency and in those with type 1 diabetes mellitus who develop adrenal insufficiency. Sensitivity to exogenous insulin is increased due to the loss of the gluconeogenic effect of cortisol and the hyperglycemic effects of epinephrine. Although rare, hypercalcemia, rather than hypocalcemia, may be associated with acute renal insufficiency.

166. C) Leukocytosis

Patients with Cushing syndrome may present with leukocytosis, an elevated white blood count. Glucocorticoid excess inhibits immune function and increases the risk and frequency of opportunistic infections. Glucose intolerance is common in Cushing syndrome, and poorly controlled hyperglycemia in a patient with obesity may be suggestive of Cushing syndrome. Hypokalemia may result from adrenal hypersecretion of mineralocorticoids, such as deoxycorticosterone and corticosterone. Osteoporosis is common in Cushing syndrome due to decreased intestinal calcium absorption, decreased bone formation, increased bone resorption, and decreased renal calcium reabsorption. Increased bone resorption can lead to hypercalciuria and renal calculi, but hypercalcemia is very rare.

167. A) ACTH

The diagnosis and determination of cause of adrenal insufficiency can be made by measuring and obtaining the results of both serum cortisol and plasma ACTH immediately at the time of patient presentation. Primary adrenal insufficiency can be characterized by an inappropriately low serum cortisol and a very high simultaneous plasma ACTH concentration. A patient has secondary (pituitary disease) or tertiary (hypothalamic disease) adrenal insufficiency when both serum cortisol and plasma ACTH concentrations are inappropriately low. The corticotropin-releasing hormone test can be used to differentiate between secondary and tertiary adrenal insufficiency. While valid, the insulin-induced hypoglycemia test is not widely used due to the risks associated with hypoglycemia. It is a rational test of hypothalamic-pituitary-adrenal response to stress; however, there is little reason to perform the test in patients with a suspected recent ACTH deficiency.

168. D) Serum cortisol concentration at 6 a.m. less than 3 mcg/dL

The patient is presenting with symptoms concerning for peripheral vascular collapse and electrolyte abnormalities often found in adrenal insufficiency. Because the predominant manifestation of adrenal crisis is shock, adrenal crisis should be considered and ruled out in any patient with symptoms of vasodilatory shock. The diagnosis of adrenal insufficiency of any cause involves the presentation of inappropriately low cortisol production. In patients without an adrenal insufficiency, serum cortisol concentrations are higher in the early morning (about 6 a.m.) and range from about 10 to 20 mcg/dL. Therefore, an early-morning low serum cortisol concentration of less than 3 mcg/dL strongly suggests adrenal insufficiency. Note, however, that while it is suggestive of an adrenal insufficiency, a low morning serum cortisol concentration alone is not a reliable indicator for diagnosis. An ACTH stimulation test should also be performed in all patients in whom the diagnosis of adrenal insufficiency is being considered (unless the diagnosis has been ruled out by a normal serum cortisol value). Adrenal insufficiency can be excluded with a salivary cortisol concentration at 8 a.m. above 5.8 ng/mL, whereas a level of about 1.8 ng/mL is suggestive of adrenal insufficiency. At 4 p.m., the normal range for serum cortisol concentrations is 3 to 10 mcg/dL; serum concentrations are at their lowest (less than 5 mcg/dL) 1 hour after the usual time of sleep due to the circadian rhythm in ACTH secretion. Therefore, measuring serum cortisol at these times is not recommended for the diagnosis of adrenal insufficiency.

169. C) Tertiary

Based on the clinical manifestations (weakness, fatigue, muscle and joint pain), this patient is likely experiencing secondary or tertiary adrenal insufficiency. Hyperpigmentation is the most characteristic physical finding in nearly all patients with primary adrenal insufficiency. This finding is not present in patients with secondary or tertiary adrenal insufficiency because corticotropin secretion is not increased. This patient is not presenting with the predominant manifestation of adrenal crisis, which is shock (e.g., tachycardia, hypotension, cool extremities, dehydration); therefore, this diagnosis is less likely. Hypoglycemia is more common in secondary adrenal insufficiency. Hyponatremia and volume expansion are often present in secondary and tertiary adrenal insufficiency, but hyperkalemia is not present, reflecting the presence of aldosterone. CRH can be used to differentiate between secondary and tertiary adrenal insufficiency. In patients with secondary or pituitary-related adrenal insufficiency, there is little or no ACTH response; in patients with tertiary disease secondary to lack of CRH from the hypothalamus, an exaggerated and prolonged ACTH response can be observed.

170. B) Corticotropin-releasing hormone test

The patient is likely experiencing secondary or tertiary adrenal insufficiency. A patient has secondary (pituitary disease) or tertiary (hypothalamic disease) adrenal insufficiency when both the serum cortisol and the plasma ACTH concentrations are inappropriately low. Further, the patient presentation of weakness, fatigue, and muscle and joint pain is more characteristic of secondary or tertiary adrenal insufficiency. Hyponatremia and volume expansion are often present, but hyperkalemia is not present, reflecting the presence of aldosterone. Hypoglycemia is more common in secondary adrenal insufficiency. The corticotropin-releasing hormone test can be used to differentiate between secondary and tertiary adrenal insufficiency. The standard high-dose (250 mcg) ACTH stimulation test excludes primary adrenal insufficiency and most patients with secondary adrenal insufficiency. In patients with primary adrenal insufficiency, an inappropriately low serum cortisol and a very high simultaneous plasma ACTH concentration can be observed. Urinary cortisol measurements are not often used to screen for adrenal insufficiency because basal urinary cortisol excretion is low in patients with severe adrenal insufficiency but may be low to normal in patients with partial adrenal insufficiency. While valid, the insulin-induced hypoglycemia test is not widely used due to the risks associated with hypoglycemia. It is a rational test of hypothalamic-pituitary-adrenal response to stress; however, there is little reason to perform the test in patients with a suspected recent ACTH deficiency.

171. B) Serum cortisol measurement

The patient presents with signs and symptoms concerning for a myxedema coma—severe hypothyroidism leading to slowing of function in multiple organs. The hallmark presentation includes decreased mental status, hypothermia, hypotension, bradycardia, hyponatremia, hypoglycemia, and hypoventilation. Aggressive treatment is needed for this medical emergency. The diagnosis should be suspected in any patient presenting with these symptoms and with other important clues, such as the presence of a thyroidectomy scar or a history of radioiodine therapy or hypothyroidism. If suspected, workup for the diagnosis includes measurement of thyroid-stimulating hormone (TSH), free thyroxine, and serum cortisol levels. The serum thyroxine concentration is usually very low, and the serum TSH concentration may be high (indicating primary hypothyroidism), or low, normal, or slightly high (indicating central hypothyroidism). Patients with hypothyroidism may have associated adrenal insufficiency; therefore, it is important to assess the cortisol level. The corticotropin-releasing hormone test may be needed for further workup to differentiate between secondary and tertiary adrenal insufficiency, but that would not be necessary right now nor aid in the diagnosis of myxedema coma. Performing an insulin-induced hypoglycemia test on a patient with suspected myxedema would not be safe because the patient is likely already hypoglycemic, and further decrease in blood glucose can cause additional harm. Urinary cortisol measurements would not be indicated because they are not often used as a screening test for adrenal insufficiency (basal urinary cortisol excretion is low in patients with severe adrenal insufficiency but may be low to normal in patients with partial adrenal insufficiency).

172. A) Primary

The patient is likely experiencing primary adrenal insufficiency. While often nonspecific, the presenting clinical manifestations of primary adrenal insufficiency frequently include fatigue, weight loss, nausea, vomiting, and muscle and joint pain. Hyperpigmentation is the most characteristic physical finding in nearly all patients with primary adrenal insufficiency. This finding is not present in patients with secondary or tertiary adrenal insufficiency because corticotropin secretion is not increased. Additionally, postural hypotension and salt craving are more specific for primary adrenal insufficiency. Common laboratory findings include hyponatremia, hyperkalemia, and anemia. In patients with primary adrenal insufficiency, an inappropriately low serum cortisol and a very high simultaneous plasma ACTH concentration can be observed. A patient has secondary (pituitary disease) or tertiary (hypothalamic disease) adrenal insufficiency when both serum cortisol and plasma ACTH concentrations are inappropriately low. This patient is not presenting with the predominant manifestation of adrenal crisis, which is shock (e.g., tachycardia, hypotension, cool extremities, dehydration), so this diagnosis is less likely.

173. D) Plasma fractionated metanephrines

The patient presents with the classic triad of episodic headache, sweating, and tachycardia, which is concerning for a pheochromocytoma. Most patients present with sustained or paroxysmal hypertension. This patient is considered at high risk for a pheochromocytoma due to the incidentally discovered adrenal mass on a previous CT scan that has imaging characteristics consistent with pheochromocytoma. Other indications for high risk include family history of pheochromocytoma, genetic syndrome that predisposes to pheochromocytoma, or history of resected pheochromocytoma. When there is a high index of suspicion for pheochromocytoma, the first-line test is to measure plasma fractionated metanephrines. A low risk of suspicion includes patients with resistant hypertension and hyperadrenergic spells (e.g., self-limited episodes of palpitations, diaphoresis, tremor) in which case 24-hour urine fractionated metanephrines and catecholamines would be indicated. While most catecholamine-secreting tumors are sporadic, many are part of a familial disorder, so genetic testing may be indicated, but usually only after a pathologic diagnosis has been confirmed.

174. C) High serum thyroid-stimulating hormone (TSH) concentration

This patient is presenting with signs and symptoms concerning for a myxedema coma, which is severe hypothyroidism leading to slowing of function in multiple organs. The hallmark presentation includes decreased mental status, hypothermia, hypotension, bradycardia, hyponatremia, hypoglycemia, and hypoventilation. The diagnosis should be suspected in any patient presenting with these symptoms and with other indications, such as the presence of a thyroidectomy scar or a history of radioiodine therapy or hypothyroidism. If suspected, workup for the diagnosis includes measurement of TSH, free thyroxine, and serum cortisol levels. Most patients with myxedema coma have primary hypothyroidism; the serum T4 concentration is usually very low, and the serum TSH concentration is often high. Note, however, that a patient with myxedema coma may present with central hypothyroidism and have a low, normal, or slightly high TSH concentration as well. Patients are often hypoglycemic, so their blood glucose is often low. Patients with both primary and central hypothyroidism may have associated adrenal insufficiency in which case the serum cortisol level is often low.

175. A) CT of the abdomen and pelvis

Radiological evaluation to confirm and localize the tumor is indicated after biochemical tests establish the diagnosis of a pheochromocytoma. A CT scan or MRI of the abdomen and pelvis are both reasonable first-line tests because both detect almost all sporadic symptomatic tumors (as most are 3 cm or larger in diameter). The choice between CT and MRI relies on facility availability, certain patient specifics (e.g., the presence of MRI-compatible pacemaker), and cost. An x-ray would not be indicated as it would not be able to yield the detailed imaging needed for further evaluation and treatment. A total body nuclear imaging study may be indicated if the initial CT or MRI was negative and the patient had symptoms and biochemical evidence of a pheochromocytoma. It may also be indicated in patients with large adrenal pheochromocytomas (e.g., greater than 8 cm) that have been originally identified on initial imaging. An image-guided needle biopsy should be avoided in those with a suspected pheochromocytoma due to the high rate of biopsy-related complications.